SIXTH EDITION

PUBLIC HEALTH

What It Is and How It Works

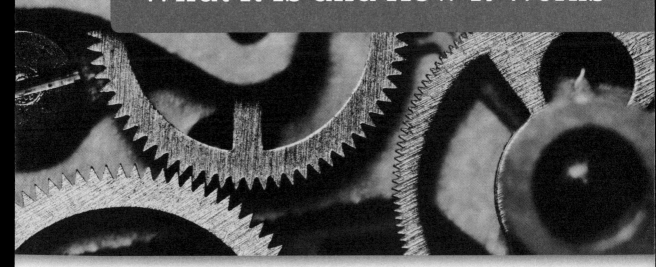

Bernard J. Turnock, MD, MPH

Clinical Professor of Community Health Sciences
School of Public Health
University of Illinois at Chicago
Chicago, Illinois

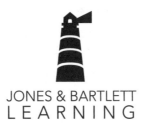

JONES & BARTLETT
LEARNING

World Headquarters
Jones & Bartlett Learning
5 Wall Street
Burlington, MA 01803
978-443-5000
info@jblearning.com
www.jblearning.com

Jones & Bartlett Learning books and products are available through most bookstores and online booksellers. To contact Jones & Bartlett Learning directly, call 800-832-0034, fax 978-443-8000, or visit our website, www .jblearning.com.

Substantial discounts on bulk quantities of Jones & Bartlett Learning publications are available to corporations, professional associations, and other qualified organizations. For details and specific discount information, contact the special sales department at Jones & Bartlett Learning via the above contact information or send an email to specialsales@jblearning.com.

07669-1

Production Credits

VP, Executive Publisher: David D. Cella
Publisher: Michael Brown
Associate Editor: Lindsey Mawhiney
Associate Editor: Nicholas Alakel
Production Manager: Tracey McCrea
Senior Marketing Manager: Sophie Fleck Teague
Manufacturing and Inventory Control
  Supervisor: Amy Bacus
Composition: Cenveo® Publisher Services
Cover Design: Kristin E. Parker
Rights and Media Research Coordinator: Mary Flatley
Cover Image: © OlegDoroshin/Shutterstock
Printing and Binding: Edwards Brothers Malloy
Cover Printing: Edwards Brothers Malloy

Library of Congress Cataloging-in-Publication Data

Turnock, Bernard J., author.
  Public health: what it is and how it works / Bernard J. Turnock. — Sixth edition.
    p.; cm
  Includes bibliographical references and index.
  ISBN 978-1-284-06941-9 (pbk.)
  I. Title.
  [DNLM: 1. Public Health Administration—United States. 2. Public Health Practice—United States. WA 540 AA1]
  RA445
  362.10973—dc23
                                                                                    2015014287

6048

Printed in the United States of America
19 18 17 16 15   10 9 8 7 6 5 4 3 2 1

Dedication

To Terry, Scott, and Linda—my dearly missed siblings.

Table of Contents

Preface

The early decades of a new century provide a unique opportunity to reflect on where we have been and what we have accomplished as a nation and as a society. For public health, it is truly an opportunity to examine what we might call, for lack of a better phrase, a century of progress. What a spectacular century it has been!

My grandparents were children at the turn of the previous century. At that time, they lived in a young and rapidly developing nation whose 75 million people held not unreasonable hopes of a long and healthy life. They also faced an alarmingly large number of health hazards and risks that, when taken together, offered them the prospect of an average life expectancy of only approximately 47 years. Small-pox, tuberculosis, pneumonia, diphtheria, and a variety of diarrheal diseases were frequent, although unwelcome, visitors. It was not uncommon for families to bury several of their children before they reached adulthood.

By the time my parents were children in the 1920s and 1930s, a variety of economic, social, and scientific advances offered more than one additional decade of average life expectancy, even despite the massive social and economic disruption of the Great Depression. Still, tuberculosis, scarlet fever, whooping cough, measles, and other diseases were common. Fewer childhood deaths occurred, but many families still experienced one or more deaths among their children.

Members of the post–World War II Baby Boom Generation, like me and my four siblings, enjoyed the prospect of living to and even beyond the age of 65 and the so-called Golden Years. When I was a child, polio was one of the few remaining childhood infectious disease threats. Some of my most vivid childhood memories are of the mass immunization programs that took place in my hometown. Childhood deaths were an uncommon experience and more likely the result of causes other than infectious diseases.

As the 21st century unfolds, more than 310 million Americans, my children and yours, now look forward to an average life expectancy of about 80 years. Today, there are no fewer than two dozen different conditions for which immunizations are available—more than a dozen of which are recommended for use in all children—to prevent virtually all of the conditions that threatened previous generations.

Today, our children are even being immunized against cervical and liver cancers! Overall, childhood deaths have declined more than 95% from their levels a century earlier. That means that 19 of the 20 deaths that used to occur to children in this country no longer take place!

To many of us, a century seems like a long time. In the grand scheme of things, however, it is not, and it seems even shorter when we consider how lifetimes and generations are so interconnected. Just look at the connections linking each of us with our grandparents and our children and even our children's children, each of whom held, hold, or will hold quite different expectations for their lives and health. These links and connections play critical roles when it comes to understanding the value and benefits of the work of public health. At the turn of the next century, an estimated 570 million Americans will be enjoying the fruits of public health's labors over the preceding centuries. The vast majority of the people who will benefit from what public health does are yet to be born!

As someone who has spent 15 years in public health practice and another 20 years in teaching and researching the field, I have been concerned about why those who work in the field and those who benefit from its work do not better understand something so important and useful. Throughout my career as a public health professional, I have developed a profound respect for the field, the work, and the workers. I must admit, however, that even while serving as director of a large state health department, I lacked a full understanding and appreciation of this unique enterprise.

What has become clear to me is that the story of public health is not simple to tell. There is no one official at the helm, guiding it through the turbulence that is constantly encountered. There is no clear view of its intended destination and of what work needs to be done, and by whom, to get there. We cannot turn to our family physicians, to elected officials, or even to distinguished public health officials, such as our Surgeon General, for vision and direction. Surely, these people play important roles, but public health is so broadly involved with the biologic, environmental, social, cultural, behavioral, and service utilization factors associated with health that no one is accountable for addressing everything. Still, we all share in the successes and failures of our collective decisions and actions, making us all accountable to one another for the results of these efforts. My hope is that this book presents a broad view of the public health system and deters current and future public health workers from narrowly defining public health in terms of only what they do. At its core, the purpose of this book is to describe public health simply and clearly in terms of what it is, what it does, how it works, and why it is important to all of us.

Although there is no dearth of fine books in this field, there is a shortage of understanding, appreciation, and support for public health and its various manifestations. Many of the current texts on public health attempt to be comprehensive in covering the field without the benefit of a conceptual framework understandable to insiders and outsiders alike. The dynamism and complexity of the field suggest that public health texts are likely to become even larger and more comprehensive as the field advances. In contrast, this book aims to present the basic concepts of public health practice with an emphasis on comprehensibility rather than comprehensiveness. It offers fundamental concepts but links those concepts to practice in the real world through a series of case studies that supplement and complement the main chapters.

Many of the core competencies established by the Association of Schools of Public Health for graduates of master's in public health degree programs are addressed in this book, especially those in the professionalism, leadership, systems thinking, health policy and management, and program planning categories.

Whatever wisdom might be found in this book has filtered through to me from my mentors, colleagues, coworkers, students, and friends. For those about to toil in this vineyard of challenge and opportunity, this is meant to be a primer on public health in the United States. It is a book that seeks to reduce the vast scope, endless complexities, and ever-expanding agenda to a format simple enough to be understood by first-year students and state health commissioners alike.

New to This Edition

The sixth edition of *Public Health: What It Is and How It Works* offers several new features and incorporates information on a variety of recent developments in public health practice and the health sector. Implementation of the Affordable Care Act, strategic planning, accreditation of public health organizations, and credentialing of public health workers are among the recent developments covered in this revision. Extensive information on state and local public health practice derived from national surveys conducted since 2012 is included throughout the book. Community public health practice and emergency preparedness topics have been expanded. New conceptual frameworks for the public health system, overall health system, and public health workforce have been added. Public health workforce topics have been expanded in a new chapter, and public health infrastructure topics are addressed from a management perspective. Most notably, a series of case studies constitutes the second part of the book. More than 60 new or revised charts and tables are incorporated into the new edition, and a series of "outside-the-book" thinking exercises appears in each chapter.

Acknowledgments

Many people have shaped the concepts and insights provided in this text. This book evolved from an introductory course on public health concepts and practice that I have been teaching at the University of Illinois at Chicago School of Public Health since 1991. During that time, more than 5,000 current and aspiring public health professionals have influenced the material included in this book. Their enthusiasm and expectations have challenged me to find ways to make this subject interesting and valuable to learners at all levels of their careers.

Many parts of this book rely heavily on the work of public health practitioners and public health practice organizations. Over the years, I have had the opportunity to work with public health practice leaders at the Centers for Disease Control and Prevention, several of whom deserve special acknowledgment for their encouragement and contributions, especially Ed Baker, Paul Halverson, and Bill Dyal. Other valuable contributions came from public health colleagues, including John Lumpkin, Chris Atchison, Laura Landrum, Judith Munson, and Patrick Lenihan. Arden Handler has long been my colleague and collaborator on many public health capacity-building projects. Emily Ahonen did a masterful job of developing the case study focusing on the aftermath of the Gulf oil spill. In several chapters, I have drawn on the work of two public health agencies at which I have worked during my career, the Illinois Department of Public Health and the Chicago Department of Public Health. The influence of some outstanding public health figures who have served as mentors and role models—Jean Pakter, Paul Peterson, Quentin Young, George Pickett, and C. Arden Miller—is also apparent in this book.

Lloyd Novick provided early encouragement and support for this undertaking, as well as useful suggestions on the scope and focus of this text. Mike Brown, Lindsey Mawhiney, and Tracey McCrea at Jones & Bartlett Learning have consistently provided valuable suggestions and guidance throughout the editing and production stages. I am grateful for the many and varied contributions from all of these sources.

About the Author

Bernard J. (Barney) Turnock, MD, MPH, is currently clinical professor of community health sciences in the School of Public Health at the University of Illinois at Chicago (UIC). Since joining the UIC School of Public Health in 1990, he has also served as acting dean and associate dean for public health practice, as well as director of the Division of Community Health Sciences, director of the Center for Public Health Practice, and founder of the Illinois Public Health Preparedness Center. His major areas of interest include performance measurement, capacity building, and workforce development within the public health system. He is board certified in preventive medicine and public health and has extensive practice experience, having served as director of the Illinois Department of Public Health from 1985 to 1990, deputy commissioner and acting commissioner of the Chicago Department of Health, and state program director for Maternal and Child Health and Emergency Medical Services during his distinguished career. He has played major roles in a wide variety of public policy and public health issues in Illinois since 1978. He frequently consults on a range of public health and healthcare issues and has served as a member of the Illinois State Board of Health and as president of the Illinois Public Health Association. He is also the author of two other recently published works: *Public Health: Career Choices That Make a Difference* and *Essentials of Public Health, Third Edition*. He has received two prestigious awards from the American Public Health Association: one for excellence in health planning and practice and another for excellence in health administration. He is also a recipient of the UIC School of Public Health's "Golden Apple" award for excellence in teaching, and he was the developer and instructor for UIC's first completely online course (based on this book): Public Health Concepts and Practice—CHSC 400.

Part I

Public Health: What It Is and How It Works

The 10 chapters in Part I of this book aim to present the essentials of public health from a public health system perspective. These chapters introduce fundamental concepts and link those concepts to practice. The case studies in Part II offer a different perspective on public health practice through the lens of real-world events and challenges.

The Part I topics are essential for public health students early in their academic careers, and they have become increasingly important for students in the social and political sciences and other health professions as well. This book is intended as much for public health practitioners as it is for students. It represents the belief that public health cannot be adequately taught through a text and that it is best learned through exploration and practice of its concepts and methods. In that light, this book should be viewed as a framework for learning and understanding public health rather than the definitive catalog of its principles and practices. Its real value will be its ability to encourage thinking "outside the book."

The first four chapters cover topics of interest to general audiences. Basic concepts underlying public health systems are presented in Chapter 1, including definitions, historical highlights, and unique features of public health. This and subsequent chapters focus largely on public health in the United States, although information on global public health and comparisons among nations appear in Chapters 2 and 3. Health and illness and the various factors that influence health and quality of life are presented from an ecological perspective in Chapter 2. This chapter also presents data and information on health status and risk factors in the United States and introduces a method for analyzing health problems to identify their precursors. Chapter 3 addresses the overall health system and its intervention strategies, with a special emphasis on trends and developments, including implementation of the Affordable Care Act, that are important to public health. This chapter highlights interfaces between public health and a rapidly changing health system. Chapter 4 examines the organization of public health responsibilities in the United States by reviewing its legal basis and the current structure of public health agencies at the federal, state, and local levels. Together, these first four chapters serve as a primer on what public health is and how it relates to health interests in modern America.

The next five chapters flesh out the skeleton of public health introduced in the first half of the book. They examine how public health does what it does, exploring issues of the inner workings of public health that are critical for the more serious students of the field. Chapter 5 reviews the core functions and essential services of public health and how these concepts organize 21st-century community public health practice. This chapter identifies key processes or practices that operationalize public health's core functions and tools that have been developed to improve public health practice. Chapter 6 offers a comprehensive examination of the public health system's most important asset, its workforce. Chapter 7 builds on the governmental structure of American public health (from Chapter 4) and the public health workforce (from Chapter 6) and examines how the basic building blocks of the public health system, including human, informational, organizational, and fiscal resources, can be managed to improve performance. Outputs of the public health system and intervention strategies in the form of programs and services are the focus of Chapter 8. Evidence-based public health practice is examined in terms of its population-based community prevention services and clinical preventive services, and an approach to program planning and evaluation for public health interventions is presented. Chapter 9 describes the emergency preparedness and response roles of public health, including the opportunities afforded by increased public health expectations and a substantial influx of federal funding. The final chapter looks to the future of public health in the second decade of a new century and beyond, building on the lessons learned from the preceding century. Emerging problems, opportunities afforded by the expansion of collaborations and partnerships, and obstacles impeding public health responses are also examined in the concluding chapter.

Each chapter uses a variety of figures and tables to illustrate the concepts and provide useful resources for public health practitioners. A glossary of public health terminology is provided for the benefit of those unfamiliar with some of the commonly used terms, as well as to convey the intended meaning for terms that may have several different connotations in practice. Each chapter includes discussion questions and exercises, which require "outside-the-book thinking" to complement the topics presented and provide a framework for thought and discussion. These allow the text to be used more flexibly in public health courses at various levels, using different formats for learners at different levels of their training and careers.

Together, the 10 chapters in Part I offer a systems perspective to public health, grounded in a conceptual model that characterizes public health by its mission, functions, capacity, processes, and outcomes. This model is the unifying construct for this text. It provides a framework for examining and questioning the wisdom of our current investment strategy that directs 20 times more resources toward medical services than it spends for public health and prevention strategies—even though treatment strategies contributed only 5 of the 30 years of increased life expectancy at birth that have been achieved in the United States since 1900.

Chapter 1

What Is Public Health?

LEARNING OBJECTIVES

Given the historical phenomena that have shaped the development of public health responses, formulate a working definition and logic model for public health in the 21st century. Key aspects of this competency expectation include being able to

- Articulate several different definitions of public health
- Describe the origins and content of public health responses over history
- Trace the development of the public health responses system in the United States
- Broadly characterize the contributions and value of public health
- Identify three or more distinguishing features of public health
- Describe public health as a system using a logic model with inputs, processes, outputs, and results, emphasizing the role of core functions and essential public health services
- Identify five or more Internet web sites that provide useful information on the public health system in the United States

---

The passing of one century and the early decades of the next afford a rare opportunity to look back at where public health has been and forward to the challenges that lie ahead. Imagine a world 100 years from now where life expectancy is 30 years more and infant mortality rates are 95% lower than they are today. The average human life span would be more than 107 years, and less than one of every 2,000 infants would die before their first birthday. These seem like unrealistic expectations and unlikely achievements; yet, they are no greater than the gains realized during the 20th century in the United States. In 1900, few envisioned the century of progress in public health that lay ahead. Yet by 1925 public health leaders such as C.E.A. Winslow were noting a nearly 50% increase in life expectancy (from 36 years to 53 years) for residents of New York City between the years 1880 and 1920.[1] Accomplishments such as these caused Winslow to speculate what might be possible through widespread application of scientific knowledge. With the even more spectacular achievements over the rest of the 20th century, we all should wonder what is possible in the century that has just begun.

This year may be remembered for many things, but it is unlikely that many people will remember it as a spectacular year for public health in the United States. No major discoveries, innovations, or triumphs set this year apart from other years in recent memory. Yet, on closer examination, maybe there were! Like the story of the wise man who invented the game of chess for his king and asked for payment by having the king place one grain of wheat on the first square of the chessboard, two on the second, four on the third, eight on the fourth, and so on, the small victories of public health over the past century have resulted in cumulative gains so vast in scope that they are difficult to comprehend.

This year, there will be nearly 900,000 fewer cases of measles reported than in 1941, 200,000 fewer cases of diphtheria than in 1921, more than 250,000 fewer cases of whooping cough than in 1934, and 21,000 fewer cases of polio than in 1951.[2] The early decades of the new century witnessed 50 million fewer smokers than would have been expected, given trends in tobacco use through 1965. More than 2 million Americans were alive who otherwise would have died from heart disease and stroke, and nearly 100,000 Americans were alive as a result of automobile seat belt use. Protection of the U.S. blood supply had prevented more than 1.5 million hepatitis B and hepatitis C infections and more than 50,000 human immuno-deficiency virus (HIV) infections, as well as more than $5 billion in medical costs associated with these three diseases.[3] Today, average blood lead levels in children are less than one-third of what they were a quarter century ago. This catalog of accomplishments could be expanded many times over. Figure 1-1 summarizes this progress, including two of the most widely followed measures of a population's health status—life expectancy and infant mortality.

These results did not occur by themselves. They came about through decisions and actions that represent the essence of what is public health. It is the story of public health and its immense value and importance in our lives that is the focus of this text. With this impressive litany of accomplishments, it would seem that public health's story would be easily told. For many reasons, however, it is not. As a result, public health remains poorly understood by its prime beneficiary—the public—as well as many of its dedicated practitioners. Although public health's results, as measured in terms of improved health status, diseases prevented, scarce resources saved, and improved quality of life, are more apparent today than ever before, society seldom links the activities of public health with its results. This suggests that the public health community must more effectively communicate what public health is and what it does, so that its results can be readily traced to their source.

This chapter is an introduction to public health that links basic concepts to practice. It considers three questions:

- What is public health?
- Where did it come from?
- Why is it important in the United States today?

To address these questions, this chapter begins with a sketch of the historical development of public health activities in the United States. It then examines

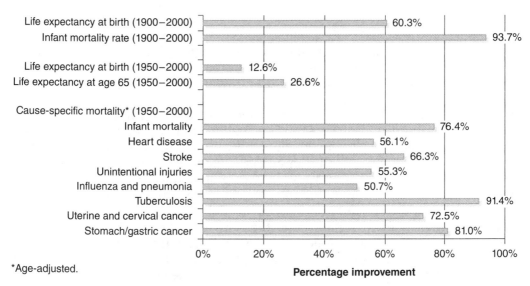

Figure 1-1 Percentage improvement in selected measures of life expectancy and age-adjusted, cause-specific mortality for the time periods 1900–2000 and 1950–2000, United States.

Data from Centers for Disease Control and Prevention, National Center for Health Statistics. *Health, United States 2009.* Hyattsville, MD: NCHS; 2009 and Rust G, Satcher D, Fryer GE, Levine RS, Blumenthal DS. Triangulating on success: innovation, public health, medical care, and cause-specific US mortality over a half century (1950–2000). *Am J Public Health.* 2010;100:S95–S104.

several definitions and characterizations of what public health is and explores some of its unique features. Finally, it offers insight into the value of public health in biologic, economic, and human terms.

Taken together, these topics provide a foundation for understanding what public health is and why it is important. A conceptual framework that approaches public health from a systems perspective is introduced to identify the dimensions of the public health system and facilitate an understanding of the various images of public health that coexist in the United States today. We will see that, as in the story of the blind men examining the elephant, various sectors of our society have mistaken separate components of public health for the entire system.

A BRIEF HISTORY OF PUBLIC HEALTH IN THE UNITED STATES

Early Influences on American Public Health

Although the complete history of public health is a fascinating saga in its own right, this section presents only selected highlights. When ancient cultures perceived illness as the manifestation of supernatural forces, they felt that little in the way of either personal or collective action was possible. For many centuries, disease was synonymous with epidemic. Diseases, including horrific epidemics of infectious diseases such as the Black Death (plague), leprosy, and cholera, were phenomena to be accepted. It was not until the so-called Age of Reason and the Enlightenment that scholarly inquiry began to challenge the "givens" or accepted realities of the time. Eventually expansion of the science and knowledge base would reap substantial rewards.

With the advent of industrialism and imperialism, the stage was set for epidemic diseases to increase their terrible toll. As populations shifted to urban centers for the purpose of commerce and industry, public health conditions worsened. The mixing of dense populations living in unsanitary conditions and working long hours in unsafe and exploitative industries with wave after wave of cholera, smallpox, typhoid, tuberculosis, yellow fever, and other diseases was a formula for disaster. Such disaster struck again and again across the globe, but most seriously and most often at the industrialized seaport cities that provided the portal of entry for diseases transported as stowaways alongside commercial cargo. The experience, and subsequent susceptibility, of different cultures to these diseases partly explains how relatively small bands of Europeans were able to overcome and subjugate vast Native American cultures. Seeing the Europeans unaffected by scourges such as smallpox served to reinforce beliefs that these light-skinned visitors were supernatural figures, unaffected by natural forces.[4]

The British colonies in North America and the new American republic certainly bore their share of the burden. American diaries of the 17th and 18th centuries chronicle one infectious disease onslaught after another. These epidemics left their mark on families, communities, and even history. For example, the national capital had to be moved out of Philadelphia because of a devastating yellow fever epidemic in 1793. This epidemic also prompted the city to develop its first board of health in that same year.

The formation of local boards of distinguished citizens, the first boards of health, was one of the earliest organized responses to epidemics. This response was revealing in that it represented an attempt to confront disease collectively. Because science had not yet determined that specific microorganisms were the causes of epidemics, avoidance had long been the primary tactic used. Avoidance meant evacuating the general location of the epidemic until it subsided or isolating diseased individuals or those recently exposed to diseases on the basis of a mix of fear, tradition, and scientific speculation. Several developments, however, were swinging the pendulum ever closer to more effective counteractions.

The work of public health pioneers such as Edward Jenner, John Snow, and Edwin Chadwick illustrates the value of public health, even when its methods are applied amidst scientific uncertainty. Well before Koch's postulates established scientific methods for linking bacteria with specific diseases and before Pasteur's experiments helped to establish the germ theory, both Jenner and Snow used deductive logic and common sense to do battle with smallpox and cholera, respectively. In 1796, Jenner successfully used vaccination for a disease that ran rampant through communities across the globe. This was the initial shot in a long and arduous campaign that, by the year 1977, had totally eradicated smallpox from all of its human hiding places in every country in the world. The potential for its reemergence through the actions of terrorists is a topic left to a fuller discussion of public health emergency preparedness and response.

Snow's accomplishments even further advanced the art and science of public health. In 1854, Snow traced an outbreak of cholera to the well water drawn from the pump at Broad Street and helped to prevent hundreds, perhaps thousands, of cholera cases. In that same year, he demonstrated that another large outbreak could be traced to one particular water company that drew its water from the Thames River, downstream from London, and that another company that drew its water upstream from London was not linked with cholera cases. In both efforts, Snow's ability to collect and analyze data allowed him to determine causation, which, in turn, allowed him to implement corrective actions that prevented additional cases. All of this occurred without benefit of the knowledge that there was an odd-shaped little bacterium that was carried in water and spread from person to person by hand-to-mouth contact!

England's General Board of Health conducted its own investigations of these outbreaks and concluded that air, rather than contaminated water, was the cause.[5] Its approach, however, was one of collecting a vast amount of information and accepting only that which supported its view of disease causation. Snow, on the other hand, systematically tested his hypothesis by exploring evidence that ran contrary to his initial expectations.

Chadwick was a more official leader of what has become known as the sanitary movement of the latter half of the 19th century. In a variety of official capacities, he played a major part in structuring government's role and responsibilities for protecting the public's health. Because of the growing concern over the social and sanitary conditions in England, a National Vaccination Board was established in 1837. Shortly thereafter, Chadwick's *Report on an Inquiry into the Sanitary Conditions of the Laboring Population of Great Britain* articulated a framework for broad public actions that served as a blueprint for the growing sanitary movement. One result was the establishment in 1848 of a General Board of Health. Interestingly, Chadwick's interest in public health had its roots in Jeremy Bentham's utilitarian movement. For Chadwick, disease was viewed as causing poverty, and poverty was responsible for the great social ills of the time, including societal disorder and high taxation to provide for the general welfare.[6] Public health efforts were necessary to reduce poverty and its wider social effects. This view recognizes a link between poverty and health, although in an opposite direction to current thinking as to the social determinants of health and role of fundamental causes of societal ills. Today, it is more common to consider poor health as a result of poverty, rather than as its cause.

Chadwick was also a key participant in the partly scientific, partly political debate that took place in British government as to whether deaths should be attributed to pathological conditions or to their underlying factors, such as hunger and poverty. It was Chadwick's view that pathologic, as opposed to less proximal social and behavioral, factors should be the basis for classifying deaths.[6] Chadwick's arguments prevailed, although aspects of this debate continue to the present day. William Farr, sometimes called the father of modern vital statistics, championed the opposing view.

OUTSIDE-THE-BOOK THINKING 1-1

Access the website of the national honorary society for public health (www.deltaomega.org) and select one of the classic documents available there. Then describe the significance of this classic in the history of public health and its relevance for public health practitioners today.

In the latter half of the 19th century, as sanitation and environmental engineering methods evolved, more effective interventions became available against epidemic diseases. Further, the scientific advances of this period paved the way for modern disease control efforts targeting specific microorganisms.

Growth of Local and State Public Health Activities in the United States

Lemuel Shattuck's *Report of the Sanitary Commission of Massachusetts* in 1850 outlined existing and future public health needs for that state and became America's roadmap for development of a public health system. Shattuck called for the establishment of state and local health departments to organize public efforts aimed at sanitary inspections, communicable disease control, food sanitation, vital statistics, and services for infants and children. Although Shattuck's report closely paralleled Chadwick's efforts in Great Britain, acceptance of his recommendations did not occur for several decades. In the latter part of the century, his farsighted and far-reaching recommendations came to be widely implemented. With greater understanding of the value of environmental controls for water and sewage and of the role of specific control measures for specific diseases (including quarantine, isolation, and vaccination), the creation of local health agencies to carry out these activities supplemented—and, in some cases, supplanted—local boards of health. These local health departments developed rapidly in the seaports and other industrial urban centers, beginning with a health department in Baltimore in 1798, because these were the settings where the problems were reaching unacceptable levels.

Because infectious and environmental hazards are no respecters of local jurisdictional boundaries, states began to develop their own boards and agencies after 1870. These agencies often had very broad powers to protect the health and lives of state residents, although the clear intent at the time was that these powers be used to battle epidemics of infectious diseases. In examining how law impacts governmental public health roles, we will revisit these powers and duties because they serve as both a stimulus and a limitation for what can be done to address many contemporary public health issues and problems.

Federal Public Health Activities in the United States

This sketch of the development of public health in the United States would be incomplete without a brief introduction to the roles and powers of the federal government. Federal health powers, at least as enumerated in the U.S. Constitution, are minimal. It is surprising to some to learn that the word "health" does not even appear in the Constitution. As a result of not being a power explicitly granted to the federal government (such as defense, foreign diplomacy, international and inter-state commerce, or printing money), health was a power to be exercised by states or reserved to the people themselves.

Two sections of the Constitution have been interpreted over time to allow for federal roles in health, in concert with the concept of the so-called implied powers necessary to carry out explicit powers. These are the ability to tax in order to provide for the "general welfare" (a phrase appearing in both the preamble and body of the Constitution) and the specific power to regulate commerce, both international and interstate. These provisions allowed the federal government to establish a beach-head in health, initially through the Marine Hospital Service (eventually to become the Public Health Service). After the ratification of the 16th Amendment in 1916, authorizing a national income tax, the federal government acquired the ability to raise substantial sums of money, which could then be directed toward promoting the general welfare. The specific means to this end were a variety of grants-in-aid to state and local governments. Beginning in the 1960s, federal grant-in-aid programs designed to fill gaps in the medical care system nudged state and local governments further and further into the business of medical service provision. Federal grant pro-grams for other social, substance abuse, mental health, and community prevention services soon followed. The expansion of federal involvement into these areas, how-ever, was not accomplished by these means alone.

Prior to 1900, and perhaps not until the Great Depression, Americans did not believe that the federal government should intervene in their social circumstances. Social values shifted dramatically during the Depression, a period of such great social insecurity and need that the federal government was now permitted—indeed, expected—to intercede. Other chapters will expand on the growth of the federal government's influence on public health activities and its impact on the activities of state and local governments.

OUTSIDE-THE-BOOK THINKING 1-2

Research the history of public health in your state or locality and then describe how public health strategies and responses have changed over time. What influences were most responsible for these changes? Does this suggest that public health roles and functions have changed over time, as well?

To explain more easily the broad trends of public health in the United States, it is useful to delineate distinct eras in its history. One simple scheme, outlined in Table 1-1, uses the years 1850, 1950, and 2000 as approximate dividers. Prior to 1850, the system was characterized by recurrent epidemics of infectious diseases, with little in the way of collective response possible. During the sanitary movement in the second half of the 19th and first half of the 20th century, science-based con-trol measures were organized and deployed through a public health infrastructure that was developing in the form of local and state health departments. After 1950, gaps in the medical care system and federal grant dollars acted together to increase

Table 1-1   Major Eras in Public Health History in the United States

Prior to 1850	Battling epidemics
1850–1949	Building state and local infrastructure
1950–1999	Filling gaps in medical care delivery
After 1999	Preparing for and responding to community health threats

public provision of a wide range of medical services. That increase set the stage for the current reexamination of the links between medical and public health practice. Some retrenchment from the direct service provision role has occurred since about 1990. As chronicled throughout this text, a new era for public health that seeks to balance community-driven public health practice with preparedness and response for public health emergencies is underway.

IMAGES AND DEFINITIONS OF PUBLIC HEALTH

The historical development of public health activities in the United States provides a case study for understanding what public health is today. Nonetheless, the term public health evokes several different images among the general public and those dedicated to its improvement. To only a relatively small number, the term describes a broad social enterprise or system.

To others, the term describes the professionals and workforce whose job it is to solve certain important health problems. At a meeting in the early 1980s to plan a community-wide education and outreach campaign in order to reduce infant mortality, a community relations director of a large television station made some comments that reflected this view. When asked whether his station had been involved in infant mortality reduction efforts in the past, he responded, "Yes, but that's not our job. If you people in public health had been doing your job properly, we wouldn't be called on to bail you out!" Obviously, this man viewed public health as an effort of which he was not a part.

Still another image of public health is that of a body of knowledge and techniques that can be applied to health-related problems. Here, public health is seen as what public health does. Snow's investigations exemplify this perspective.

Similarly, many people perceive public health primarily as the activities ascribed to governmental public health agencies. For the majority of the public, this latter image represents public health in the United States, resulting in the common view that public health primarily involves the provision of medical care to indigent populations. Since 2001, however, public health has also emerged as a front line defense against bioterrorism and other threats to personal security and safety.

A final image of public health is that of the intended results of these endeavors. In this image, public health is literally the health of the public, as measured in terms of health and illness in a population. The term population health, often defined as health outcomes and their distribution in a population, is increasingly used for this image of public health.[7]

Table 1-2 Images of Public Health

> - Public health: the system and social enterprise
> - Public health: the profession
> - Public health: the methods (knowledge and techniques)
> - Public health: governmental services (especially medical care for the poor)
> - Public health: the health of the public

This chapter will focus primarily on the first of these images, public health as a social enterprise or system. It is important to understand what people mean when they speak of public health. As summarized in Table 1-2, the profession, the methods, the governmental services, the ultimate outcomes, and even the broad social enterprise itself are all commonly encountered images of what public health is today.

With varying images of what public health is, we would expect no shortage of definitions. There have been many, but three definitions, each separated by a generation, provide especially important insights into what public health is. These are highlighted in Table 1-3.

In 1988 the prestigious Institute of Medicine (IOM) provided a useful definition in its landmark study of public health in the United States, *The Future of Public Health*. The IOM report characterized public health's mission as "fulfilling society's interest in assuring conditions in which people can be healthy."[8] This definition directs attention to the many conditions that influence health and wellness, underscoring the broad scope of public health and legitimizing its interest in social, environmental, economic, political, and medical care factors that affect health and illness. The definition's premise that society has an interest in the health of its members implies that improving conditions and health status for others is acting in our own self-interest. The assertion that improving the health status of others provides benefits to all is a core value of public health.

Another core value of public health is reflected in the IOM definition's use of the term *assuring*. Assuring conditions in which people can be healthy means vigilantly promoting and protecting everyone's interests in health and well-being. This value echoes the wisdom in the often-quoted African aphorism that "it takes a village to raise a child." Former Surgeon General David Satcher, the first African American

Table 1-3 Selected Definitions of Public Health

> - "the science and art of preventing disease, prolonging life, and promoting health and efficiency through organized community effort"[9]
> - "Successive re-definings of the unacceptable"[10]
> - "fulfilling society's interest in assuring conditions in which people can be healthy"[8]
>
> Data from Institute of Medicine, National Academy of Sciences. *The Future of Public Health*. Washington, DC: National Academy Press: 1988; Winslow CEA. The untilled field of public health. *Mod Med*. 1920; 2:183–191, and Vickers G., What sets the goals of public health? *Lancet*. 1958;1:599–604.

to head this country's most respected federal public health agency, the Centers for Disease Control and Prevention (CDC), once described a visit to Africa in which he met with African teenagers to learn firsthand of their personal health attitudes and behaviors. Satcher was struck by their concerns over the rapid urbanization of the various African nations and the changes that were threatening their culture and sense of community. These young people felt lost and abandoned; they questioned Satcher as to what America and the world community were willing to do to help them survive these changes. As one young man put it, "Where will we find our village?" In many respects, public health serves as everyone's village, whether we are teens in Africa or adults in the United States. The IOM report's characterization of public health advocated for just such a social enterprise and stands as a bold philosophical statement of mission and purpose.

The IOM report also sought to define the boundaries of public health by identifying three core functions of public health: assessment, policy development, and assurance. In one sense, these functions are comparable to those generally ascribed to the medical care system involving diagnosis and treatment. Assessment is the analogue of diagnosis, except that the diagnosis, or problem identification, is made for a group or population of individuals. Similarly, assurance is analogous to treatment and implies that the necessary remedies or interventions are put into place. Finally, policy development is an intermediate role of collectively deciding which remedies or interventions are most appropriate for the problems identified (the formulation of a treatment plan is the medical system's analogue). These core functions broadly describe what public health does—as opposed to what it is.

The concepts embedded in the IOM definition are also reflected in Winslow's definition, developed nearly a century ago. His definition describes both what public health does and how this gets done. It is a comprehensive definition that has stood the test of time in characterizing public health as:

> ... the science and art of preventing disease, prolonging life, and promoting health and efficiency through organized community effort for the sanitation of the environment, the control of communicable infections, the education of the individual in personal hygiene, the organization of medical and nursing services for the early diagnosis and preventive treatment of disease, and for the development of the social machinery to insure everyone a standard of living adequate for the maintenance of health, so organizing these benefits as to enable every citizen to realize his birthright of health and longevity.[9]

There is much to consider in Winslow's definition. The phrases, "science and art," "organized community effort," and "birthright of health and longevity" capture the substance and aims of public health. Winslow's catalog of methods illuminates the scope of the endeavor, embracing public health's initial targeting of infectious and environmental risks, as well as current activities related to the organization, financing, and accountability of medical care services. His allusion to the "social machinery to insure everyone a standard of living adequate for the maintenance of health" speaks to the relationship between social conditions and health in all societies.

There have been many other attempts to define public health, although these have received less attention than either the Winslow or IOM definitions. Several build on the observation that, over time, public health activities reflect the interaction of disease with two other phenomena that can be roughly characterized as science and social values: (1) what do we know, and (2) what do we choose to do with that knowledge?

A prominent British industrialist, Geoffrey Vickers, provided an interesting addition to this mix more than a half century ago while serving as Secretary of the Medical Research Council. In identifying the forces that set the agenda for public health, Vickers noted, "The landmarks of political, economic, and social history are the moments when some condition passed from the category of the given into the category of the intolerable. I believe that the history of public health might well be written as a record of successive re-definings of the unacceptable."[10]

The essence of Vickers' formulation lies in its focus on social justice and the delicate and shifting interface between science and social values. Through this lens, we can view a tracing of public health over history, facilitating an understanding of why and how different societies have reacted to health risks differently at various points in time and space. In this light, the history of public health is one of harnessing scientific knowledge to shape responses to problems that have crossed the boundary into social unacceptability.

OUTSIDE-THE-BOOK THINKING 1-3

Which of the definitions of public health presented in this chapter best describes public health in the 21st century? Why?

Each of these definitions offers important insights into what public health is and what it does. Individually and collectively, they describe a social enterprise and system that is both important and unique, as we will see in the sections that follow.

PUBLIC HEALTH AS A SYSTEM

So what is public health? Maybe no single answer will satisfy everyone. There are, in fact, several dimensions of public health that must be considered. Viewing public health as a system of interconnected components, such as the population health system illustrated in Figure 1-2, is one approach. Yet, the public health system described in this chapter is more complex than the simple network of participants presented in this figure. The public health described in this chapter is a broad social enterprise, more akin to a movement, that seeks to extend the benefits of current knowledge in ways that will have the maximum impact on the health status of a population. It does so by identifying problems that call for collective action to protect, promote, and improve health, primarily through preventive strategies. This public health is unique in its interdisciplinary approach and methods, its emphasis on preventive strategies, its linkage with government and political decision making, and its dynamic adaptation to new problems placed on its agenda. Above all else, it is a collective effort to identify and address the unacceptable realities that result in

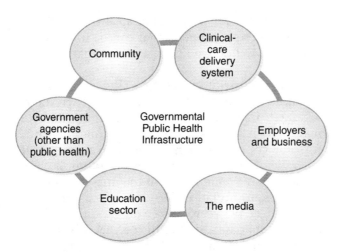

Figure 1-2 Population health system.

Reproduced from Institute of Medicine, Committee on Public Health Strategies to Improve Health, Board on Population Health and Public Health Practice (June 2011). For the public's health: Revitalizing law and policy to meet new challenges, Figure 1–1, page 17. Washington, DC: The National Academies Press.

preventable and avoidable health and quality of life outcomes, and it is the composite of efforts and activities that are carried out by people and organizations committed to these ends.

With this broad view of public health as a social enterprise, the question shifts from what public health is to what these other images of public health represent and how they relate to each other. Logic models are widely used in modern public health practice to illustrate how the various dimensions of a program relate to each other and achieve their intended results. Basically, logic models indicate what occurs as a result of the preceding step using a basic "if... then" rationale. Programs have structural elements, sometimes referred to as input or capacity, (e.g., workers, information, relationships, facilities, funding, etc.) that are blended to carry out specific activities or processes, which then produce certain outputs that lead in turn to various effects or outcomes. The underlying logic for programs is that inputs → processes → outputs → outcomes. Logic models are also useful in characterizing and analyzing more complex entities, including organizations and systems.

OUTSIDE-THE-BOOK THINKING 1-4

Develop a map or some other graphic representation of the national public health system. Your map can take any form you choose. Which components or dimensions of the public health system are most important to capture in such a map?

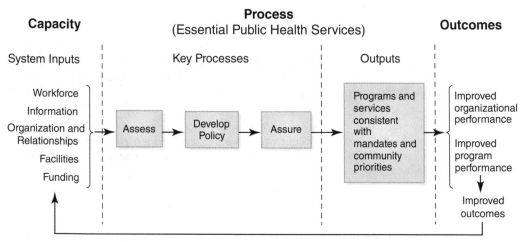

Figure 1-3 Logic model representation of the public health system.

Figure 1-3 characterizes the public health system in the form of such a logic model, demonstrating the utility of this approach. For example, it is useful to consider inputs as resource investments. The efficiency of a program or system reflects the ratio of outputs to inputs. The effectiveness of a program or system reflects the degree to which intended outcomes are achieved. Equity reflects the degree to which outcomes are distributed fairly or proportionally. Overall satisfaction with results in terms of effectiveness, (efficiency and equity) contributes to whether a program or system is valued by its stakeholders, which in turn contributes to the level of resources made available. This important feedback loop is apparent in the lower part of this logic model.

This logic model framework integrates the mission and functions of public health in relation to the inputs, processes, outputs, and outcomes of the system. Although descriptions for these system components are offered in Table 1-4, it is sometimes easier to appreciate this model when a more familiar industry, such as the automobile industry, is used as an example. The mission or purpose might be expressed as meeting the personal transportation needs of the population. This industry carries out its mission by providing appropriate vehicles to its customers; this characterizes its function. In this light, we can now examine the inputs, processes, outputs, and outcomes of the system set up to carry out this function. Inputs would include steel, rubber, plastic, and so forth, as well as the workers, know-how, technology, facilities, machinery, and support services necessary to allow the raw materials to become cars and trucks. The key processes necessary to carry out the primary function might be characterized as designing vehicles, making or acquiring parts, assembling parts into vehicles, moving vehicles to dealers, and selling and servicing vehicles after purchase. No doubt this is an incomplete listing of this industry's processes; it is oversimplified here to make the point. In any event, these processes translate the abstract concept of getting vehicles to people into the operational steps necessary to carry out this basic function. The outputs of these processes

Table 1-4   Dimensions of the Public Health System

Capacity (Inputs):
- The resources and relationships necessary to carry out the core functions and essential services of public health (e.g., human resources, information resources, fiscal and physical resources, appropriate relationships among the system components)

Process (Practices and Outputs):
- Those collective practices or processes that are necessary and sufficient to ensure that the core functions and essential services of public health are being carried out effectively, including the key processes that identify and address health problems and their causative factors and the interventions intended to prevent death, disease, and disability, and to promote quality of life

Outcomes (Results):
- Indicators of health status, risk reduction, and quality-of-life enhancement outcomes are long-term objectives that define optimal, measurable future levels of health status; maximum acceptable levels of disease, injury, or dysfunction; or prevalence of risk factors

Data from Centers for Disease Control and Prevention, Public Health Program Office, 1990.

are vehicles located where people can purchase them. The outcomes include satisfied customers and company profits.

Applying this same general framework to the public health system is also possible but may not be so obvious. The mission and functions of public health are well described in the IOM report's framework. The core functions of assessment, policy development, and assurance are somewhat more abstract functions than making vehicles but still can be made operational through descriptions of their key steps or processes.[11,12] The inputs of the public health system include its human, organizational, informational, fiscal, and other resources. These resources and relationships are structured to carry out public health's core functions through a variety of processes that are termed essential public health practices or services. These processes produce outputs in the form of interventions (policies, programs, and services) that derive from assessing health and planning effective strategies.[13] These outputs or interventions are designed to produce the desired results, which, with public health, might well be characterized as health or quality-of-life outcomes. The logic model representation of the public health system illustrates these relationships.

In this model, not all components are as readily understandable and measurable as others. Several of the inputs are easily counted or measured, including human, fiscal, and organizational resources. Outputs are also generally easy to recognize and count (e.g., prenatal care programs, number of immunizations provided, health messages on the dangers of tobacco, laws and regulations). Health outcomes are also readily understood in terms of mortality, morbidity, functional disability, time lost from work or school, and even more sophisticated measures, such as years of potential life lost and quality-of-life years lost. The elements that are most difficult to understand and visualize are the processes or essential services of the public health system. Identifying these operational aspects of the public health system allow us

Table 1-5   Public Health in America

Vision:
Healthy People in Healthy Communities
Mission:
*Promote Physical and Mental Health
and Prevent Disease, Injury, and Disability*

Public Health

- Prevents epidemics and the spread of disease
- Protects against environmental hazards
- Prevents injuries
- Promotes and encourages healthy behaviors
- Responds to disasters and assists communities in recovery
- Assures the quality and accessibility of health services

Essential Public Health Services

- Monitor health status to identify community health problems
- Diagnose and investigate health problems and health hazards in the community
- Inform, educate, and empower people about health issues
- Mobilize community partnerships to identify and solve health problems
- Develop policies and plans that support individual and community health efforts
- Enforce laws and regulations that protect health and ensure safety
- Link people with needed personal health services and assure the provision of health care when otherwise unavailable
- Assure a competent public health and personal health care workforce
- Evaluate effectiveness, accessibility, and quality of personal and population-based health services
- Research for new insights and innovative solutions to health problems

Reproduced from Essential Public Health Services Working Group of the Core Public Health Functions Steering Committee, U.S. Public Health Service, 1994.

to better understand public health practice, measure it, and relate it to its outputs and outcomes. A national work group assembled by the U.S. Public Health Service in 1994 developed a consensus statement of what public health is and does in language understandable to those both inside and outside the field of public health. Table 1-5 presents the result of that effort, a statement entitled "Public Health in America."[14] The conceptual framework identified in the logic model representation of the public health system and the narrative representation in the "Public Health in America" statement are useful models for understanding the public health system and how it works. Figure 1-4 demonstrates how the 10 essential public health services operationalize the three core public health functions identified in the 1988 IOM report.

This framework attempts to bridge the gap between what public health is, what it does, and how it does what it does (through its capacity, processes, and outcomes). It also allows us to examine the various components of the system so that we can better appreciate how the pieces fit together.

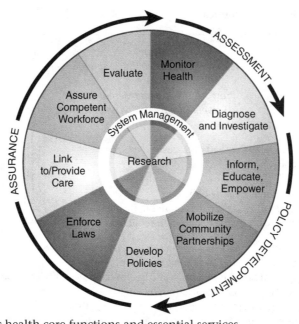

Figure 1-4   Public health core functions and essential services.

Reproduced from Centers for Disease Control and Prevention, National Public Health Performance Standards. Available at http://www.health.gov/phfunctions/public.htm. Accessed June 17, 2014.

UNIQUE FEATURES OF PUBLIC HEALTH

Several unique features are apparent in the public health system. These are spotlighted in Table 1-6 and include the underlying social justice philosophy of public health; its inherently political nature; its ever-expanding agenda, with new problems and issues being assigned over time; its link with government; its grounding in a broad base of evidence-based biologic, physical, quantitative, social, and behavioral sciences; its focus on prevention as a prime intervention strategy; and the unique bond and sense of mission that links its key stakeholders.

Table 1-6   Selected Unique Features of Public Health

- Basis in social justice philosophy
- Inherently political nature
- Dynamic, ever-expanding agenda
- Link with government
- Grounding in the sciences
- Use of prevention as a prime strategy
- Uncommon culture and bond

Social Justice Philosophy

It is vital to recognize the social justice orientation of public health and even more critical to understand the potential for conflict and confrontation that it generates. Social justice is the foundation of public health. The concept first emerged around 1848, a time that might be considered the birth of modern public health. Social justice argues that public health is properly a public matter and that its results in terms of death, disease, health, and well-being reflect the decisions and actions that a society makes, for good or for ill.[15] Justice is an abstract concept that determines how each member of a society is allocated his or her fair share of collective burdens and benefits. Societal benefits to be distributed may include happiness, income, or social status. Burdens include restrictions of individual action and taxation. Justice dictates that there is fairness in the distribution of benefits and burdens; injustices occur when persons are denied some benefit to which they are entitled or when some burden is imposed unduly. If access to health services, or even health itself, is considered to be a societal benefit (or if poor health is considered to be a burden), the links between the concepts of justice and public health become clear. Market justice and social justice represent two forms of modern justice.

Market justice emphasizes personal responsibility as the basis for distributing burdens and benefits. Other than respecting the basic rights of others, individuals are responsible primarily for their own actions and are free from collective obligations. Individual rights are highly valued, whereas collective responsibilities are minimized. In terms of health, individuals assume primary responsibility for their own health. There is little expectation that society should act to protect or promote the health of its members beyond addressing risks that cannot be controlled through individual action.

Social justice argues that significant factors within the society can impede the fair distribution of benefits and burdens.[16] Examples of such impediments include social class distinctions, heredity, and discrimination on the basis of race, ethnicity, gender, or sexual preference. Collective action, often leading to the assumption of additional burdens, is necessary to neutralize or overcome those impediments. In the case of public health, the goal of extending the potential benefits of the physical and behavioral sciences to all groups in the society, especially when the burden of disease and ill health within that society is unequally distributed, is largely based on principles of social justice. It is clear that many modern public health (and other public policy) problems disproportionately affect some groups, usually a minority of the population, more than others. As a result, their resolution requires collective actions in which those less affected take on greater burdens, while not commensurately benefiting from those actions. When the necessary collective actions are not taken, even the most important public policy problems remain unsolved, despite periodically becoming highly visible.[16] This scenario explains our inadequate responses to such intractable American problems as inadequate housing, poor public education systems, unemployment, racial discrimination, and poverty. However, it is also true for public health problems such as tobacco-related illnesses, infant mortality, substance abuse, mental health services, long-term care, and environmental pollution. The failure to effect comprehensive national health reform in 1994 is an example of this phenomenon. At that time, middle-class Americans deemed the modest price tag of health reform to be excessive, refusing to pay more out of their own pockets when they perceived that their own access and services were not likely to improve. The bitter political conflict accompanying the enactment of national health reform legislation in the form of the Affordable Care Act of 2010 reflected these same themes.

These and similar examples suggest that a critical challenge for public health as a social enterprise lies in overcoming the social and ethical barriers that prevent us from doing more with the knowledge and tools already available to us.[16] Extending the frontiers of science and knowledge may not be as effective for improving public health as shifting the collective values of our society to act on what we already know. Recent public health successes, such as public attitudes toward smoking in both public and private locations and operating motor vehicles after alcohol consumption, provide evidence in support of this assertion. These advances came through changes in social norms, rather than through bigger and better science.

Inherently Political Nature

The social justice underpinnings of public health serve to stimulate political conflict. Public health is both public and political in nature. It serves populations, which are composites of many different communities, cultures, and values. Politics allows for issues to be considered, negotiated, and finally determined within societies. At the core of political processes are differing values and perspectives as to both the ends to be achieved and the means for achieving those ends. Advocating causes and agitating various segments of society to identify and address unacceptable conditions that adversely affect health status often lead to increased expectations and demands on society, generally through government. As a result, public health advocates appear at times as antigovernment and anti-institutional. Governmental public health agencies seeking to serve the interests of both government and public health are frequently caught in the middle. This creates tensions and conflict that can put these public health professionals at odds with governmental leaders on the one hand and external public health advocates on the other.

Expanding Agenda

A third unique feature of public health is its broad and ever-increasing scope. Traditional domains of public health interest include biology, environment, lifestyle, and health service organization. Within each of these domains are many factors that affect health status; in recent decades, many new public policy problems have been moved onto the public health agenda as their predisposing factors have been identified and found to fall into one or more of these domains. A multilevel, multidimensional view of the determinants of population health, often termed a social-ecological model of health, represented in Figure 1-5, has emerged to guide public health practice.

The assignment of new problems to the public health agenda is an ever-evolving phenomenon. For example, prior to 1900, the primary problems addressed by public health were infectious diseases and related environmental risks. After 1900, the focus expanded to include problems and needs of children and mothers to be addressed through health education and maternal and child health services as public

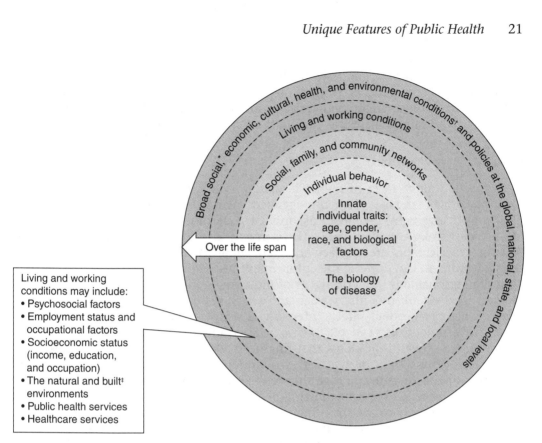

Living and working conditions may include:
• Psychosocial factors
• Employment status and occupational factors
• Socioeconomic status (income, education, and occupation)
• The natural and built‡ environments
• Public health services
• Healthcare services

Notes:
Adapted from Whitehead M and Dahlgren G. What can be done about inequalities in health? Lancet. 1991;338(8774): 1059–63. The dashed lines between levels of the model denote interaction effects between and among the various levels of health determinants (Worthman, CM. Epidemiology of human development. In Hormones, Health and Behavior: A Socio-Ecological and Lifespan Perspective. Panter-Brink C and Worthman CM (eds), 47–104. Cambridge: Cambridge University Press.).

*Social conditions include, but are not limited to, economic inequality, urbanization, mobility, cultural values, attitudes, and policies related to discrimination and intolerance on the basis of race, gender, and other differences.
†Other conditions at the national level might include major sociopolitical shifts, such as recession, war, and governmental collapse.
‡The built environment includes transportation, water and sanitation, housing, and other dimensions of urban planning.

Figure 1-5   A social-ecological framework for thinking about the determinants of population health.

Reproduced from The Committee on Assuring the Health of the Public in the 21st Century, Institute of Medicine. *The Future of the Public's Health in the 21st Century.* Washington, DC: National Academy Press; 2003. Reprinted with permission, copyright 2003, National Academy of Sciences.

---

lic sentiment over the health and safety of children increased. In the middle of the century, chronic disease prevention and medical care fell into public health's realm as an epidemiologic revolution began to identify causative agents for chronic diseases and links between use of health services and health outcomes. Later, substance abuse, mental illness, teen pregnancy, long-term care, and other issues fell to public health, as did several emerging problems, most notably the epidemics of violence and HIV infections. The public health agenda expanded even further as a result of the recent national dialogue over health reform and how health services will be organized and managed. Bioterrorism preparedness is an even more recent addition to this agenda amidst heightened concerns and expectations after the events of September 11, 2001, and the anthrax attacks the following month.

Link with Government

A fourth unique facet of public health is its link with government. Although public health is far more than the aggregate activities of federal, state, and local health agencies, many people think only of governmental public health agencies when they think of public health. Government does play a unique role in seeing that the key elements are in place and that public health's mission gets addressed. Only government can exercise the enforcement provisions of our public policies that limit the personal and property rights of individuals and corporations in areas such as retail food establishments, sewage and water systems, occupational health and safety, consumer product safety, infectious disease control, and drug efficacy and safety. Government also can play the convener and facilitator role for identifying and prioritizing health problems that might be addressed through public resources and actions. These roles derive from the underlying principle of beneficence, in that government exists to improve the well-being of its members. Beneficence often involves a balance between maximizing benefits and minimizing harms on the one hand and doing no harm on the other.

Two general strategies are available for governmental efforts to influence public health. At the broadest level, governments can modify public policies that influence health through social and environmental conditions, such as policies for education, employment, housing, public safety, child welfare, pollution control, workplace safety, and family support. In line with the IOM report's definition of public health, these actions seek to ensure conditions in which people can be healthy. Another strategy of government is to directly provide programs and services that are designed to meet the health needs of the population. It is often easier to garner support for relatively small-scale programs directed toward a specific problem (such as tuberculosis or HIV infections) than to achieve consensus around broader health and social issues. This strategy is basically a "command-and-control" approach, in which government attempts to increase access to and utilization of services largely through deployment of its own resources rather than through working with others. A variation of this strategy for government is to ensure access to healthcare services through public financing approaches (Medicare and Medicaid are prime examples) or through specialized delivery systems (such as the Veterans Administration facilities, the Indian Health Service, and federally funded community health centers).

Whereas the United States has largely opted for the latter of these strategies, other countries have acted to place greater emphasis on broader social policies. Both the overall level of investment for and relative emphasis between these strategies contribute to the widely varying results achieved in terms of health status indicators among different nations.

Many factors dictate the approaches used by a specific government at any point in time. These factors include history, culture, the structure of the government in question, and current social circumstances. There are also several underlying motivations that support government intervention. For paternalistic reasons, governments may act to control or restrict the liberties of individuals to benefit a group, whether or not that group seeks these benefits. For utilitarian reasons, governments intervene because of the perception that the state as a whole will benefit in some important way. For equality considerations, governments act to ensure that benefits and burdens are equally distributed among individuals. For equity considerations, governments justify interventions in order to distribute the benefits of society in proportion to need. These motivations reflect the views of each society as to whether health itself or merely access to health services is to be considered a right of individuals and populations within that society. Many societies, including the United States, act through government to ensure equal access to a broad array of preventive and treatment services. Equity in health status for all groups within the society may not be an explicit aspiration however, even where efforts are in place to ensure equality in access. Even more important for achieving equity in health status are concerted efforts to improve health status in population groups with the greatest disadvantage, mechanisms to monitor health status and contributing factors across all population groups, and participation of disadvantaged population groups in the key political decision-making processes within the society.[17] To the extent that equity in health status among all population groups does not guide actions of a society's government, these other elements will be only marginally effective.

As noted previously, the link between government and public health makes for a particularly precarious situation for governmental public health agencies. The conflicting value systems of public health and the wider community generally translate into public health agencies having to document their failure in order to make progress. It is said that only the squeaky wheel gets the grease; in public health, it often takes an outbreak, disaster, or other tragedy to demonstrate public health's value. Since 1985, increased funding for basic public health protection programs quickly followed outbreaks related to bacteria-contaminated milk in Illinois, tainted hamburgers in Washington State, and contaminated public water supplies in Milwaukee. Following concerns over preparedness of public health agencies to deal with bioterrorism and other public health threats, a massive infusion of federal funding occurred.

The assumption and delegation of public health responsibilities are quite complex in the United States, with different patterns in each of the 50 states. Over recent decades, the concept of a governmental presence in health has emerged and gained widespread acceptance within the public health community. This concept characterizes the role of local government, often, but not necessarily always, operating through its official health agencies, which serve as the residual guarantors that needed services will actually be there when needed. In practice it means that, no matter how duties are assigned locally, there is a presence that ensures that health needs are identified and considered for collective action. How this concept is operationalized will become apparent in chapters focusing on the role that government plays in carrying out the core functions of public health.

Grounded in Science

One of the most unique aspects of public health—and one that continues to separate public health from many other social movements is its grounding in science. This relationship is clear for the medical and physical sciences that govern our understanding of the biologic aspects of humans, microorganisms, and vectors, as well as the risks present in our physical environments. However, it is also true for the social sciences of anthropology, sociology, psychology, and economics that affect our understanding of human culture and behaviors influencing health and illness. The quantitative sciences of epidemiology and biostatistics remain essential tools and methods of public health practice. Often five basic sciences of public health are identified: epidemiology, biostatistics, environmental science, management sciences, and behavioral sciences. These constitute the core education of public health professionals.

The importance of a solid and diverse scientific base is both a strength and weakness of public health. Surely there is no substitute for evidence-based science in the modern world. The public remains curiously attracted to scientific advances, at least in the physical and biologic sciences, and this base is important to market and promote public health interventions. For many years, epidemiology has been touted as the basic science of public health practice, suggesting that public health itself is applied epidemiology. Modern public health thinking views epidemiology less as the basic science of public health than as one of many contributors to a complex undertaking. In recent decades, knowledge from the social sciences has greatly enriched and supplemented the physical and biologic sciences. Yet these are areas less familiar to and perhaps less well appreciated by the public, making it difficult to garner public support for newer, more socially and behaviorally mediated public health interventions. The old image of public health based on the hard sciences underlying environmental sanitation and communicable disease control is being superseded by a new image of public health approaches more grounded in what the public perceives to be "softer" science. This transition, at least temporarily, lessens public understanding and confidence in public health and its methods.

Focus on Prevention

If public health professionals were pressed to provide a one-word synonym for public health, the most frequent response would probably be prevention. In general, prevention characterizes actions that are taken to reduce the possibility that something will happen or in hopes of minimizing the damage that may occur if it does happen. Prevention is a widely appreciated and valued concept that is best understood when its object is identified. Although prevention is considered by many to be the purpose of public health, the specific intentions of prevention can vary greatly. Prevention can target deaths, hospital admissions, days lost from school, consumption of human and fiscal resources, and many other ends. There are as many targets for prevention as there are various health outcomes and effects to be avoided.

Prevention efforts often lack a clear constituency because success results in unseen consequences. Because these consequences are unseen, people are less likely to develop an attachment for or support the efforts preventing them. Advocates for such causes as mental health services, care for individuals with developmental disabilities, and organ transplants often make their presence felt. However, few state capitols have seen candlelight demonstrations by thousands of people who did not get diphtheria.

This invisible constituency for prevention is partly a result of the interdisciplinary nature of public health. With no predominant discipline, it is even more difficult for people to understand and appreciate the work of public health. From one perspective, the undervaluation of public health is understandable; the majority of the beneficiaries of recent and current public health prevention efforts have not yet been born! Despite its lack of recognition, prevention as a strategy has been remarkably successful and appears to offer great potential for future success, as well.

Uncommon Culture

The final unique feature of public health to be discussed here appears to be both a strength and weakness. The tie that binds public health professionals is neither a common preparation through education and training nor a common set of work experiences and work settings. Public health is unique in that the common link is a set of intended outcomes toward which many different sciences, arts, and methods can contribute. As a result, public health professionals include anthropologists, sociologists, psychologists, physicians, nurses, nutritionists, lawyers, economists, political scientists, social workers, laboratory workers, managers, sanitarians, engineers, epidemiologists, biostatisticians, gerontologists, disability specialists, and dozens of other professions and disciplines. All are bound to common ends, and all employ somewhat different perspectives from their diverse education, training, and work experiences. "Whatever it takes to get the job done" is the theme, suggesting that the basic task is one of problem solving around health issues. This aspect of public health is the foundation for strategies and methods that rely heavily on collaborations and partnerships.

This multidisciplinary and interdisciplinary approach is unique among professions, calling into question whether public health is really a unified profession at all. An argument can be made that public health is not a profession. There is no minimum credential or training that distinguishes public health professionals from either other professionals or nonprofessionals. Only a tiny proportion of those who work in organizations dedicated to improving the health of the public possess one of the academic public health degrees (the master's of public health degree and several other master's and doctoral degrees granted by schools of public health and other institutions). With the vast majority of public health workers not formally trained in public health, it is difficult to characterize its workforce as a profession.

OUTSIDE-THE-BOOK THINKING 1-5

Which of its unique features distinguish public health from medicine as a profession? Which distinguish it from social work? From law?

Until only recently, public health has lacked key characteristics that distinguish professions from occupations. Significant progress has been made such that public health now meets several of these defining criteria, including: (1) a distinct body of knowledge, (2) an educational credential offered by schools and programs accredited by a specialized accrediting body, (3) career paths that include autonomous practice, and (4) a separate credential, Certified in Public Health (CPH), indicative of self-regulation based on the newly launched examination of the National Board of Public Health Examiners.[18]

Nonetheless, several obstacles will continue to challenge independent professional status, including the viability of the new credential and variability in the content of graduate training programs. The impact of complete professionalization could be considerable in terms of recruitment into the field, autonomy of practice, ultimate strengthening of the public health infrastructure, and impact on public health policy and outcomes.

VALUE OF PUBLIC HEALTH

How can we measure the value of public health efforts? This question is addressed both directly and indirectly throughout this text. Later chapters will examine the dimensions of public health's value in terms of lives saved and diseases prevented, as well as in dollars and cents. Nonetheless, some initial information will set the stage for greater detail later.

Public opinion polls conducted in recent years suggest that public health is already highly valued in the United States.[19] The overwhelming majority of the public rate a variety of key public health services as "very important." Substantially more Americans believe that "public health/protecting populations from disease" is more important than "medicine/treating people who are sick." Public opinion surveys such as these suggest that public health's contributions to health and quality of life have not gone unnoticed. Other assessments of the value of public health support this contention.

In 1965, McKeown concluded, "health has advanced significantly only since the late 18th century and until recently owed little to medical advances."[20] This conclusion is bolstered by more recent studies concluding that public health's prevention efforts are responsible for 25 years of the nearly 30-year improvement in life expectancy at birth in the United States since 1900. This bold claim is based on evidence that only 5 years of the 30-year improvement were the result of medical care.[21] Even for these 5 years, medical treatment accounted for 3.7 years, and clinical preventive services (such as immunizations and screening tests) accounted for 1.5 years. The remaining 25 years have resulted largely from prevention efforts in the form of social policies, community actions, and personal decisions. Many of these decisions and actions targeted infectious diseases affecting infants and children early in the 20th century. The dramatic reduction in deaths due to infectious diseases between 1900 and 1950 is evident in Figure 1-6. Later in that century, gains in life expectancy were largely achieved through reductions in chronic diseases affecting adults, including cardiovascular disease as demonstrated in Figure 1-1. A study of life years gained from modern health disease treatments and changes in population risk factors in England and Wales from 1981 to 2000 concluded that 79% of the increase in life years gained was attributed to reductions in major risk factors. Only 21% of the life years gained could be attributed to medical and surgical treatments of coronary heart disease.[22]

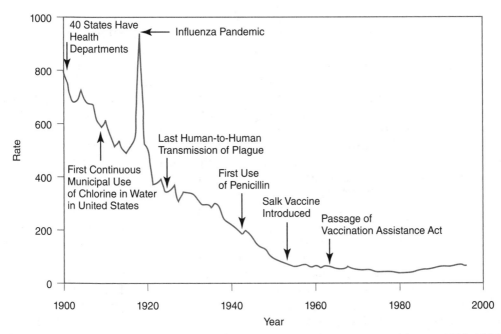

Figure 1-6 Crude death rate (per 100,000) for infectious diseases, United States, 1900–1996.

Reproduced from Centers of Disease Control and Prevention. Public health achievments, United States, 1900–1999: control of infectiious diseases. *MMWR.* 1999;48:621–629.

The value of public health is further reflected in Table 1-7, which identifies 10 great public health achievements that occurred during the 20th century. These may appear to be distant and sterile accomplishments, but they also tell the story of public health in very human terms. A poignant example dates from the 1950s, when the United States was in the midst of a terrorizing polio epidemic. Few communities

Table 1-7 Ten Great Public Health Achievements—United States, 1900–1999

- Vaccination
- Motor-vehicle safety
- Safer workplaces
- Control of infectious diseases
- Decline in deaths from coronary heart disease and stroke
- Safer and healthier foods
- Healthier mothers and babies
- Family planning
- Fluoridation of drinking water
- Recognition of tobacco use as a health hazard

Data from Centers for Disease Control and Prevention. Ten great public health achievements—United States, 1900–1999. *MMWR.* 1999; 48(12):241–243.

were spared during the periodic onslaughts of this serious disease during the first half of the 20th century in America. Public fear was so great that public libraries, community swimming pools, and other group activities were closed during the summers when the disease was most feared. Biomedical research had discovered a possible weapon against epidemic polio in the form of the Salk vaccine, however, which was developed in 1954 and licensed for use 1 year later. A massive and unprecedented campaign to immunize the public was quickly undertaken, setting the stage for a triumph of public health. The real triumph came in a way that might not have been expected, however, because soon into the campaign, isolated reports of vaccine-induced polio were identified in Chicago and California. Within 2 days of the initial case reports, action by governmental public health organizations at all levels resulted in the determination that these cases could be traced to one particular manufacturer. This conclusion was reached only a few hours before the same vaccine was to be provided to hundreds of thousands of California children. The result was prevention of a disaster and rescue of the credibility of an immunization campaign that has virtually cut this disease off at its knees. The campaign proceeded on schedule and, 5 decades later, wild poliovirus has been eradicated from the western hemisphere.

Similar examples have occurred throughout history. The battle against diphtheria is a case in point. A major cause of death in 1900, diphtheria infections are virtually unheard of today. This achievement cannot be traced solely to advances in bacteriology and the antitoxins and immunizations that were deployed against this disease. Neither was this disease defeated by brilliant political and programmatic initiatives led by public health experts. It was the confluence of scientific advances and public perception of the disease itself that resulted in diphtheria's demise as a threat to entire populations.[23] These forces shaped public health policies and the effectiveness of intervention strategies. This is a story of science and social values as the major forces shaping public health.

OUTSIDE-THE-BOOK THINKING 1-6

Search for and become familiar with the web sites of the American Public Health Association (APHA), Association of State and Territorial Health Officials (ASTHO), National Association of County and City Health Officials (NACCHO, Public Health Foundation (PHF), U.S. Environmental Protection Agency (EPA), U.S. Department of Homeland Security (DHS), U.S. Department of Health and Human Services (DHHS) and its various Public Health Services Agencies, such as the Centers for Disease Control and Prevention (CDC), Food and Drug Administration (FDA), Health Resources and Services Administration (HRSA), National Institutes of Health (HIH), and Agency for Healthcare Research and Quality (AHRQ). Each site offers useful insights into the central question for this chapter, "What Is Public Health?"

CONCLUSION

Public health evokes different images for different people, and, even to the same people, it can mean different things in different contexts. The intent of this chapter has been to describe some of the common perceptions of public health in the United States. Is it a complex, dynamic, social enterprise, akin to a movement? Or is it best characterized as a goal of the improved health outcomes and health status that can be achieved by the work of all of us, individually and collectively? Or is public health some collection of activities that move us ever closer toward our aspirations? Or is it the profession that includes all of those dedicated to its cause? Or is public health merely what we see coming out of our official governmental health agencies—a strange mix of safety-net medical services for the poor and a variety of often-invisible community prevention services?

Although it is tempting to consider expunging the term public health from our vocabularies because of the baggage associated with these various images, this would do little to address the obstacles to accomplishing our central task, because public health encompasses all of these images and perhaps more!

Based on principles of social justice, inherently political in its processes, addressing a constantly expanding agenda of problems, inextricably linked with government, grounded in science, emphasizing preventive strategies, and with a workforce bound by common aspirations, public health is unique in many ways. Its value, however, transcends its uniqueness. Public health efforts have been major contributors to recent improvements in health status and can contribute even more in a new century with new challenges.

By carefully examining the various dimensions of the public health system in terms of its inputs, practices, outputs, and outcomes, we can gain insight into what it does, how it works, and how it can be improved. Better results do not come from setting new goals; they come from understanding and improving the processes that will then produce better outputs, in turn leading to better outcomes. Understanding the public health system as a necessary step toward its improvement is a theme that recurs throughout this text.

REFERENCES

1. Winslow CEA. Public health at the crossroads. *Am J Public Health*. 1926; *16*: 1075–1085.
2. Hinman A. Eradication of vaccine-preventable diseases. *Ann Rev Public Health*. 1999; *20*: 211–229.
3. U.S. Public Health Service. *For a Healthy Nation: Returns on Investment in Public Health*. Washington, DC: PHS; 1994.
4. McNeil WH. *Plagues and Peoples*. New York: Doubleday; 1977.
5. Paneth N, Vinten-Johansen P, Brody H. A rivalry of foulness: official and unofficial investigations of the London cholera epidemic of 1854. *Am J Public Health*. 1998; *88*: 1545–1553.
6. Hamlin C. Could you starve to death in England in 1839? The Chadwick-Farr controversy and the loss of the "social" in public health. *Am J Public Health*. 1995; *85*: 856–866.
7. Kindig DA. Understanding population health terminology. *Milbank Q*. 2007; *85*: 139–161.
8. Institute of Medicine, National Academy of Sciences. *The Future of Public Health*. Washington, DC: National Academy Press; 1988.
9. Winslow CEA. The untilled field of public health. *Mod Med*. 1920; *2*: 183–191.
10. Vickers G. What sets the goals of public health? *Lancet*. 1958; *1*: 599–604.
11. Baker EL, Melton RJ, Stange PV, et al. Health reform and the health of the public. *JAMA*. 1994; *272*: 1276–1282.
12. Harrell JA, Baker EL. The essential services of public health. *Leadership Public Health*. 1994; *3*: 27–30.
13. Handler A, Issel LM, Turnock BJ. A conceptual framework to measure performance of the public health system. *Am J Public Health* 2001; *91*: 1235–1239.

14. Public Health Functions Steering Committee. *Public Health in America.* Washington, DC: U.S. Public Health Service; 1995.

15. Krieger N, Brin AE. A vision of social justice as the foundation of public health: commemorating 150 years of the spirit of 1848. *Am J Public Health.* 1998; *88*: 1603–1606.

16. Beauchamp DE. Public health as social justice. *Inquiry.* 1976; *13*: 3–14.

17. Susser M. Health as a human right: an epidemiologist's perspective on public health. *Am J Public Health.* 1993; *83*: 418–426.

18. Evashwick CJ, Begun JW, Finnegan JR. Public health as a distinct profession: has it arrived? *J Public Health Management Practice.* 2013; *19*(5): 412–419.

19. Harris Polls. Public Opinion about Public Health, United States. 1999.

20. McKeown T. *Medicine in Modern Society.* London, England: Allen & Unwin; 1965.

21. Bunker JP, Frazier HS, Mosteller F. Improving health: measuring effects of medical care. *Milbank Q.* 1994; *72*: 225–258.

22. Unal B, Critchley JA, Fidan D, Capewell S. Life-years gained from modern cardiological treatments and population risk factor changes in England and Wales, 1981–2000. *Am J Public Health.* 2005; *95*: 103–108.

23. Hammonds EM. *Childhood's Deadly Scourge: The Campaign to Control Diphtheria in New York City, 1880–1930.* Baltimore, MD: Johns Hopkins University Press; 1999.

Measuring Population Health

The 21st century began much as its predecessor did, with immense opportunities to advance the health of the public through actions that ensure conditions favorable for health and quality of life. All systems direct their efforts toward certain outcomes; they track progress by ensuring that these outcomes are clearly defined and measurable. In public health, this calls for clear definitions and measures of health and quality of life in populations. That task is the focus of this chapter. Key questions to be addressed are:

- What is health?
- What factors influence health and illness?

- How can health status and quality of life be measured?
- What do current measures tell us about the health status and quality of life of Americans in the early decades of the 21st century?
- How can this information be used to assess population and community health status and develop effective public health interventions and public policy?

The relevance of these questions resides in their focus on factors that cause or influence particular health outcomes. Efforts to identify and measure key aspects of health and factors influencing health have relied largely on traditional approaches over the past century, although there are signs that this pattern may be changing. The key questions identified above will be addressed slightly out of order, for reasons that should become apparent as this chapter unfolds.

HEALTH IN THE UNITED STATES

Many important indicators of health status in the United States have improved considerably over the past century, although there is evidence that health status could be even better than it is. At the turn of the 20th century, nearly 2% of the U.S. population died each year. The crude mortality rate in 1900 was about 1,700 deaths per 100,000 population. Life expectancy at birth was 47 years. Additional life expectancy at age 65 was another 12 years. Medicine and health care were largely proprietary in 1900 and of questionable benefit to health. More extensive information on the health status of the population at that time would be useful, but very little exists.

Indicators of health status improved in the United States throughout the 20th century.[1] Between the years 1900 and 2000, the crude mortality rate was cut in half to 872 per 100,000. By the year 2000, life expectancy at birth was nearly 77 years and life expectancy at age 65 was another 18 years.

The leading causes of death also changed dramatically over the 20th century, as demonstrated in Figure 2-1 depicting causes of death in 1900 and 2000. In 1900, the 10 leading causes of death were influenza and pneumonia, tuberculosis, diarrhea and related diseases, heart disease, stroke, chronic nephritis, accidents, cancer, perinatal conditions, and diphtheria. By the year 2000, tuberculosis, gastroenteritis, and diphtheria dropped off the list of the top 10 killers, and deaths from influenza and pneumonia fell from first to seventh position on the list. Diseases of aging and other chronic conditions superseded these infectious disease processes as changes in the age structure of the population, especially the increase in persons over age 65, resulted in higher overall crude rates for heart disease and cancer and the appearance of diabetes, Alzheimer's disease, chronic kidney conditions, and septicemia on the modern list of the top 10 killers.

Changes in crude death rates substantially understate the gains in life expectancy realized for all age groups over the 20th century. On an age-adjusted basis, improvements were even more impressive. Age-adjusted mortality rates fell about 75% between 1900 and 2000, with infant and child mortality rates 95% lower, adolescent and young adult mortality rates 80% lower, rates for 25–64 year-old adults lower by 60%, and rates for adults older than age 65 falling 35%.

These gains were not solely the result of better prevention and control of infectious diseases and advances in antibiotics and vaccinations in the first half of the

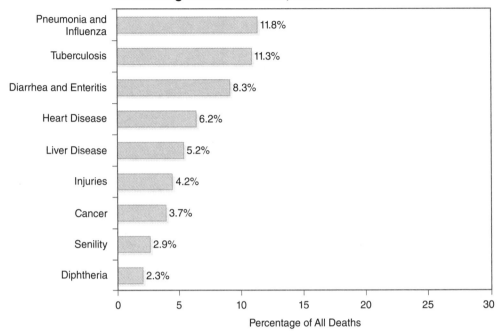

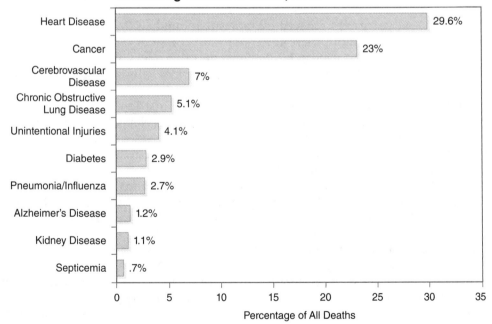

Figure 2-1 The 10 leading causes of death as a percentage of all deaths in the United States, 1900 and 2000.

Reproduced from the Office of Disease Prevention and Health Promotion. *Healthy People 2010: Understanding and Improving Health.* Rockville, MD: ODPHP; 2000 and National Center for Health Statistics. *Health, United States,* 2002. Hyattsville, MD: NCHS; 2002.

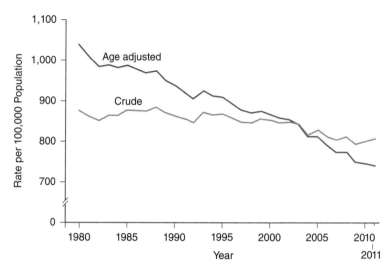

Figure 2-2   Crude and age-adjusted mortality rates, United States, 1980–2011.

Reproduced from Centers for Disease Control and Prevention, National Center for Health Statistics, National Vital Statistics System.

century. During the second half of the 20th century, overall age-adjusted mortality rates fell about 50%, while infant mortality rates declined more than 75%. During that period, mortality rates among children and young adults (ages 1–24 years) and adults 45–64 years were reduced by more than one-half. Mortality rates among adults 25–44 years fell more than 40%, and rates for elderly persons (age 65 and older) fell about one-third. Figure 2-2 demonstrates that age-adjusted mortality rates continued to fall faster than overall crude mortality rates through the first decade of the 21st century.

Gains for adult age groups in recent decades have outstripped those for younger age groups, a trend that began about 1960 as progress accelerated toward reduction of mortality from injuries and certain major chronic diseases that largely affected adults. Over the second half of the 20th century, dramatic reductions in the death rates for heart disease, stroke, unintentional injuries, influenza and pneumonia, and infant mortality have been joined by more recent reductions in rates for human immunodeficiency virus (HIV) infections, liver diseases, and suicide. On the other hand, death rates have increased for diabetes, Alzheimer's disease, and chronic lung and kidney conditions, signaling the new morbidities associated with longer life spans. Homicide rates have improved somewhat over the past decade but still reflect a substantial increase since 1950.[1]

Despite this progress, considerable disparities persist for many of the major causes of death. Differences among races are notable, but there are also significant differences by gender for the various causes of death. These differences are often dramatic and run from top to bottom through the chain of causation. Disparities are found not only in indicators of poor health outcomes, such as mortality, but also in the levels of risk factors in the population groups most severely affected. A sobering example of these disparities is reflected in the 10-year difference in life expectancy between white females and black males.

OUTSIDE-THE-BOOK THINKING 2-1

Examine each of these websites. Which ones are most useful for the major topics examined in this chapter? Why?

- Healthfinder (www.healthfinder.gov), a Department of Health and Human Services (DHHS)-sponsored gateway site that provides links to more than 550 websites (including more than 200 federal sites and 350 state, local, not-for-profit, university, and other consumer health sources), nearly 500 selected online documents, frequently asked questions on health issues, and databases and web search engines by topic and agency
- Fedstats (fedstats.sites.usa.gov/), a gateway to a variety of federal agency data and information, including health statistics
- National Center for Health Statistics (NCHS) (www.cdc.gov/nchs/index.htm), an invaluable resource for data and information, especially "Health, United States," which can be downloaded from this site
- Centers for Disease Control and Prevention (CDC) Mortality and Morbidity Weekly Report (www.cdc.gov/mmwr/) and MMWR morbidity and mortality data by time and place (www.cdc.gov/mmwr/distrnds.html)
- U.S. Census data (www.census.gov), the best general denominator data anywhere

There is also evidence that disability levels are declining in the general population over time. Disability levels among individuals aged 55–70 years who were offspring of the famous Framingham Heart Study cohort were substantially lower, in comparison with their parents' experience at the same age.[2] In addition, fewer offspring had chronic diseases or perceived their health as fair or poor. Self-reported health status and activity limitations because of chronic conditions changed little during the 1990s, and injuries with lost workdays steadily declined during the 1990s.

In sum, U.S. health indicators tell two very different tales. By many measures, the American population has never been healthier. By others, much more needs to be done for specific racial, ethnic, and gender groups. The gains in health status over the past century have not been shared equally by all subgroups of the population. In fact, relative differences have been increasing. This widening gap in health status creates both a challenge and a dilemma for future health improvement efforts. The greatest gains can be made through closing these gaps and equalizing health status within the population. Yet the burden of greater risk and poorer health status resides in a relatively small part of the total population, calling for efforts that target those minorities with increased resources. An alternative approach is to continue current strategies and resource deployment levels in order to sustain steady overall improvement among all groups in the population. This strategy, however, is likely to continue or worsen existing gaps. In the early years of the new century, the major health challenge facing the United States appears to be less related to the need to improve population-wide health outcomes than the need to eliminate or reduce disparities. This challenges the nation's commitment to its principles of equality and social justice as addressing inequities in measures of health and quality of life requires a greater understanding of health and the measures used to describe it than afforded by death rates and life expectancies.

HEALTH, ILLNESS, AND DISEASE

Relationships among health outcomes and the factors that influence them are complex, often confounded by different understandings of the concepts in question and how they are measured. Health is difficult to define and more difficult yet to measure. For much of history, the notion of health has been negative. This was due in part to the continuous onslaught of epidemic diseases. With disease a frequent visitor, health became the disease-free state. One was healthy by exclusion.

As knowledge of disease increased and methods of prevention and control improved, health has come to be considered from a more positive perspective. The World Health Organization (WHO) seized this opportunity in its 1946 constitution, defining health as not merely the absence of disease but a state of complete physical, mental, and social well-being.[3] This definition of health emphasizes that there are different, complexly related forms of wellness and illness, and suggests that a wide range of factors can influence the health of individuals and groups. It also suggests that health is not an absolute concept.

Although health and well-being may be synonyms, health and disease are not necessarily opposites. Most people view health and illness as existing along a continuum and as opposite and mutually exclusive states. However, this simplistic, one-dimensional model of health and illness does not comport very well with the real world. A person can have a condition or injury and still be healthy and feel well. There are many examples, but certainly Olympic wheelchair racers would fit into this category. It is also possible for someone without a specific disease or injury to feel ill or not well. If health and illness are not mutually exclusive, then they exist in separate dimensions, with wellness and illness in one dimension and the presence or absence of disease or injury in another.

These distinctions are important because disease is a relatively objective, pathologic phenomenon, whereas wellness and illness represent subjective experiences. This allows for several different states to exist: wellness without disease or injury, wellness with disease or injury, illness with disease or injury, and illness without physical disease or injury. This multidimensional view of health states is consistent with the WHO delineation of physical, mental, and social dimensions of health or well-being. Health or wellness is more than the absence of disease alone. Furthermore, one can be physically but not mentally and socially well.

With health measurable in several different dimensions, the question arises as to whether there is some maximum or optimal end point of health or well-being or whether health is something that can always be improved through changes in its physical, mental, and social facets. This suggests that the goal should be a minimal acceptable level of health, rather than a state of complete and absolute health. Due in part to these considerations, WHO revised its definition in 1978, calling for a level of health that permits people to lead socially and economically productive lives.[4] This shifts the focus of health from an end in itself to a resource for everyday life, linking physical to personal and social capacities. It also suggests that it will be easier to identify measures of illness than of health.

Disease and injury are often viewed as phenomena that may lead to significant loss or disability in social functioning, making one unable to carry out one's main personal or social functions in life, such as parenting, schooling, or employment. In this perspective, health is equivalent to the absence of disability; individuals able to carry out their basic functions in life are healthy. This characterization of health as the absence of significant functional disabilities is perhaps the most common one for this highly sought state. Still, this definition is a negative one in that it defines health as the absence of disability.

The concept of well-being advanced in the WHO definition goes beyond the physical aspects of health that are the usual focus of measurements and comparisons. Including the mental and social aspects of well-being or health legitimizes the examination of factors that affect mental and social health. Together, these themes underscore the need to consider carefully what is being measured in order to understand what these measures tell us about health, illness, and disease states in a population and the factors that influence these outcomes.

MEASURING HEALTH

The plethora of information on health outcomes suggests that measuring the health status of populations is a simple task. However, although often interesting and sometimes even dramatic, the commonly used measures of health status fail to paint a complete picture of health. Many of the reasons are obvious. The commonly used measures actually reflect disease and mortality, rather than health itself. The long-standing misperception that health is the absence of disease is reinforced by the relative ease of measuring disease states, in comparison with states of health. Actually, the most commonly used indicators focus on a state that is neither health nor disease—namely, death.

Despite the many problems with using mortality as a proxy for health, mortality data are generally available and widely used to describe the health status of populations. This is ironic because such data only indirectly describe the health status of living populations. Unfortunately, data on morbidity (illnesses, injuries, and functional limitations of the population) are neither as available nor as readily understood as are mortality data. This situation is improving, however, as new forms and sources of information on health conditions become more readily available. Sources for information on morbidities and disabilities now include medical records from hospitals, managed care organizations, and other providers, as well as information derived from surveys, businesses, schools, and other sources. Assessments of the health status of populations are increasingly utilizing measures from these sources. An excellent compilation of data and information on both health status and health services, *Health United States*, is published annually by the National Center for Health Statistics.[1] Much of the data used in this chapter is derived from this source.

Mortality-Based Measures

Although mortality-based indicators of health status are both widely used and useful, there are some important differences in their use and interpretation. The most commonly used are crude mortality, age-specific and age-adjusted mortality, life expectancy, and years of potential life lost (YPLL). Although all are based on the same events, each provides somewhat different information as to the health status of a population.

Crude mortality rates count deaths within the entire population and are not sensitive to differences in the age distribution of different populations. The mortality comparisons presented in Figure 2-2 comparing crude and age-adjusted death rates illustrate the limitations of using crude death rates to assess the mortality experience of the U.S. population. On the basis of these data, we might conclude that mortality rates in the United States had declined about 10% since 1980. However, because there has been an increasing proportion of population in the higher age categories over recent decades, these are not truly comparable populations. The 10% reduction actually understates the differences in mortality experience over this 30-year period after changes in the age structure of the population are controlled. The 10% reduction then becomes a 30% reduction! Because differences in the age characteristics of the two populations are a primary concern, we look for methods to correct or adjust for the age factor. Age-specific and age-adjusted rates do just that. The second half of the 20th century witnessed decreases of 50% or more for age-adjusted mortality rates for stroke, heart disease, infant deaths, tuberculosis, influenza and pneumonia, syphilis, unintentional injuries, HIV infections, and gastric, uterine, and cervical cancers.[1] Improvements in age-adjusted mortality rates for the leading causes of death are continuing in the early years of the new century.[1]

Age-specific mortality rates relate the number of deaths to the number of persons in a specific age group. The infant mortality rate is probably the best-known example, describing the number of deaths of live-born infants occurring in the first year of life per 1,000 live births. Public health studies often use age-adjusted mortality rates to compensate for different mixes of age groups within a population (e.g., a high proportion of children or elderly). Age-adjusted rates are calculated by applying age-specific rates to a standard population (we now use the 2000 U.S. population). This adjustment permits more meaningful comparisons of mortality experience between populations with different age distribution patterns. Differences between crude and age-adjusted mortality rates can be substantial.

Life expectancy, also based on the mortality experience of a population, is a computation of the number of years between any given age (e.g., birth or age 65) and the average age of death for that population. Figure 2-3 presents recent data and trends for life expectancy at birth in the United States; Figure 2-4 provides international comparisons for life expectancy. Together with infant mortality rates, life expectancies are commonly used in comparisons of health status among nations. These two mortality-based indicators are often considered to be general indicators of the overall health status of a population. Infant mortality and life expectancy measures for the United States are lackluster in comparison with those of other developed nations. The figure presenting international comparisons of life expectancy at birth by gender suggests that the United States is far from being the healthiest nation in the world.

YPLL is a mortality-based indicator that places greater weight on deaths that occur at younger ages. Years of life lost before some arbitrary age (often age 65 or 75) are computed and used to measure the relative impact on society of different causes of death. If age 65 is used as the threshold for calculating YPLL, an infant death would contribute 65 YPLL, and a homicide at age 25 would contribute 40 YPLL. A death due to stroke at age 70 would contribute no years of life lost before age 65, and so on. Until relatively recently, age 65 was widely used as the threshold age.

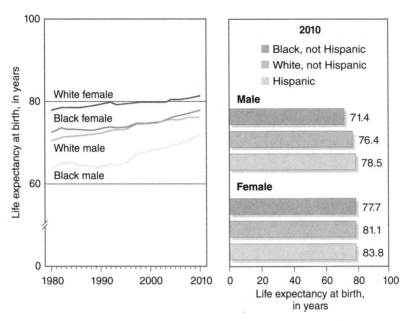

Figure 2-3   Life expectancy at birth by race and gender, United States, 1980–2010.

Reproduced from CDC/NCHS, *Health, United States,* 2013, Figure 1. Data from the National Vital Statistics System.

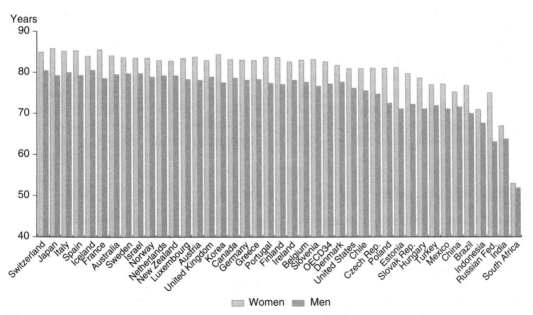

Figure 2-4   Life expectancy at birth, by sex, United States and selected countries and territories, 2011 (or nearest year).

Reproduced from OECD Health Statistics 2013, http://dx.doi.org/10.1787/health-data-en; World Bank for non-OECD countries. [OECD: International Organization for Economic Cooperation and Development].

Table 2-1   Age-Adjusted Years of Potential Life Lost (YPLL) Before Age 75 by Cause of Death and Ranks for YPLL and Number of Deaths, United States, 2000

Causes of Death	YPLL	Rank by YPLL	Rank by Number of Deaths
Cancer	1,698,500	1	2
Heart disease	1,270,700	2	1
Unintentional injuries	1,052,500	3	5
Suicide	343,300	4	11
Homicide	274,200	5	14
Cerebrovascular diseases	226,500	6	3
Chronic obstructive lung disease	190,700	7	4
Diabetes mellitus	181,200	8	6
HIV infections	178,900	9	18
Chronic liver disease and cirrhosis	141,700	10	12

Data from National Center for Health Statistics. *Health, United States,* 2002. Hyattsville, MD: NCHS; 2002.

With life expectancies now exceeding 75 years at birth, YPLL calculations using age 75 as the threshold have become more common. Data on YPLL before age 75 is presented in Table 2-1, illustrating the usefulness of this approach in providing a somewhat different perspective as to which problems are most important in terms of their magnitude and impact. The use of YPLL ranks cancer, HIV infections, and various forms of injury-related deaths higher than does the use of crude numbers or rates. Conversely, the use of crude rates ranks heart disease, stroke, pneumonia, diabetes, and chronic lung and liver diseases higher than does the use of YPLL. Four of the top 10 causes of death, as determined by the number of deaths, do not appear in the list of the top 10 causes of YPLL. Each of these various mortality indicators can be examined for various racial and ethnic subpopulations to identify disparities among these groups.

Morbidity, Disability, and Quality Measures

Mortality indicators can also be combined with other health indicators that describe quality considerations to provide a measure of the span of healthy life. These indicators can be an especially meaningful measure of health status in a population because they also consider morbidity and disability from conditions that impact on functioning but do not cause death (e.g., cerebral palsy, schizophrenia, arthritis). A commonly used measure of aggregate disease burden is the disability-adjusted life-year or DALY. Other variants on this theme are span-of-healthy-life indicators (called years of healthy life) that combine mortality data with self-reported health status and activity limitation data acquired through the National Health Interview Survey. Depending on the healthy life expectancy measure,

Americans average about 10 years of poor health, 15 years of activity limitation, and 30 years of living with a chronic disease. Women have better health status than men, and whites do better than blacks on virtually all of these measures. For healthy life expectancies at age 65, a similar picture appears. The implication is that extending healthy life expectancy can be achieved through several pathways. One would be to extend life expectancy without increasing the measures of poor health, activity limitation, and chronic disease burden. Another would be to reduce the measures of poor health, activity limitation, and chronic disease burden within a constant life expectancy. The optimal approach would accomplish both by extending life expectancy and reducing the burden of poor health, activity limitation, and chronic disease.

Although less frequently encountered, indicators of morbidity and disability are also quite useful in measuring health status. Both prevalence (the number or rate of cases at a specific point or period in time) and incidence (the number or rate of new cases occurring during a specific period) are widely used measures of morbidity.

Increasingly, information on self-reported health status and on days lost from work or school because of acute or chronic conditions is collected through surveys of the general population. The National Center for Health Statistics also conducts ongoing surveys of health providers on complaints and conditions requiring medical care in outpatient settings. These surveys provide direct information on self-reported health status and illuminate some of the factors, such as household income levels, that are associated with health status.

INFLUENCES ON HEALTH

In 1996, public health surveillance in the United States took a historic step. At that time, the Centers for Disease Control and Prevention (CDC) added prevalence of cigarette smoking to the list of diseases and conditions to be reported by states to CDC.[5] This action marked the first time that a health behavior, rather than an illness or disease, was considered nationally reportable—a groundbreaking step for surveillance efforts. How the focus of public health efforts shifted from conventional disease outcomes to reporting on underlying causes amenable to public health intervention is an important story.

Risk Factors

The recognition of tobacco use as a major health hazard was no simple achievement, partly because many factors directly or indirectly influence the level of a health outcome in a given population. For example, greater per capita tobacco use in a population is associated with higher rates of heart disease and lung cancer, and lower rates of early prenatal care are associated with higher infant mortality rates. Because these factors are part of the chain of causation for health outcomes, tracking their levels provides an early indication as to the direction in which the health outcome is likely to change. These factors increase the likelihood or risk of particular health outcomes occurring and can be characterized broadly as risk factors.

The types and number of risk factors are as varied as the influences themselves. Depending on how these factors are lumped or split, traditional categories include

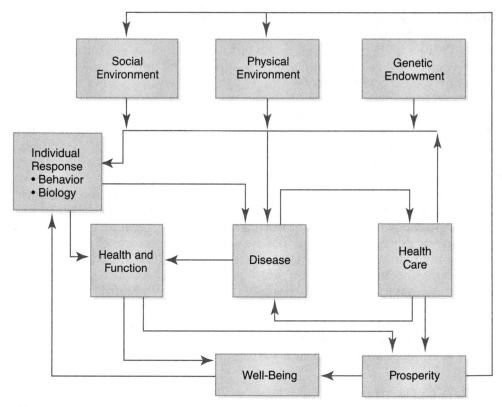

Figure 2-5   Determinants of health.

Reproduced from Evans RG, Stoddard GL. Producing health, consuming health. *Soc Sci Med.* 1990;31:1359.

---

biologic factors (from genetic endowment to aging), environmental factors (from food, air, and water to communicable diseases), lifestyle factors (from diet to injury avoidance and sexual behaviors), psychosocial factors (from poverty to stress, personality, and cultural factors), and use of and access to health-related services. Refinements of this framework are reflected in Figure 2-5, which differentiates several outcomes of interest, including disease, functional capacity, prosperity, and well-being that can be influenced by various risk factors. These various components are often interrelated (e.g., stress, a social environmental factor, may stimulate individual responses, such as tobacco or illicit drug use, which, in turn, influence the likelihood of disease, functional capacity, and well-being). In addition, variations in one outcome, such as disease, may influence changes in others, such as well-being, depending on the mix of other factors present. This complex set of interactions, consistent with the social-ecological model, draws attention to fundamental factors or causes that can result in many diseases, rather than focusing on specific factors that contribute little to population-wide health status.

Although many factors are causally related to health outcomes, some are more direct and proximal causes than others. Specific risk factors have been clearly linked to specific adverse health states through epidemiologic studies. For example,

Table 2-2 Selected Behavioral Risk Factors Related to Leading Causes of Deaths in the United States, 2000

Cause of Death and Percentage of all Deaths	Smoking	High Fat/ Low Fiber	Sedentary Lifestyle	High Blood Pressure	Elevated Cholesterol	Obesity	Alcohol Use
Heart disease (30%)	✗	✗	✗	✗	✗	✗	✗
Cancer (23%)	✗	✗	✗			✗	✗
Stroke (7%)	✗	✗		✗	✗	✗	
Chronic lung disease (5%)	✗						
Unintentional injuries (4%)	✗						✗
Pneumonia & influenza (3%)	✗						
Diabetes (3%)		✗	✗			✗	
HIV infection (1%)							
Suicide (1%)							✗
Chronic liver disease (1%)							✗
Atherosclerosis (1%)	✗	✗	✗		✗		

Data from causes and percent death from National Center for Health Statistics, *Health, United States,* 2002. Hyattsville, MD: NCHS; 2002. Risk factors related to causes from Brownson RC, Remington PL, Davis JR, et al. *Chronic Disease Epidemiology and Control.* 2nd ed. Washington, DC: American Public Health Association; 1998; and U.S. Public Health Service. *The Surgeon General's Report on Nutrition and Health.* Washington, DC: PHS, 1988.

numerous studies have linked unintentional injuries with a variety of risk factors, including the accessibility to firearms and the use of alcohol, tobacco, and seat belts. Tobacco, hypertension, over-nutrition, and diabetes are well-known risk factors for heart disease. As documented in Table 2-2, epidemiologic research and studies over the past 50 years have linked numerous behavioral risk factors to many common diseases and conditions.[6] Ongoing behavioral risk factor surveys (often through telephone interviews) are conducted by governmental public health agencies to track trends in the prevalence of many important risk behaviors within the population. These surveys document that the health-related behaviors of tens of millions of Americans place them at risk for developing chronic disease and injuries.

Despite the recent emphasis on behavioral factors, risk factors in the physical environment remain important influences on health. Air pollution, for example, is directly related to a wide range of diseases, including lung cancer, pulmonary emphysema, chronic bronchitis, and bronchial asthma. National standards exist for many of the most important air pollutants and are tracked to determine the extent of these risks in the general population. The proportion of the U.S. population residing in counties that have exceeded national standards for these pollutants suggests that air pollution risks, like behavioral risks, affect tens of millions of Americans.[7] The physical environment influences health through several pathways, including facilitating risk-taking behaviors, influencing social relationships, and even exposing residents to visual cues that can arouse fear, anxiety, and depression.

Behavioral and environmental risk factors are clearly germane to public health interest and efforts. Focusing on these factors provides a different perspective of the enemies of personal and public health than that conveyed by disease-specific incidence or mortality data. Such a focus also promotes more rational policy development and interventions. Unfortunately, determining which underlying factors are most important is more difficult than it appears because of differences in the outcomes under study and measures used. For example, a study using 1980 data found tobacco, hypertension, and over-nutrition responsible for about three-fourths of deaths before age 65 and injury risks, alcohol, tobacco, and gaps in primary prevention accounting for about three-fourths of all YPLL before age 65.[8] Further complicating these analyses is the finding that individual risk factors may result in several different health outcomes. For example, alcohol use is linked with motor vehicle injuries, other injuries, cancer, and cirrhosis; tobacco use can result in heart disease, stroke, ulcers, fire and burn injuries, and low birth weight, as well as cancer.[6,8]

Despite problems with their measurement, the identification of antecedent causes is important for public health policy and interventions. Table 2-3 compares

Table 2-3   Listed and Actual Causes of Death, United States, 2000

10 Leading Causes of Death	Number	Actual Causes of Death	Number
Heart disease	710,760	Tobacco	435,000
Malignant neoplasm	553,091	Poor diet and physical inactivity	400,000
Cerebrovascular disease	167,661	Alcohol consumption	85,000
Chronic lower respiratory tract diseases	122,009	Microbial agents	75,000
Unintentional injuries	97,900	Toxic agents	55,000
Diabetes mellitus	69,301	Motor vehicle	43,000
Influenza and pneumonia	65,313	Firearms	29,000
Alzheimer's disease	49,558	Sexual behavior	20,000
Nephritis, nephrotic syndrome, and nephrosis	37,251	Illicit drug use	17,000
Septicemia	31,224	**Total**	**1,159,000**
Other	499,283		
Total	**2,403,351**		

Data from Mokdad AM, Marks JS, Stoup DF, Gerberding JL. Actual causes of death in the United States, 2000. *JAMA.* 2004;291:1238–1245.

deaths in the year 2000 by their listed causes of death and their actual causes (major risk factors).[9] The two lists provide contrasting views as to the major health problems and needs of the U.S. population.

Coroners and medical examiners report immediate and underlying causes of death through death certificates, which have two parts, one for entering the immediate and underlying conditions that caused the death and a second for identifying conditions or injuries that contributed to death but did not cause death. For example, a death attributed to cardiovascular disease might list cardiac tamponade as the immediate cause, due to or as a consequence of a ruptured myocardial infarction, which itself was due to or a consequence of coronary arteriosclerosis. For this death, hypertensive cardiovascular disease might be listed as a significant condition contributing to, but not causing, the immediate and underlying causes. So where do smoking, obesity, diet, and physical inactivity get identified as the real causes of such deaths? Perhaps the Chadwick-Farr debate of the mid-19th century continues today in terms of whether deaths in the year 2000 should be attributed to tobacco use, just as many of those in England in 1839 might have been attributed to starvation.

OUTSIDE-THE-BOOK THINKING 2-2

Visit the Internet web site of several national print media and use the search features to identify articles on public health for a recent month. Catalog the health problems (both conditions and risks) from that search and compare this with the listing of health problems and issues on Table 2-3. Are the types of conditions and risks you encountered in the print media similar? Were some conditions and risks either overrepresented or underrepresented in the media, in comparison with their relative importance as suggested by Table 2-3? What are the implications for the role of the media in informing and educating the public regarding public health issues?

Social and Cultural Influences

Understanding the health effects of biologic, behavioral, and environmental risk factors is straightforward in comparison with understanding the effects of social, economic, and cultural factors on the health of populations. This is due in part to a lack of agreement as to what is being measured. Socioeconomic status and poverty are two factors that generally reflect position in society. There is considerable evidence that social position is an overarching fundamental determinant of health status, even though the indicators used to measure social standing are imprecise, at best.

Social standing affects lifestyle, environment, and the utilization of services; it remains an important predictor of good and poor health in our society. Social class differences in mortality have long been recognized around the world. In 1842, Chadwick reported that the average ages at death for occupationally stratified groups in England were as follows: "gentlemen and persons engaged in the professions, 45 years; tradesmen and their families, 26 years; mechanics, servants and laborers, and their families, 16 years."[10] Life expectancies and other health indicators have improved considerably in England and elsewhere since 1842, but differences in mortality rates among the various social classes persist to the present day.

OUTSIDE-THE-BOOK THINKING 2-3

Great Debate: There are three propositions to be considered. Proposition A: Disease entities should be listed as official causes of death. Proposition B: Underlying factors that result in these diseases should be listed as official causes of death. Proposition C: No causes of death should be listed on death certificates. Select one of these positions and develop a position statement with your rationale.

Several countries, including Great Britain and the United States, have identifiable social strata that permit comparisons of health status by social class. Britain conducts ongoing analyses of socioeconomic differences according to official categorizations based on general social standing within the community. For the United States, educational status, race, and family income are often used as indirect or proxy measures of social class. Despite the differences in approaches and indicators, there is little evidence of any real difference between Britain and the United States in terms of what is being measured. In both countries, explanations for the differences in mortality appear to relate primarily to inequalities in social position and material resources.[11,12] This effect operates all up and down the hierarchy of social standing; at each step improvements in social status are linked with improvements in measures of health status. For example, a study based on 1971 British census follow-up data found that a relatively affluent, home-owning group with two cars had a lower mortality risk than did a similar relatively privileged group with only one car.[11]

In the United States, epidemiologists have studied socioeconomic differences in mortality risk since the early 1900s. Infant mortality has been the subject of many studies that have consistently documented the effects of poverty. Findings from the National Maternal and Infant Health Survey, for example, demonstrated that the effects of poverty were greater for infants born to mothers with no other risk factors than for infants born to high-risk mothers.[13] Poverty status was associated with a 60% higher rate of neonatal mortality and a 200% higher rate for postneonatal mortality than for those infants of higher-income mothers.

Poverty affects many health outcomes. Low-income families in the United States have an increased likelihood (or relative risk) of a variety of adverse health outcomes, often two to five times greater than that of higher-income families. The percentage of persons reporting fair or poor health is about four times as high for persons living below the poverty level as for those with family income at least twice the poverty level.[1]

The implications of the consistent relationship between measures of social standing and health outcomes suggest that studies need to consider how and how well social class is categorized and measured. Imprecise measures may understate the actual differences that are the result of socioeconomic position in society. Importantly, if racial or ethnic differences are simply attributed to social class differences, factors that operate through race and ethnicity, such as racism or ethnic discrimination, will be overlooked. These additional factors also affect the difference between the social position one has and the position one would have attained, were it not for one's race or ethnicity. Race in the United States, independent of socioeconomic status, is linked to mortality, although these effects vary across age and disease categories.[14] Nevertheless, anthropologists concluded long ago that race is not an appropriate generic category for comparing health outcomes. Its usefulness does not derive from any biologic or genetic differences, but rather, it derives from its social, cultural, political, and historical meanings.

Studies of the effect of social factors on health status across nations add some interesting insights. In general, health appears to be closely associated with income differentials within countries, but there is only a weak link between national mortality rates and average income among the developed countries.[15] This pattern suggests that health is affected less by changes in absolute material standards across affluent populations than by relative income differences and the resulting disadvantage in each country. It is not the richest countries that have the greatest life expectancy. Rather, it is those developed nations with the narrowest income differentials between rich and poor. This finding argues that health in the developed world is less a matter of a population's absolute material wealth than of how the population's circumstances compare with those of other members of their society. A similar perspective views income to be related to health through two pathways: a direct effect on the material conditions necessary for survival, and an effect on social participation and the opportunity to control one's own life circumstances.[16] In settings or societies that provide little in the way of material conditions (e.g., clean water, sanitation services, ample food, adequate housing), income is more important for health. Where material conditions are conducive to good health, income acts through social participation.

The effects of culture on health and illness are also becoming better understood. To medical anthropologists, diseases are not purely independent phenomena. Rather, they are to be viewed and understood in relation to ecology and culture. Certainly, the type and severity of disease varies by age, sex, social class, and ethnic group. For example, Puerto Rican children overall have a higher prevalence of asthma than Mexican American, non-Hispanic white, and African American children.[17] Differences in poverty status do not explain the disparities for Puerto Rican and African American children, two populations that have higher asthma rates than non-Hispanic white and Mexican American children regardless of poverty status. The reason for the higher rate among Puerto Rican children overall is unknown, but the different distributions and social patterns suggest differences in culture-mediated behaviors. Such insights are essential to developing successful prevention and control programs. Culture serves to shape health-related behaviors, as well as human responses to diseases including changes in the environment, which, in turn, affect health. As a mechanism of adapting to the environment, culture has great potential for both positively and negatively affecting health.

There is evidence that different societies shape the ways in which diseases are experienced and that social patterns of disease persist, even after risk factors are identified and effective interventions become available.[18,19] For example, the link between poverty and various outcomes has been well established, yet even after advances in medicine and public health and significant improvement in general living and working conditions, the association persists. One explanation is that as some risks were addressed, others developed, such as health-related behaviors, including violent behavior and alcohol, tobacco, and drug use. In this way, societies create and shape the diseases that they experience. This makes sense, especially if we view the social context in which health and disease reside—the setting and social networks. For problems such as HIV infections, sexually transmitted diseases, and illicit drug use, spread is heavily influenced by the links between those at risk.[20] This also helps to explain why people in disorganized social structures are more likely to report their own health as poor than are similar persons with more social capital.[21,22]

Societal responses to diseases are also socially constructed. Efforts to prevent the spread of typhoid fever by limiting the rights of carriers (such as Typhoid Mary) differed greatly from those to reduce transmission risks from diphtheria carriers. Because many otherwise normal citizens would have been subjected to extreme measures in order to avoid the risk of transmission, it was not socially acceptable to invoke similar measures for these similar risks.

If these themes of social and cultural influences are on target, they place the study of health disparities and inequities at the top of the public health agenda. They also argue that health should be viewed as a social phenomenon. Rather than attempting to identify each and every risk factor that contributes only marginally to disparate health outcomes of the lower social classes, a more effective approach would be to directly address the broader social policies (distribution of wealth, education, employment, discrimination, and the like) that foster the social disparities that cause the observed differences in health outcomes.[19] This social-ecological view of health and its determinants is critical to understanding and improving health status in the United States and other nations.

Global Health Influences

Considerable variation exists among the world's nations on virtually every measure of health and illness currently in use. The principal factors responsible for observed trends and obvious inequities across the globe fall into the general categories of the social and physical environment, personal behavior, and health services. Given the considerable variation in social, economic, and health status among the developed, developing, and underdeveloped nations, it is naive to make broad generalizations. Countries with favorable health status indicators, however, generally have a well-developed health infrastructure, ample opportunities for education and training, relatively high status for women, and economic development that counterbalances population growth. Nonetheless, countries at all levels of development share some problems, including the escalating costs involved in providing a broad range of health, social, and economic development services to disadvantaged subgroups within the population. Social and cultural upheaval associated with urbanization is another problem common to countries at all levels of development. Over the course of the 20th century, the proportion of the world's population living in urban areas tripled—to about 40%; this trend is expected to continue throughout the new century.

The principal environmental hazards in the world today appear to be those associated with poverty. This is true for developed as well as developing and under-developed countries. Some international epidemiologists predict that, in the 21st century, the effects of overpopulation and production of greenhouse gases will join poverty as major threats to global health. These factors represent human effects on the world's climate and resources and are easily remembered as the "3 Ps" of global health (pollution, population, and poverty):

- Pollution of the atmosphere by greenhouse gases, which will result in significant global warming, affecting both climate and the occurrence of disease
- Worldwide population growth, which will result in a population of 10–12 billion people within the next century
- Poverty, which is always associated with ill health and disease[23,24]

It surprises many Americans that population is a major global health concern. Birth rates vary inversely with the level of economic development and the status of women among the nations of the world. Continuing high birth rates and declining death rates will mean even more rapid growth in population in developing countries. It has taken all of history to reach the world's current population level, but it will take less than half a century to double that. Many factors have influenced this growth, including public health, which has increased the chances of conception by improving the health status of adults, increasing infant and child survival, preventing premature deaths of adults in the most fertile age groups, and reducing the number of marriages dissolved by one partner's premature death.

Global warming represents yet another phenomenon with considerable potential for health effects. Climate change has direct temperature effects on humans and increases the likelihood of extreme weather events. A number of infectious diseases are also climate sensitive, some because of effects on mosquitoes, ticks, and other vectors in terms of their population size and density and changes in population movement, forest clearance and land use practices, surface water configurations, and human population density.[25] Global warming will also contribute to air quality-related health conditions and concerns.

In general, public health approaches to dealing with world health problems must overcome formidable obstacles, including the unequal and inefficient distribution of health services, lack of appropriate technology, poor management, poverty, and inadequate or inappropriate government programs to finance needed services. Much of the preventable disease in the world is concentrated in the developing and underdeveloped countries, where the most profound differences exist in terms of social and economic influences.

Although many of these factors appear to stem from low levels of national wealth, the link between national health status and national wealth is not firm, and comparisons across nations are seldom straightforward. Improved health status correlates more closely with changes in standards of living, advances in the politics of human relations, and a nation's literacy, education, and welfare policies than with specific preventive interventions. The complexities involved in identifying and understanding these forces and their interrelationships often confound comparisons of health status between the United States and other nations.

ANALYZING HEALTH PROBLEMS FOR CAUSATIVE FACTORS

The ability to identify risk factors and pathways for causation is essential for rational public health decisions and actions to address important health problems in a population. First, however, it is necessary to define what is meant by health problem. Here, health problem means a condition of humans that can be represented in terms of measurable health status or quality-of-life indicators. It is important to note that this basic definition must be modified for the purposes of community problem solving and the development of interventions. This characterization of a health problem as something measured only in terms of outcomes is difficult for some to accept. They point to important factors, such as access to care or poverty itself, and feel that these should rightfully be considered as health problems. Important problems they may be, but if they are truly important in the causation of some unacceptable health outcome, they can be dealt with as related factors rather than health problems.

The factors linked with specific health problems are often generically termed risk factors and can exist at one of three levels. Those risk factors most closely associated with the health outcome in question are often termed determinants. Risk factors that play a role further back in the chain of causation are called direct and indirect contributing factors. Risk factors can be described at either an individual or a population level. For example, tobacco use for an individual increases the chances of developing heart disease or lung cancer, and an increased prevalence of tobacco use in a population increases that population's incidence of (and mortality rates from) these conditions.

Determinants are scientifically established factors that relate directly to the level of a health problem. As the level of the determinant changes, the level of the health outcome changes. Determinants are the most proximal risk factors through which other levels of risk factors act. The link between the determinant and the health outcome should be well established through scientific or epidemiologic studies. For example, for neonatal mortality rates, two well-established determinants are the low-birth-weight rate (the number of infants born weighing less than 2,500 g, or about 5.5 pounds, per 100 live births) and weight-specific mortality rates. Improvement in the neonatal mortality rate cannot occur unless one of these determinants improves. Health outcomes can have one or many determinants.

Direct contributing factors are scientifically established factors that directly affect the level of a determinant. Again, there should be solid evidence that the level of the direct contributing factor affects the level of the determinant. For the neonatal mortality rate example, the prevalence of tobacco use among pregnant women has been associated with the risk of low birth weight. A determinant can have many direct contributing factors. For low birth weight, other direct contributing factors include low maternal weight gain and inadequate prenatal care.

Indirect contributing factors affect the level of the direct contributing factors. Although several steps distant from the health outcome in question, these factors are often proximal enough to be modified. The indirect contributing factor affects the level of the direct contributing factor, which, in turn, affects the level of the determinant. The level of the determinant then affects the level of the health outcome. Many indirect contributing factors can exist for each direct contributing factor. For prevalence of tobacco use among pregnant women, indirect contributing factors might include easy access to tobacco products for young women, lack of health education, and lack of smoking cessation programs.

OUTSIDE-THE-BOOK THINKING 2-4

Select a health outcome and analyze that outcome for its determinants and contributing factors, using the method described in the text. Identify at least two major determinants for the problem that you select. For each determinant, identify at least two direct contributing factors, and for each direct contributing factor, identify at least two indirect contributing factors.

The health problem analysis framework begins with the identification of a health problem (defined in terms of health status indicators) and proceeds to establish one or more determinants; for each determinant, one or more direct contributing factors; and for each direct contributing factor, one or more indirect contributing factors. Intervention strategies at the community level generally involve addressing these indirect contributing factors. When completed, an analysis identifies as many of the causal pathways as possible to determine which contributing factors exist in the setting in which an intervention strategy is planned. The framework for this approach is presented in Table 2-4 and Figure 2-6. This framework forms the basis for developing meaningful interventions; it is used in several of the processes and instruments to assess community health needs that are currently in wide use at the local level. Community health improvement processes and tools are topics for another chapter.

Table 2-4 Risk Factors

Determinant	Scientifically established factor that relates directly to the level of the health problem. A health problem may have any number of determinants identified for it.	Example: Low birth weight is a prime determinant for the health problem of neonatal mortality.
Direct contributing factor	Scientifically established factor that directly affects the level of the determinant.	Example: Use of prenatal care is one factor that affects the low-birth-weight rate.
Indirect contributing factor	Community-specific factor that affects the level of a direct contributing factor. Such factors can vary considerably from one community to another.	Example: Availability of day care or transportation services within the community may affect the use of prenatal care services.

Data from Centers for Disease Control and Prevention, Public Health Practice Program Office, 1991.

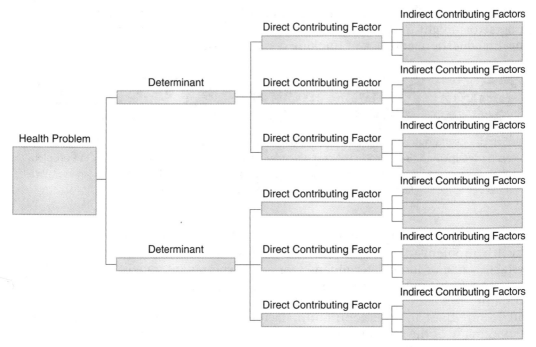

Figure 2-6   Health problem analysis worksheet.

Reproduced from Centers for Disease Control and Prevention, Public Health Practice Program Office, 1991.

Although this framework is useful, it does not fully account for the relationships among the various levels of risk factors. Some direct contributing factors may affect more than one determinant, and some indirect contributing factors may influence more than one direct contributing factor. For example, illicit drug use during pregnancy influences both the likelihood of low birth weight and birth weight-specific survival rates. To account fully for these interactions, some direct and indirect contributing factors may need to be included in several different locations on the worksheet. Despite the advancement of epidemiologic methods, many studies ignore the contributing factors that affect the level of these major risk factors, leading to simplistic formulations of multiple risk factors for health problems that exist at the community level.[26]

ECONOMIC DIMENSIONS OF HEALTH OUTCOMES

The ability to measure and quantify outcomes and risks is essential for rational decisions and actions. Specific indicators, as well as methods of economic analysis, are available to provide both objective and subjective valuations. Several health indicators attempt to value differentially health status; outcomes, including age-adjusted rates; span of healthy life; and YPLL. For example, YPLL represents a method of weighting or valuing health outcomes by placing a higher value on deaths that occur at earlier ages. Years of life lost thus become a common denominator or, in one sense, a common currency. Health outcomes can be translated into this currency or into an actual currency, such as dollars. This translation allows for comparisons to be made among outcomes in terms of which costs more per person, per episode, or per another reference point. Cost comparisons of health outcomes and health events have become common in public health. Approaches include cost-benefit, cost-effectiveness, and cost-utility studies.

Cost-benefit analyses provide comprehensive information on both the costs and the benefits of an intervention. All health outcomes and other relevant impacts are included in the determination of benefits. The results are expressed in terms of net costs, net benefits, and time required to recoup an initial investment. If the benefits are expressed in health outcome terms, years of life gained or quality-adjusted life-years (QALYs) may be calculated. This provides a framework for comparing disparate interventions. QALYs are calculated from a particular perspective that determines which costs and consequences are included in the analysis. For public health analyses, societal perspectives are necessary. When comprehensively performed, cost-benefit analyses are considered the gold standard of economic evaluations.

Cost-effectiveness analyses focus on one outcome to determine the most cost-effective intervention when several options are possible. Cost-effectiveness examines a specific option's costs to achieve a particular outcome. Results are often specified as the cost per case prevented or cost per life saved. For example, screening an entire town for a specific disease might identify cases at a cost of $150 per new case, whereas a screening program directed only at high-risk groups within that town might identify cases at a cost of $50 per new case. Although useful for evaluating different strategies for achieving the same result, cost-effectiveness approaches are not very helpful in evaluating interventions intended for different health conditions.

Cost-utility analyses are similar to cost-effectiveness studies, except that the results are characterized as cost per QALY. These are most useful when the intervention affects both morbidity and mortality, and there are a variety of possible outcomes that include quality of life.

These approaches are especially important for interventions based on preventive strategies. The argument is frequently made that "an ounce of prevention is worth a pound of cure." If this wisdom is true, preventive interventions should result in savings equal to 16 times their actual cost. Not many preventive interventions measure up to this standard, but even crude information on the costs of many health outcomes suggests that prevention has economic as well as human savings. The U.S. Public Health Service has estimated that as much as 11% of health expenditures for the year 2000 could have been averted through investments in public health for six conditions: motor vehicle injuries, occupationally related injuries, stroke, coronary heart disease, firearms-related injuries, and low-birth-weight infants.[27] Beyond the direct medical effects, there are often nonmedical costs related to lost wages, taxes, and productivity.

Economists assert that the future costs for care and services that result from prevention of mortality must be considered a negative benefit of prevention. For example, the costs of preventing a death from motor vehicle injuries should include all subsequent medical care costs for that individual over his or her lifetime, because these costs would not have occurred otherwise. They also argue that it is unfair to compare future savings to the costs of current prevention programs and that those savings must be discounted to their current value. If a preventive program will save $10 million 20 years from now, that $10 million must be translated into its current value in computing cost benefits, cost-effectiveness, or cost utility. It may be that the value of $10 million 20 years from now is only $4 million now. If the program costs $1 million, its benefit/ cost ratio would be 4:1 instead of 10:1 before we even added any additional costs associated with medical care for the lives that were saved. These economic considerations contribute to the difficulty of marketing preventive interventions.

Two additional economic considerations are important for public health policy and practice. The first of these is what is known as opportunity costs, which represents the costs involved in choosing one course of action over another. Resources spent for one purpose are not available to be spent for another. As a result, there is a need to consider the costs of not realizing the benefits or gains from paths not chosen. A second economic consideration important for public health is related to the heavy emphasis of public health on preventive strategies. The savings or gains from successful prevention efforts are generally not reinvested in public health or even other health purposes. These savings or gains from investments in prevention are lost. Maybe this is proper, because the overall benefits accrue more broadly to society, and public health remains, above all else, a social enterprise. However, imagine the situation for American industry and businesses if they could not reinvest their gains to grow their businesses. This is often the situation faced by public health, further exacerbating the difficulty of arguing for and securing needed resources.

HEALTHY PEOPLE 2020

The data and discussion in this chapter only broadly describe health status measures in the United States in the early decades of the new century. Several common themes emerge, however, that form the basis for national health objectives focusing on the year 2020.[28] Figure 2-7 (consistent with the social-ecological model described earlier) presents a *Healthy People* process grounded in a broad view of the many factors influencing health. The year 2020 objectives build on the nation's experience with three previous panels of health objectives established for the years 1990, 2000, and 2010.

Assessments of the *Healthy People 2000* and *Healthy People 2010* efforts yielded similar findings. In general, progress was apparent for many of the broader goals, especially the age-adjusted mortality targets for age groups under age 70. Nonetheless, a substantial proportion of the objectives targeting special populations, especially African Americans and Native Americans, were found to be moving in the wrong direction. These findings fueled concerns that health inequities and disparities were persisting, if not increasing, in the United States. In addition, with nearly 500 objectives established in both the 2000 and 2010 efforts, tracking became a complex undertaking. Many objectives could not be tracked because of the unavailability of or lack of consensus for the tracking measures.

Healthy People 2020 (HP2020), summarized in Table 2-5, provides a comprehensive set of 10-year, national goals and objectives for improving the health of all Americans. HP2020 contains 42 topic areas with over 1,200 objectives. A smaller set of objectives, called Leading Health Indicators, is identified in Table 2-6; these were selected to communicate high-priority health issues and actions that can be taken to address them.

Healthy People 2020
A society in which all people live long, healthy lives

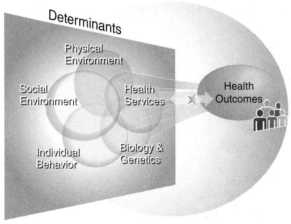

Overarching Goals:

- Attain high-quality longer lives free of preventable disease, disability, injury, and premature death.
- Achieve health equity, eliminate disparities, and improve the health of all groups.
- Create social and physical environments that promote good health for all.
- Promote quality of life, healthy development, and healthy behaviors across all life stages.

Figure 2-7 The *Healthy People 2020* model.

Reproduced from U.S. Department of Health and Human Services, *Healthy People 2020 Framework*. Available at www.healthypeople.gov website. Accessed March 15, 2014.

Table 2-5 *Healthy People 2020* Vision, Mission, Goals, and Focus Areas

Vision
A society in which all people live long, healthy lives.

Mission
Healthy People 2020 strives to:
- Identify nationwide health improvement priorities.
- Increase public awareness and understanding of the determinants of health, disease, and disability and the opportunities for progress.
- Provide measurable objectives and goals that are applicable at the national, state, and local levels.
- Engage multiple sectors to take actions to strengthen policies and improve practices that are driven by the best available evidence and knowledge.
- Identify critical research, evaluation, and data collection needs.

Overarching Goals
- Attain high-quality, longer lives free of preventable disease, disability, injury, and premature death.
- Achieve health equity, eliminate disparities, and improve the health of all groups.
- Create social and physical environments that promote good health for all.
- Promote quality of life, healthy development, and healthy behaviors across all life stages.

(continues)

Table 2-5   *Healthy People 2020* Vision, Mission, Goals, and Focus Areas   (*Continued*)

Focus Areas
1. Access to health services
2. Adolescent health
3. Arthritis, osteoporosis, and chronic back conditions
4. Blood disorders and blood safety
5. Cancer
6. Chronic kidney diseases
7. Dementia, including Alzheimer's disease
8. Diabetes
9. Disability and secondary conditions
10. Early and middle childhood
11. Educational and community-based programs
12. Environmental health
13. Family planning
14. Food safety
15. Genomics
16. Global health
17. Health communication and health information technology
18. Healthcare-associated infections
19. Hearing and other sensory or communication disorders (ear, nose, throat—voice, speech, and language)
20. Heart disease and stroke
21. HIV
22. Immunization and infectious diseases
23. Injury and violence prevention
24. Lesbian, gay, bisexual, and transgender health
25. Maternal, infant, and child health
26. Medical product safety
27. Mental health and mental disorders
28. Nutrition and weight status
29. Occupational safety and health
30. Older adults
31. Oral health
32. Physical activity
33. Preparedness
34. Public health infrastructure
35. Quality of life and well-being
36. Respiratory diseases
37. Sexually transmitted diseases
38. Sleep health
39. Social determinants of health
40. Substance abuse
41. Tobacco use
42. Vision

Reproduced from U.S. Department of Health and Human Services. *Healthy People 2020* website. Available at www.healthypeople.gov. Accessed June 3, 2014.

Table 2-6   *Healthy People 2020* Leading Indicators

Access to Health Services
- Persons with medical insurance
- Persons with a usual primary care provider

Clinical Preventive Services
- Adults who receive a colorectal cancer screening based on the most recent guidelines
- Adults with hypertension whose blood pressure is under control
- Adult diabetic population with an A1c value greater than 9 percent
- Children aged 19 to 35 months who receive the recommended doses of DTaP, polio, MMR, Hib, hepatitis B, varicella, and PCV vaccines

Environmental Quality
- Air Quality Index (AQI) exceeding 100
- Children aged 3 to 11 years exposed to secondhand smoke

Injury and Violence
- Fatal injuries
- Homicides

Maternal, Infant, and Child Health
- Infant deaths
- Preterm births

Mental Health
- Suicides
- Adolescents who experience major depressive episodes

Nutrition, Physical Activity, and Obesity
- Adults who meet current Federal physical activity guidelines for aerobic physical activity and muscle-strengthening activity
- Adults who are obese
- Children and adolescents who are considered obese
- Total vegetable intake for persons aged 2 years and older

Oral Health
- Persons aged 2 years and older who used the oral health care system in past 12 months

Reproductive and Sexual Health
- Sexually active females aged 15 to 44 years who received reproductive health services in the past 12 months
- Persons living with HIV who know their serostatus

Social Determinants
- Students who graduate with a regular diploma 4 years after starting 9th grade

Substance Abuse
- Adolescents using alcohol or any illicit drugs during the past 30 days
- Adults engaging in binge drinking during the past 30 days

Tobacco
- Adults who are current cigarette smokers
- Adolescents who smoked cigarettes in the past 30 days

Reproduced from U.S. Department of Health and Human Services. *Healthy People 2020* website. Available at www.healthypeople.gov. Accessed June 3, 2014.

The graphic framework for HP2020 offered in Figure 2-7 illustrates the fundamental interrelationships among the social determinants of health and emphasizes their collective impact and influence on health outcomes and conditions. The HP2020 framework also underscores a continued focus on population disparities, including those categorized by race/ethnicity, socioeconomic status, gender, age, disability status, sexual orientation, and geographic location. Four foundational health measures serve as indicators of progress toward achieving these goals: general health status, health-related quality of life, determinants of health, and disparities. Table 2-7 provides additional details on these measures.

Table 2-7   Measures of Progress Toward *Healthy People 2020* Goals

General Health Status
- Life expectancy (with international comparison)
- Healthy life expectancy
- Years of potential life lost (YPLL) (with international comparison)
- Physically and mentally unhealthy days
- Self-assessed health status
- Limitation of activity
- Chronic disease prevalence

Health-Related Quality of Life (HRQoL) and Well-Being
- Patient Reported Outcomes Measurement Information System (PROMIS) Global Health Measure — assesses global physical, mental and social HRQoL through questions on self-rated health, physical HRQoL, mental HRQoL, fatigue, pain, emotional distress, social activities, and roles.
- Well-Being Measures — assess the positive evaluations of people's daily lives — when they feel very healthy and satisfied or content with life, the quality of their relationships, their positive emotions, resilience, and realization of their potential.
- Participation Measures — reflect individuals' assessments of the impact of their health on their social participation within their current environment. Participation includes education, employment, civic, social and leisure activities. The principle behind participation measures is that a person with a functional limitation — for example, vision loss, mobility difficulty, or intellectual disability — can live a long and productive life and enjoy a good quality of life.

Determinants of Health
- Policymaking
- Social factors
- Health services
- Individual behavior
- Biology and genetics

Disparities
- Race and ethnicity
- Gender
- Sexual identity and orientation
- Disability status or special health care needs
- Geographic location (rural and urban)

Reproduced from U.S. Department of Health and Human Services. *Healthy People 2020* website. Available at www.healthypeople.gov. Accessed June 3, 2014.

Central to the *Healthy People 2020* effort are four overarching goals, two of which focus on:

1. Attaining high-quality, longer lives free of preventable disease, disability, injury, and premature death; and
2. Achieving health equity, eliminating disparities, and improving the health of all groups.

Although these two overarching goals appear appropriate, they are only arguably linked. From one perspective, they represent two very different approaches to improving outcomes for the population as a whole. If we view the health status of the entire population as a Gaussian curve, one approach would be to shift the entire curve further toward better outcomes, and a second approach would be to change the shape of the curve, reducing the difference between the extremes. These represent quite different strategies that would be associated with quite different policies and interventions. Focusing on the tail end of the distribution of health requires investment in questionably effective attempts that benefit relatively few and fail to promote the health of the majority. On the other hand, even small improvements in overall society-wide health measures have provided greater gains for society than very perceptible improvements in the health of a few.[29] The choice is one that can be viewed as focusing on "epiphenomena," such as risk factors or on the larger context and social environment. *Healthy People 2020* ambitiously seeks to do both.

OUTSIDE-THE-BOOK THINKING 2-5

Projections call for a continuing increase in life expectancy through the first half of the 21st century. What effect will increased life expectancy have on the major goals of *Healthy People 2020*—increasing the quality and years of healthy life and eliminating health disparities?

Monitoring all national health objectives is not considered feasible at the state and local level. Instead, only priorities linked to the national health objectives will likely be tracked. An Institute of Medicine committee in 1997 identified a basic set of indicators for use in community health improvement processes (Table 2-8). Together with the catalog of leading health indicators from the current Healthy People process, these measures provide a useful starting point for population-based community health assessment and improvement initiatives.

OUTSIDE-THE-BOOK THINKING 2-6

Your community is about to undertake a community health assessment and you have been tasked to review and improve the list of community health profile indicators proposed for this process. These include the *Healthy People 2020* Leading Health Indicators (Table 2-6) and the basic community health indictors proposed by the IOM (Table 2-8). Identify and justify three indicators you would add to this list, based on what you know about the health status and needs of your community.

Table 2-8   Proposed Indicators for a Community Health Profile

Sociodemographic Characteristics
1. Distribution of the population by age and race/ethnicity
2. Number and proportion of persons in groups such as migrants, homeless, or the non-English speaking for whom access to community services and resources may be a concern
3. Number and proportion of persons aged 25 and older with less than a high school education
4. Ratio of the number of students graduating from high school to the number of students who entered ninth grade 3 years previously
5. Median household income
6. Proportion of children less than 15 years of age living in families at or below the poverty level
7. Unemployment rate
8. Number and proportion of single-parent families
9. Number and proportion of persons without health insurance

Health Status
10. Infant mortality rate by race/ethnicity
11. Numbers of deaths or age-adjusted death rates for motor vehicle crashes, work-related injuries, suicide, homicide, lung cancer, breast cancer, cardiovascular diseases, and all causes, by age, race, and gender, as appropriate
12. Reported incidence of AIDS, measles, tuberculosis, and primary and secondary syphilis, by age, race, and gender, as appropriate
13. Births to adolescents (ages 10–17) as proportion of total live births
14. Number and rate of confirmed abuse and neglect cases among children

Health Risk Factors
15. Proportion of 2-year-old children who have received all age-appropriate vaccines, as recommended by the Advisory Committee on Immunization Practices
16. Proportion of adults aged 65 and older who have ever been immunized for pneumococcal pneumonia; proportion who have been immunized in the past 12 months for influenza
17. Proportion of the population who smoke, by age, race, and gender, as appropriate
18. Proportion of the population aged 18 or older who are obese
19. Number and type of U.S. Environmental Protection Agency air quality standards not met
20. Proportion of assessed rivers, lakes, and estuaries that support beneficial uses (e.g., fishing- and swimming-approved)

Healthcare Resource Consumption
21. Per-capita healthcare spending for Medicare beneficiaries (the Medicaid adjusted average per-capita cost)

Functional Status
22. Proportion of adults reporting that their general health is good to excellent
23. During the past 30 days, average number of days for which adults report that their physical or mental health was not good

Quality of Life
24. Proportion of adults satisfied with the healthcare system in the community
25. Proportion of persons satisfied with the quality of life in the community

Data from the Institute of Medicine. Using Performance Monitoring to Improve Community Health: A Role for Performance Monitoring. Washington, DC: National Academy Press; 1997.

CONCLUSION

From a social-ecological perspective, the health status of a population is influenced by many factors drawn from biology, behavior, the physical and social environment, and the use of health services. Social and cultural factors also play an important role in the disease patterns experienced by different populations, as well as in the responses of these populations to disease and illness. Globally, risks associated with population growth, pollution, and poverty result in mortality and morbidity that are still associated with infectious disease processes. In the United States, behaviorally mediated risks, including tobacco, diet, alcohol, and injury risks, rather than infectious disease processes, are the major contributors to health status, and the considerable gap between low-income minority populations and other Americans continues to widen. Public health activities strive to improve population health status (effectiveness) through cost-beneficial strategies and interventions (efficacy) and with equal benefits for all segments of the population (equity). Elimination and reduction of the disparities in health status among population groups have emerged as the most critical national health goal for the year 2020. With the increasing availability of data on health status, as well as on determinants and contributing factors, the potential for more rational policies and interventions has increased. Over the long term, public policies that narrow income disparities and increase access to education, jobs, and housing do far more to improve the health status of populations than do efforts to provide more healthcare services. Health improvement efforts require more than data on health problems and contributing factors, which view health from a negative perspective. Also needed is information from a positive perspective, in terms of community capacities, assets, and willingness. More important still, there must be recognition and acceptance that the right to health is a basic human right and one inextricably linked to all other human rights, lest quality of life be seriously compromised.[30] It is this right to health that energizes and challenges public health workers to measure health and quality of life in ways that promote its improvement.

REFERENCES

1. National Center for Health Statistics. *Health, United States, 2013*. Hyattsville, MD: NCHS; 2014.

2. Allaire SH, LaValley MP, Evans SR, O'Connor GT, Kelly-Hayes M, Meenan RF, Levy D, Felson DT. Evidence for decline in disability and improved health among persons aged 55 to 70 years: the Framingham heart study. *Am J Public Health*. 1999; *89*: 1678–1683.

3. Constitution of World Health Organization. In: World Health Organization. Chronicle of World Health Organization. Geneva, Switzerland: WHO; 1947; *1*: 29–43.

4. Whaley RF, Hashim TJ. *A Textbook of World Health*. New York: Parthenon; 1995.

5. Centers for Disease Control and Prevention. First reportable underlying cause of death. *MMWR*. 1996; *45*: 537.

6. Brownson RC, Remington PL, Davis JR, eds. *Chronic Disease Epidemiology and Control*. 2nd ed. Washington, DC: American Public Health Association; 1998.

7. Seitz F, Plepys C. Monitoring air quality in *Healthy People 2000*. *Healthy People 2000 Statistical Notes*. Hyattsville, MD: National Center for Health Statistics; 1995: No. 9.

8. Amler RW, Eddins DL. Cross-sectional analysis: precursors of premature death in the U.S. In: Amler RW, Dull DL, eds. Closing the Gap. Atlanta, GA: Carter Center; 1985: 181–187.

9. Mokdad AM, Marks JS, Stroup DF, Gerberding JL. Actual causes of death in the United States, 2000. *JAMA*. 2004; *291*: 1238–1245.

10. Chadwick E. *Report on the Sanitary Conditions of the Labouring Population of Great Britain 1842*. Edinburgh, Scotland: Edinburgh University Press; 1965.

11. Smith GD, Egger M. Socioeconomic differences in mortality in Britain and the United States. *Am J Public Health*. 1992; *82*: 1079–1081.

12. Schrijvers CTM, Stronks K, van de Mheen HD, Mackenbach JP. Explaining educational differences in mortality: the role of behavioral and material factors. *Am J Public Health*. 1999; *89*: 535–540.

13. Centers for Disease Control and Prevention. Poverty and infant mortality: United States, 1988. *MMWR*. 1996; *44*: 922–927.

14. Ng-Mak DS, Dohrenwend BP, Abraido-Lanza AF, Turner JB. A further analysis of race differences in the national longitudinal mortality study. *Am J Public Health*. 1999; *89*: 1748–1751.

15. Wilkenson RG. National mortality rates: the impact of inequality. *Am J Public Health*. 1992; *82*: 1082–1084.

16. Marmot M. The influence of income on health: views of an epidemiologist. *Health Affairs*. 2002; *21*: 31–46.

17. Centers for Disease Control and Prevention. Percentage of children <18 years who currently have asthma, by race/ethnicity and poverty status, United States, 2003–2005. *MMWR*. 2007; *56*(5): 99.

18. Sargent CF, Johnson TM, eds. *Medical Anthropology: Contemporary Theory and Method*. Rev ed. Westport, CT: Praeger; 1996.

19. Link BG, Phelan JC. Understanding sociodemographic differences in health: the role of fundamental social causes. *Am J Public Health*. 1996; *86*: 471–473.

20. Friedman SR, Curtis R, Neaigus A, Jose B, Des Jarlais DC. *Social Networks, Drug Injectors' Lives and HIV/AIDS*. New York: Kluwer; 1999.

21. Kawachi I, Kennedy BP, Glass R. Social capital and self-rated health: a contextual analysis. *Am J Public Health*. 1999; *89*: 1187–1193.

22. Malmstom M, Sundquist J, Johansson SE. Neighborhood environment and self-reported health status: a multilevel analysis. *Am J Public Health*. 1999; *89*: 1181–1186.

23. Doll R. Health and the environment in the 1990s. *Am J Public Health*. 1992; *82*: 933–941.

24. Winkelstein W. Determinants of worldwide health. *Am J Public Health*. 1992; *82*: 931–932.

25. Intergovernmental Panel on Climate Change. Impacts, adaptation, and vulnerability: contribution of Working Group II to the Third Assessment Report of the Intergovernmental Panel on Climate Change. In: McCarthy JJ, Canziani OF, Leary NA, Dokken DJ, White KS, eds. *Climate Change 2001*. Cambridge, UK: Cambridge University Press; 2001: 75–913.

26. Fielding JE. Public health in the twentieth century: advances and challenges. *Ann Rev Public Health*. 1999; *20*: xiii-xxx.

27. U.S. Public Health Service. *For a Healthy Nation: Return on Investments in Public Health*. Washington, DC: PHS; 1994.

28. U.S. Department of Health and Human Services. *Healthy People 2020*. Available at www.healthypeople.gov. Accessed June 16, 2014.

29. McKinlay JB, Marceau LD. A tale of 3 tails. *Am J Public Health*. 1999; *89*: 295–298.

30. Universal Declaration of Human Rights. GA res 217 A(iii), UN Doc A/810, art *25*(1);1948.

Public Health and
the Health System

After more than 5 decades of discussion, debate, and inaction later, significant health reform finally came to the health system in the United States in the second decade of the 21st century. Some believe it was too much, too quickly. Others found it too little and too late. The Patient Protection and Affordable Care Act (P.L. 111-148, more commonly known as the Affordable Care Act or "Obamacare") was enacted in 2010 with its major provisions to be implemented piecemeal over the ensuing decade. The extent to which the Affordable Care Act addresses the major problems and issues facing the health system in the United States rests in large part on what those problems and issues were, are, and will be. This chapter picks up where the previous chapter left off—with influences on health. The influences to be examined in this chapter, however, are the interventions and services available through the health system.

The relationship between public health and other health-related activities has never been clear. Some of the lack of clarity may be the result of the several different images of public health described previously, but certainly not all. In addition to the health system remaining poorly understood by the American public, there are different views among health professionals and policymakers as to whether public health is part of the health system or whether it is a separate, parallel enterprise. Most agree that these entities serve the same ends but disagree as to the balance between the two and the locus for strategic decisions and actions. The issue of ownership—which entity's leadership and strategies will predominate—underlies these different perspectives. In this text, the term health system will refer to all aspects of the organization, financing, and provision of programs and services for the prevention and treatment of illness and injury. Public health activities are an important component of this larger health system and, indeed, the entire health system serves the health of the public. This view differs from the image that most people have of our health system; the public commonly perceives the health system to include only the medical care and treatment aspects of the overall system.

Although their relationship may not be clear, there is ample cause for public health interest in the health system. Perhaps most compelling is the sheer size and scope of the U.S. health system, characteristics that have made the health system as much an ethical as an economic issue. More than 15 million workers and $3.0 trillion in resources are devoted to health-related purposes.[1] However, this huge investment in fiscal and human resources may not be accomplishing what it can and should in terms of health outcomes. Lack of access to needed health services for an alarming number of Americans and inconsistent quality have been contributing to less than optimal health outcomes. Although access and quality have long been public health concerns, costs associated with excess capacity within the health system has emerged as another important issue for public health.

This chapter examines the U.S. health system from several perspectives that consider the public health implications of costs and affordability, as well as several other important public policy and public health questions:

- Does the United States have a rational strategy for investing its resources to maintain and improve people's health?
- Does the current strategy inequitably limit access to and benefit from needed services?
- Is the health system accountable to its end-users and ultimate payers for the quality and results of its services?
- Are the changes occurring from recent health reform legislation (Affordable Care Act) bringing meaningful reform to the U.S. health system?

It is these issues of health, excess, access, accountability, and quality that make the health system a public health concern.

Complementary, even synergistic, efforts involving medicine and public health are apparent in many of the important gains in health outcomes achieved during the 20th century. Underlying these synergies is an appreciation that a successful health system deploys and integrates a variety of strategies and activities that differ in terms of their strategic intent, level of prevention, relationship to medical and public health practice, and community or individual focus. Key economic, demographic, and resource trends will then be briefly presented as a prelude to understanding important themes and emerging paradigm shifts. New opportunities afforded by sweeping changes in the health system will be apparent in the review of these issues.

OUTSIDE-THE-BOOK THINKING 3-1

Great debate: This debate examines contributors to improvement in health status in the United States since 1900. There are two propositions to be considered. Proposition A: Public health interventions are responsible for these improvements. Proposition B: Medical care interventions are responsible for these improvements. Select one—and only one—of these positions and present a compelling argument.

PREVENTION AND HEALTH SERVICES

Improved health status in the United States over the past 100+ years is due to a variety of intervention strategies and services.[2] Key relationships among health, illness, and various interventions intended to maintain or restore health are illustrated in Figure 3-1. Wellness and illness are dynamic states that are influenced by a wide

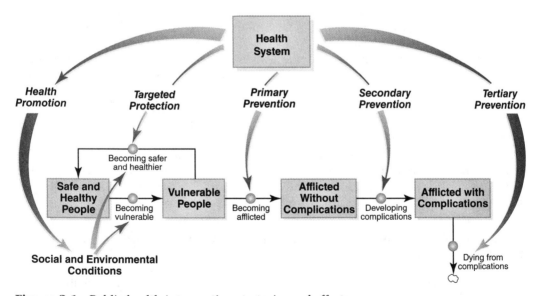

Figure 3-1   Public health intervention strategies and effects.

Adapted from U.S. Department of Health and Human Services, Centers for Disease Control and Prevention, Syndemic Prevention Network, 2008.

variety of biologic, environmental, behavioral, social, cultural, and health service factors that interact within a social-ecological framework. The complex interaction of these factors contributes to the occurrence or absence of disease or injury, which, in turn, contributes to the health status and well-being of individuals and populations.

Several different intervention points are possible, including two general strategies—health promotion and specific protection—that seek to maintain health by intervening prior to the development of disease or injury.[3] Each involves activities that alter the interaction of the various health-influencing factors in ways that either avert or alter the occurrence of disease or injury.

Health Promotion and Specific Protection

Health promotion activities attempt to modify human behaviors to reduce those known to affect adversely the ability to resist disease or injury-inducing factors, thereby eliminating exposures to harmful factors. Examples of health promotion activities include interventions such as nutrition counseling, genetic counseling, family counseling, and the myriad activities that constitute health education. However, health promotion also properly includes the provision of adequate housing, employment, and recreational conditions, as well as other forms of community development activities. What is clear from these examples is that many fall outside the common understanding of what constitutes health care. Several of these are viewed as the duty or responsibility of other societal institutions, including public safety, housing, education, and even business. It is somewhat ironic that activities that focus on the state of health and that seek to maintain and promote health are not commonly perceived to be "health services." To some extent, this is also true for the other category of health-maintaining strategies—specific protection activities.

Specific protection activities provide individuals with resistance to factors (such as microorganisms like viruses and bacteria) or modify environments to decrease potentially harmful interactions of health-influencing factors (such as toxic exposures in the workplace). Examples of specific protection include activities directed toward specific risks (e.g., the use of protective equipment for asbestos removal), immunizations, occupational and environmental engineering, and regulatory controls and activities to protect individuals from environmental carcinogens (such as exposure to secondhand or side-stream smoke) and toxins. Several of these are often identified with settings other than traditional healthcare settings. Many are implemented and enforced through governmental agencies.

Early Case Finding and Prompt Treatment, Disability Limitation, and Rehabilitation

Although health promotion and specific protection focus on the healthy state and seek to prevent disease, a different set of strategies and activities is necessary after disease or injury occurs. In such circumstances, the appropriate strategies are those facilitating early detection, prompt treatment, or rehabilitation, depending on the stage of development of the disease.

In general, early detection and prompt treatment reduce individual pain and suffering and are less costly to both the individual and society than treatment initiated after a condition has reached a more advanced state. Interventions to achieve early detection and prompt treatment include screening tests, case-finding efforts, and periodic physical exams. Screening tests are increasingly available to detect illnesses before they become symptomatic. Case-finding efforts for both infectious and non-infectious conditions are directed at populations at greater risk for the condition on the basis of criteria appropriate for that condition. Periodic physical exams and other screenings, such as those consistent with the age-specific recommendations of the U.S. Preventive Health Services Task Force, incorporate these practices and are best provided through an effective primary medical care system.[4] Primary care providers who are sensitive to disease patterns and predisposing factors can play substantial roles in the early identification and management of most medical conditions.

Another strategy targeting disease is disease management through effective and complete treatment. It is these activities that most Americans equate with the term health care, largely because this strategy constitutes the lion's share of the U.S. health system in terms of resource deployment. Quite appropriately, these efforts largely aim to arrest or eradicate disease and to limit disability and prevent death. The final intervention strategy focusing on disease—rehabilitation—is designed to return individuals who have experienced a condition to the maximum level of function consistent with their capacities.

Links with Prevention

An important aspect of this view of the health system is that it emphasizes the potential for prevention inherent in each of the five health intervention strategies. Prevention can be categorized in several ways. The best-known approach classifies prevention in relation to the stage of the disease or condition.

Preventive intervention strategies are considered primary, secondary, or tertiary. Primary prevention involves prevention of the disease or injury itself, generally through reducing exposure or risk factor levels. Secondary prevention attempts to identify and control disease processes in their early stages, often before signs and symptoms become apparent. In this case, prevention is akin to preemptive treatment. Tertiary prevention seeks to prevent disability through restoring individuals to their optimal level of functioning after damage is done.

The relationship of the five health intervention strategies to the three levels of prevention is also illustrated in Figure 3-1. Health promotion and specific protection are primary prevention strategies seeking to prevent the development of disease. Early case finding and prompt treatment represent secondary prevention, because they seek to interrupt the disease process before complications occur. Disease management and rehabilitation are considered tertiary-level prevention in that they seek to prevent or reduce disability associated with disease or injury. Although these are considered tertiary prevention, they receive primary attention under current policy and resource deployment.

Figure 3-2 further illustrates each of the three levels of prevention strategies in relation to population disease status and effect on disease incidence and prevalence. The various potential benefits from the three prevention levels derive from

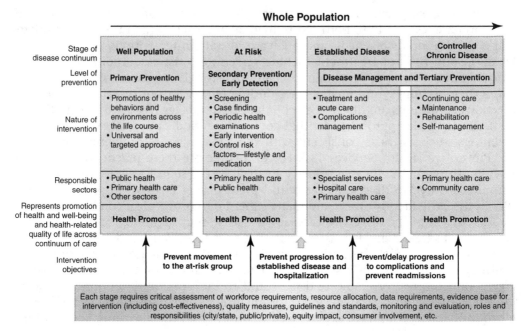

Figure 3-2   Comprehensive model of chronic disease prevention and control.

Modified from National Public Health Partnership. Preventing Chronic Disease: A Strategic Framework [Background paper]; 2001.

the basic epidemiologic concepts of incidence and prevalence. Prevalence (the rate of existing cases of illness, injury, or a health event) is a function of both incidence (the rate of new cases) and duration. Reducing either incidence or duration can lower prevalence. Primary prevention aims to reduce the incidence of conditions, whereas secondary and tertiary prevention seek to reduce prevalence by shortening duration and minimizing the effects of disease or injury. It should be apparent that there is a finite limit to how much a condition's duration can be reduced. As a result, approaches emphasizing primary prevention have greater potential benefit than do approaches emphasizing other levels of prevention. The importance of the differential impact of prevention and treatment approaches to a particular health problem or condition cannot be overstated.

These same considerations are pertinent to the concept of postponement of morbidity as a prevention strategy. Increased life expectancy without postponement of morbidity may actually increase the burden of illness within a population, as measured by prevalence. However, postponement may result in the development of a condition so late in life that it results in either no or less disability in functioning.

Within this framework for considering intervention strategies aimed at health or illness, the potential for prevention as an element of all strategies is clear. There are substantial opportunities to use primary and secondary prevention strategies to improve health in general and reduce the burden of illness for individuals and for society. As noted in the discussion of measuring population health, reducing the burden of illness carries the potential for substantial cost savings. These concepts serve to promote a more rational intervention and investment strategy for the U.S. health system.

OUTSIDE-THE-BOOK THINKING 3-2

Select an important health problem (disease or condition) and describe interventions for this problem across the five strategies of health-related and illness-related interventions (health promotion, specific protection, early detection, disability limitation, and rehabilitation) discussed in this chapter.

Links with Public Health and Medical Practice

Another useful aspect of this view of the health system is in its allocation of responsibilities for carrying out the various interventions. Three practice domains can be roughly delineated: public health practice, medical practice, and long-term care practice.[3] This framework assigns public health practice primary responsibility for health promotion, specific protection, and a good share of early case finding. It is important to note that the concept of public health practice here is a broad one that accommodates the activities carried out by many different types of health professionals and workers, not only those working in public health agencies. Although many of these activities are carried out in public health agencies of the federal, state, or local government, many are not. Public health practice occurs in voluntary health agencies, as well as in settings such as schools, social service agencies, industry, and even traditional medical care settings. In terms of prevention, public health practice embraces all of the primary prevention activities in the model, as well as some of the activities for early diagnosis and prompt treatment.

The demarcations between public health and medical practice are neither clear nor absolute. In recent decades, public health practice has been extensively involved in screening and has become an important source of primary medical care for populations with diminished access to care.

The mix of population-based and personal health services considered to represent public health practice varies over time and by location and history. The essential public health services framework largely focuses on population-based activities, including monitoring health status, investigating health problems and hazards, informing and educating people about health issues, mobilizing community partnerships, developing policies and plans, enforcing laws and regulations, ensuring a competent workforce, evaluating effectiveness and quality of services, and researching for new insights and solutions. One of these essential public health services, however, focuses on personal health services by linking people with needed health services and ensuring the provision of health care when it is otherwise unavailable.

Even as public health practice has branched into personal health services, medical practice continues to provide the major share of primary care services to most segments of the population. Medical practice—those services normally provided by or

Table 3-1   Healthcare Pyramid Levels

- Tertiary Medical Care
  - Subspecialty referral care requiring highly specialized personnel and facilities
- Secondary Medical Care
  - Specialized attention and ongoing management for common and less frequently encountered medical conditions, including support services for people with special challenges due to chronic or long-term conditions
- Primary Medical Care
  - Clinical preventive services, first-contact treatment services, and ongoing care for commonly encountered medical conditions
- Population-Based Public Health Services
  - Interventions aimed at disease prevention and health promotion that shape a community's overall health profile

Reproduced from U.S. Public Health Service. *For a Healthy Nation: Return on Investments in Public Health.* Hyattsville, MD: PHS; 1994.

under the supervision of a physician or other traditional healthcare provider—have long been viewed as including three levels as depicted in Table 3-1. Primary medical care has been variously defined but generally focuses on the basic health needs of individuals and families. It is first-contact health care in the view of the patient; provides at least 80% of necessary care; includes a comprehensive array of services, on site or through referral, including health promotion and disease prevention, as well as curative services; and is accessible and acceptable to the patient population. This comprehensive characterization of primary care differs substantially from what is commonly encountered as primary care in the U.S. health system. Often lacking from current so-called primary care services are those relating to health promotion and disease prevention.

Modern concepts of disease management have evolved from efforts to provide a more integrated approach to healthcare delivery in order to improve health outcomes and reduce costs, often for defined populations such as Medicaid enrollees. Disease management focuses on identifying and proactively monitoring high risk populations, assisting patients and providers to adhere to treatment plans that are based on proven interventions, promoting provider coordination, increasing patient education, and preventing avoidable medical complications.

Beyond primary medical care are two more specialized categories of care that are often termed secondary and tertiary care. Secondary care is specialized care serving the major share of the remaining 20% of the need that lies beyond the scope of primary care. Physicians or hospitals generally provide secondary care, ideally upon referral from a primary care source. Tertiary medical care is even more highly specialized and technologically sophisticated medical and surgical care for those with unusual or complex conditions (generally no more than a few percent of the need in any service category). Tertiary care is characteristically provided in large medical centers or academic health centers.

Long-term care is appropriately classified separately because of the special needs of the population requiring such services and the specialized settings where many of

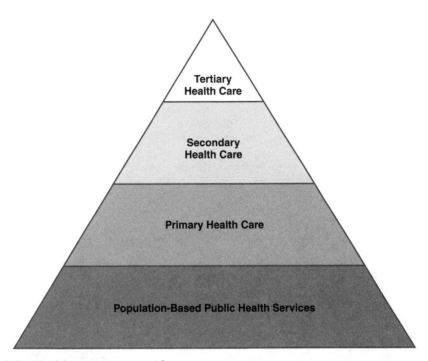

Figure 3-3   Health services pyramid.

Reproduced from U.S. Public Health Service. *For a Healthy Nation: Return on Investments in Public Health.*
Washington, DC: PHS; 1994.

these services are offered. This, too, is changing as specialized long-term care services increasingly move out of long-term care facilities and into home and community settings.

These three levels of healthcare services are often portrayed as the upper tiers of a pyramid with population-based public health services included as a fourth tier, as illustrated in Figure 3-3. In this pyramid, primary prevention is largely represented by the bottom tier and secondary prevention activities are largely included in primary medical care. Tertiary prevention activities fall largely in the secondary and tertiary medical care components of the pyramid. The use of a pyramid to represent health services implies that each level serves a different proportion of the total population. Everyone should be served by population-wide public health services, and nearly everyone should be served by primary medical care. However, increasingly smaller proportions of the total population require secondary- and tertiary-level medical care services. This formulation suggests that the medical services should be built on a foundation of population-based services and that the system of services, like a pyramid, should be constructed from the bottom up. It would not be rational to build a pyramid or a health system from the top down; there might not be enough resources to address the lower levels that served the vast majority of the population. Nonetheless, there is ample evidence in later sections of this chapter that this is exactly what has occurred with the U.S. health system. An alternative

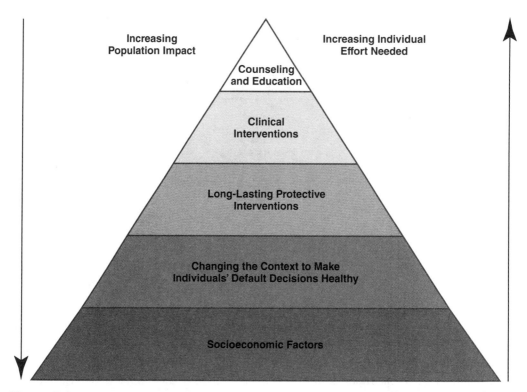

Figure 3-4 Health impact pyramid

Reproduced from A framework for public health action: the health impact pyramid. Fieden TR. *Am J Public Health*. 2010 April; 100(4): 590–595. doi: 10.2105/AJPH.2009.185652

perspective to the health services pyramid, the health impact pyramid presented in Figure 3-4, suggests a more rational design for a health system.

Targets of Health Service Strategies

A final facet of this health system framework characterizes the targets for the various strategies and activities. Generally, primary preventive services are community-based and targeted toward populations or groups rather than individuals. Early case-finding activities can be directed toward groups or toward individuals. For example, many screening activities target groups at higher risk when these are provided through public health agencies. The same screening activities can also be provided for individuals through physicians' offices and hospital out-patient departments. Much of primary and virtually all of secondary and tertiary medical care is appropriately individually oriented. It should be noted that there is a concept, termed community-oriented primary care, in which primary care pro-viders assume responsibility for all of the individuals in a community, rather than only those who seek out care from the provider. Even in this model, however, care is provided on an individual basis. Long-term care involves elements of both community-based service and individually oriented service. These services are tailored for individuals but often in a group setting or as part of a package of services for a defined number of recipients, as in a long-term care facility.

Public Health and Medical Practice Interfaces

This framework also sheds light on the potential conflicts between public health and medical practice. Although the two are described as separate domains of practice, there are many interfaces that provide a template for either collaboration or conflict. Both paths have been taken over the past century. Public health practitioners have traditionally deferred to medical practitioners for providing the broad spectrum of services for disease and injuries in individuals. Medical practitioners have generally acknowledged the need for public health practice for health promotion and specific protection strategies. The interfaces raise difficult issues. For example, for one specific protection activity—childhood immunizations—the extensive role of public health practice may actually have served to fragment health services for children. It would be logical to provide these services within a well-functioning primary care system, where they could be better integrated with other services for this population. Despite occasional differences as to roles, in most circumstances, medical practice has supported the role of public health to serve as the provider of last resort in ensuring medical care for persons who lack financial access to private health care. This, too, has varied over time and from place to place.

OUTSIDE-THE-BOOK THINKING 3-3

What are the most critical issues facing the healthcare system in the United States today? Before answering this question, see what insights you can find at the web sites of these major health organizations: American Medical Association (www.ama-assn.org), American Hospital Association (www.aha.org), American Nurses Association (www.ana.org), and the Association of American Medical Colleges (www.aamc.org).

Advances in bacteriologic diagnoses in public health laboratories, for example, fostered friction between medical practitioners and public health professionals for diseases such as tuberculosis and diphtheria that were often difficult for clinicians to identify from other common but less serious maladies. Clinicians feared that laboratory diagnoses would replace clinical diagnoses and that, in highly competitive medical markets, paying patients would abandon private physicians for public health agencies.

Some of the most serious conflicts have come in the area of primary care services, including early case-finding activities. Because of the increased yield of screening tests when these are applied to groups at higher risk, public health practice has sought to deploy more widely risk group or community case-finding methods (including outreach and linkage activities). This has, at times, been perceived by medical practitioners as encroachment on their practice domain for certain primary care services, such as prenatal care. Although there has been no rule that public health practice could not be provided within the medical practice domain and vice versa, the perception that these are separate, but perhaps unequal, territories has been widely held by both groups.

It is important to note that this territoriality is not based only on turf issues. There are significant differences in the world views and approaches of these two domains. Medical practice quite properly seeks to produce the best possible outcome through the development and execution of individualized treatment plans. Seeking the best possible outcome for an individual suggests that decisions are made primarily for the benefit of that individual. Costs and resource availability are secondary considerations. Public health practice, on the other hand, seeks to deploy its limited resources to avoid the worst outcomes at the group or population level. Some level of risk is tolerated at the collective level to prevent an unacceptable level of adverse outcomes from occurring. These are quite different approaches to practice: maximizing individual positive outcomes, as opposed to minimizing adverse collective outcomes. As a result, differences in perspective and philosophy often underlie differences in approaches that initially appear to be concerns over territoriality.

An example that illustrates these differences is apparent in approaches to widespread use of human immunodeficiency virus (HIV) antibody testing in the mid- and late 1980s. Medical practitioners perceived that HIV antibody testing would be very useful in clinical practice and that its widespread use would enhance case finding. As a result, medical practitioners generally opposed restrictions on use of these tests, such as specific written informed consent and additional confidentiality provisions. Public health practitioners perceived that widespread use of the test without safeguards and protections would actually result in fewer persons at risk being tested and decreased case finding in the community. With both groups focusing on the same science in terms of the accuracy of the specific testing regimen, these differences in practice approaches may be difficult to understand. However, in view of their ultimate aims and concerns as to individual versus collective outcomes, the conflict is more understandable.

Perspectives and roles may differ for public health and medical practice, but both are important and necessary. The real question is how best to blend these approaches for purposes of improving health status throughout the population. There is sufficient cause to question current policy and investment strategies. Table 3-2 examines the potential contributions of various strategies (personal responsibility, healthcare services, community action, and social policies) toward reducing the impact of the actual causes of death discussed previously. This table suggests that more medical care services are not as likely to reduce the toll from these causes as are public health approaches (community action and social policies). Yet, there are opportunities available through the current system and perhaps even greater opportunities in the near term as the system seeks to address the serious problems that have brought it to the brink of major reform.

Medicine and Public Health Collaborations

The need for a renewed partnership between medicine and public health generated several promising initiatives in the final years of the 20th century. Just as

Table 3-2   Actual Causes of Death in the United States and Potential Contribution to Reduction

	Deaths		Potential Contribution to Reduction*			
Causes	*Estimated No.*	*%*	*Personal*	*Healthcare System*	*Community Action*	*Social Policy*
Tobacco	435,000	19	++++	+	+	++
Diet/activity patterns	400,000	14	+++	+	+	++
Alcohol	85,000	5	+++	+	+	+
Microbial agents	75,000	4	+	++	++	++
Toxic agents	55,000	3	+	+	++	++++
Motor vehicles	43,000	1	++	+	+	++
Firearms	29,000	2	++	+	+++	+++
Sexual behavior	20,000	1	++++	+	+	+
Illicit use of drugs	20,000	<1	+++	+	++	++

*Plus sign indicates relative magnitude (4+ scale).

Data from Fielding J, Halfon L. Where is the health in health system reform? *JAMA.* 1994;272:1292–1296 and Mokdad AH, Marks JS, Stroup DF, Gerberding JL. Actual causes of death in the United States, 2000. *JAMA.* 2004:291:1238–1245.

bacteriology brought together public health professionals and practicing physicians at the turn of the 20th century to battle diphtheria and other infectious diseases, technology and economics may become the driving forces for a renewed partnership at the dawn of the 21st century. In pursuit of this vision, the American Medical Association and the American Public Health Association established the Medicine/Public Health Initiative to provide an ongoing forum to define mutual interests and promote models for successful collaborations. As a result of this initiative, a variety of collaborations developed, foreshadowing several important components of the Affordable Care Act.[5]

Collaborations between public health and hospitals have also gained momentum. Even prior to the enactment of the Affordable Care Act in 2010, hospitals and managed care organizations had begun to pursue community health goals, at times in concert with public health organizations and at other times filling voids that exist at the community level. In many parts of the United States, hospitals play a leading role in organizing community health planning activities. More frequently, however, they participate as major community stakeholders in health planning efforts organized through the local public health agency. A variety of positive interfaces with managed care organizations have been documented. Hospital boards and executives now commonly include community benefit objectives in their annual performance evaluations. Examples of community health strategies include:

- Establishing "boundary spanner" positions that report to the chief executive officer but focus on community-wide, rather than institutional, interests

- Changing reward systems in terms of salaries and bonuses that executives and board members linked to the achievement of community health goals
- Educating staff on the mission, vision, and values of the institution, and linking these with community health outcomes
- Exposing board to the work of community partners
- Engaging board members with the staff and community
- Reporting on community health performance (report cards)[6]

THE HEALTH SYSTEM IN THE UNITED STATES

This section does not attempt to provide a comprehensive view of the health system in the United States. The intent here is to examine those aspects of the health industry and health system that interface with public health or raise issues of public health significance, with a special focus on the problems of the system that are fueling reform and change. Data from the *Health United States* series, published annually by the National Center for Health Statistics, will be used throughout these sections to describe the economic, demographic, and resource aspects of the American health system.

Economic Dimensions

The health system in the United States is immense and growing steadily, as illustrated in Figure 3-5. Total national health expenditures in the United States doubled in the first dozen years of the 21st century to over $2.8 trillion, four times the sum expended in 1990 and 10 times more than in 1980. Health expenditures are on a pace to reach $4.5 trillion by the year 2020. In order to understand how public health interfaces with other components of the health system in the United

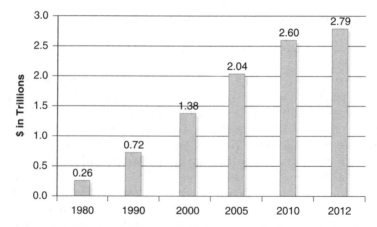

Figure 3-5 National health expenditures, United States, selected years, 1980–2012.

Data from Centers for Medicare and Medicaid Services, Office of the Actuary, National Health Statistics Group.

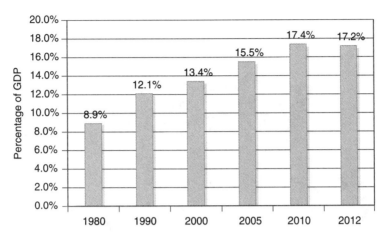

Figure 3-6 Percentage of national gross domestic product (GDP) expenditures spent for health-related purposes, United States, selected years, 1980–2012.

Data from Centers for Medicare and Medicaid Services, Office of the Actuary, National Health Statistics Group; U.S. Department of Commerce, Bureau of Economic Analysis.

States, it is important to consider the context in which these interactions take place—the health sector of modern America. The first decade of the new century witnessed weak economic growth and employment in the United States until the economy deteriorated even further into the recession of 2008–2009. Nonetheless, through periods of both economic prosperity and retrenchment, the health sector has remained a powerful component of the overall U.S. economy accounting for more than one-sixth of the total national gross domestic product (GDP) in 2012. Figure 3-6 traces the growth in health expenditures as a proportion of GDP.

The United States spends a greater share of its GDP on health care than any other industrialized nation. Health expenditures in the United Kingdom and Japan are about one-half and in Germany and Canada about two-thirds the United States figure. Per capita expenditures on health show the same pattern, with United States per capita spending on health more than twice that of Germany, Canada, Japan, and the United Kingdom. Several factors, illustrated in Figure 3-7, suggest that this is too much; such as (1) the current system is reaching the point of no longer being affordable; (2) the U.S. population is no healthier than other nations that spend far less; and (3) the opportunity costs are considerable.

Figures 3-8 and 3-9 trace where the money comes from and what it purchases in the U.S. health system. Expenditures for personal healthcare services comprise 85% of all health expenditures. A little more than one-half of the nation's health expenditures (52%) pay for hospital, physician, and other clinical services; 5% goes for nursing home care, 9% purchases prescription drugs, and 7% supports program administration. Another 24% covers a wide array of other services, including oral health, home health care, durable medical products, over-the-counter medicines, other personal care, research, and facilities, with only 3% devoted to government public health activities (about $75 billion in 2012).

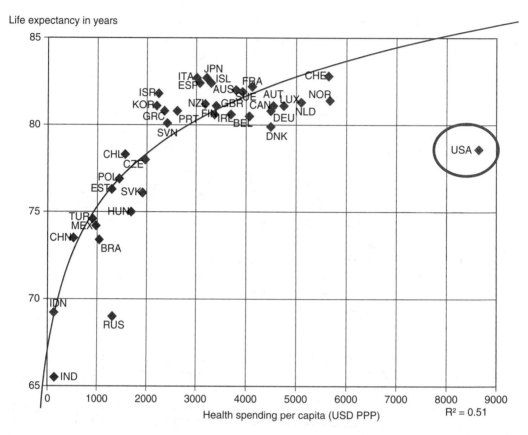

Figure 3-7   Life expectancy at birth and health spending per capita, United States and other OECD countries, 2011 (or nearest year).

Reproduced from OECD Health Statistics 2013, http://dx.doi.org/10.1787/health-data-en; World Bank for non-OECD countries.

There are three main sources for overall national health expenditures, which include government at all levels, private health insurance, and individuals paying out of pocket. Steadily increasing costs for health services have hit all three sources in their pocketbooks, and each is reaching the point at which further increases may not be affordable. The largest single purchaser of health care in the United States is the federal government, but for all three sources, the ultimate payers are individuals as taxpayers, employees, and consumers. Individuals and families covered by health insurance plans have been experiencing a steady increase in the triple burden of higher premiums, increased cost sharing, and reduced benefits. Health reform provisions of the Affordable Care Act seek to address some of these concerns as we will encounter in later sections of this chapter.

Only limited historical information is available on expenditures for prevention and population-based public health services. A study using 1988 data estimated that total national expenditures for all forms of health-related prevention (including

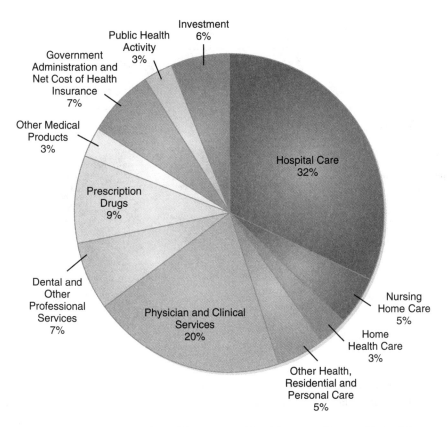

Figure 3-8   Health services purchased by national health expenditures, United States, 2012.
Data from Centers for Medicare and Medicaid Services, Office of the Actuary, National Health Statistics Group.

clinical preventive services provided to individuals and population-based public health programs, such as communicable disease control and environmental protection) amounted to $33 billion.[7] The analysis sought to include all activities directed toward health promotion, health protection, disease screening, and counseling. Included in this total, however, was $14 billion for activities not included in the calculation of national health expenditures (such as sewage systems, water purification, and air traffic safety). The remaining $18 billion in prevention-related health expenditures that was included in the calculation of total national health expenditures represented only 3.4% of all national health expenditures for that year. The share of these expenditures that represents population-based public health services cannot be determined precisely from this study but appears to be in the $6 billion to $7 billion range for 1988.

As part of the development of a national health reform proposal in 1994, federal officials developed an estimate of national health expenditures for population-based

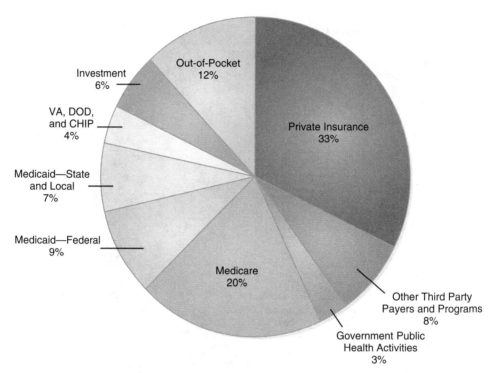

Figure 3-9   Sources of funding for national health expenditures, United States, 2012.

Data from Centers for Medicare and Medicaid Services, Office of the Actuary, National Health Statistics Group.

services.[8] On the basis of expenditures in 1993, this analysis concluded that about 1% of all national health expenditures ($8.4 billion) supported population-based programs and services. U.S. Public Health Service (PHS) agencies spent $4.3 billion for population-based services in 1993, and state and local health agencies expended another $4.1 billion. PHS officials estimated that achieving an "essential" level of population-based services nationwide would require doubling 1993 expenditure levels to $17 billion and that achieving a "fully effective" level would require tripling the 1993 levels to $25 billion.

The 1994 national health reform effort likely undercounted population-based public health activity expenditures by state and local governments. The results from a comprehensive examination of public health-related expenditures in nine states for 1994 and 1995, together with federal public health activity spending for 1995, suggest that national population-based public health spending totaled $13.8 billion in that year.

Data from the National Health Accounts identify government public health activity as a distinct category within total national health expenditures. The public health activity category captures the bulk of public health spending funded by government agencies, although it excludes spending for several personal services programs widely considered to be important public health services, such as maternal and child health, public hospitals, substance abuse prevention, and mental health services. Environmental health activities provided through environmental protection agencies are also excluded. Nonetheless, the government public health activity category within the annual national health expenditures total provides useful insights into general public health funding trends over time. Government public health activity spending was $75 billion in 2012, $11 billion from the federal level, and $64 billion from state and local governments. Figure 3-10 documents the tenfold increase in federal, state and local, and total government public health activity expenditures from 1980 through 2012.

Adjustments to public health activity expenditures are necessary in order to more accurately reflect the full array of activities included in the essential public health services framework, which includes the provision of personal health services when otherwise unavailable in addition to a battery of population-based activities. Figure 3-10 includes an estimate of total essential public health services expenditures developed by adding spending for mental health and substance abuse prevention, maternal and child health services, school health, and public hospitals to the public health activity category in the national health expenditures. For 2012, estimated essential public health services expenditures were $120 billion, about two times greater than in 2000 and three times more than in 1990.

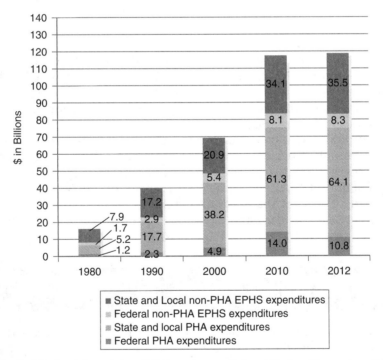

Figure 3-10 Public health activity (PHA) and essential public health services (EPHS) expenditures by government level, United States, selected years, 1980–2012.

Data from Centers for Medicare and Medicaid Services, Office of the Actuary, National Health Statistics Group.

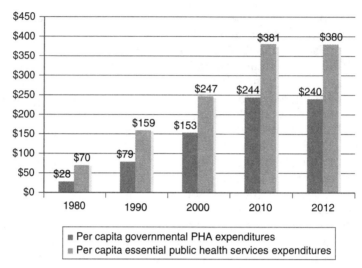

Figure 3-11   Per capita governmental public health activity and essential public health ser-vices expenditures, United States, selected years, 1980–2012.

Data from Centers for Medicare and Medicaid Services, Office of the Actuary, National Health Statistics Group.

A subset of overall public health activity expenditures supports population-based public health activities. Methods for estimating population-based public health expenditures, derived from studies completed in the mid-1990s, suggest that national population-based public health expenditures represent only about 1% of total national health expenditures.[9]

On a per capita basis, expenditures for essential public health services and over-all governmental public health activities increased by 5–8 times between 1980 and 2012 (Figure 3-11). Nonetheless, per capita public health expenditures represented only a tiny fraction of total per capita health spending ($9,500 per person) in the United States in 2012. That share was only 4.3% ($380 per capita) for total essential public health services spending and 2.6% ($240 per capita) for governmental public health activity spending in that year (Figure 3-12).

OUTSIDE-THE-BOOK THINKING 3-4

Is an ounce of prevention still worth a pound of cure in the United States? If not, what is the relative value of prevention in comparison with treatment?

Macroeconomic trends, however, tell only part of the story. The disparities between rich and poor have also been growing, leaving an increasing number of Americans without financial access to many healthcare services. These and other

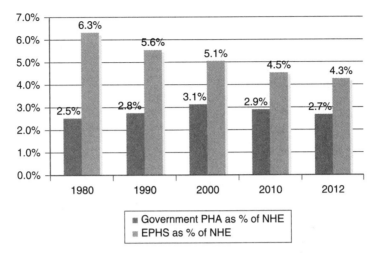

Figure 3-12 Expenditures for essential public health services and government public health activity as a percent of total health spending, United States, selected years, 1980–2012.

Data from Centers for Medicare and Medicaid Services, Office of the Actuary, National Health Statistics Group.

important aspects will be examined as we review the demands on and resources of the U.S. health system.

Demographic and Utilization Trends

Several important demographic trends affect the U.S. healthcare system. These include the slowing population growth rate, the shift toward an older population, the increasing diversity of the population, changes in family structure, and persistent lack of access to needed health services for too many Americans. The relative prevalence of particular diseases is another demographic phenomenon but will not be addressed here, although recent history with diseases such as HIV infections and H1N1 influenza illustrates how specific conditions can place increasing demands on fragile healthcare systems.

Census studies document that the growth of the U.S. population has been slowing, a trend that would be expected to restrain future growth in demand for healthcare services. However, this must be viewed in light of the projected changes in the age distribution of the U.S. population that are illustrated in Figure 3-13. Between 2000 and 2030, the population older than age 65 and older than 85 will double, whereas the younger age groups will grow little, if at all.

There is no evidence that excessive utilization or overuse of services contributes significantly to the high cost of health care in the United States. Underuse of care is actually a greater problem than overuse. Quality reviews consistently document that patients fail to receive recommended care almost half the time and that only about 10% of the time do they receive additional care that is not recommended for their specific health problem or condition.[10] Use of healthcare services, in general,

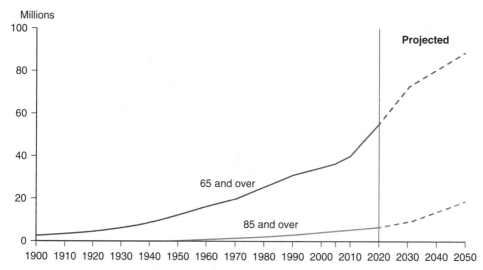

Figure 3-13 Population age 65 and over and age 85 and over, selected years, 1900–2010 and projected 2020–2050.

Reproduced from Federal Interagency Forum on Aging-Related Statistics. Available at www .agingstats.gov. Accessed June 28, 2014. Date from U.S. Census Bureau, 1900 to 1940, 1970, and 1980, U.S. Census Bureau, 1983, Table 42; 1950, U.S. Census Bureau, 1953, Table 38; 1960, U.S. Census Bureau, 1964, Table 155; 1990, U.S. Census Bureau, 1991, 1990 Summary Table File; 2000, U.S. Census Bureau, 2001, Census 2000 Summary File 1; U.S. Census Bureau, Table 1: Intercensal Estimates of the Resident Population by Sex and Age for the U.S.: April 1, 2000 to July 1, 2010 (US-EST00INT-01); U.S. Census Bureau, 2011. 2010 Census Summary File 1; U.S. Census Bureau, Table 2: Projections of the population by selected age groups and sex for the United States: 2010–2050 (NP2008-t2).

is closely correlated with the age distribution of the population. For example, adults age 75 years and older visit physicians three to four times as frequently as do children younger than age 17. Because older persons utilize more healthcare services than do younger people, their expenditures are higher. Obvious reasons for the higher utilization of healthcare resources by the elderly include the high prevalence of chronic conditions, such as arteriosclerosis, cerebrovascular disease, diabetes, senility, arthritis, and mental disorders. As the population ages, it is expected that the prevalence of chronic disorders and the treatment costs associated with them will also increase. This could be minimized through prevention efforts that either avert or postpone the onset of these chronic diseases. Nonetheless, these important demographic shifts portend greater demand for healthcare services in the future.

Another important demographic trend is the increasing diversity of the population. The nonwhite population is growing three times faster than the white population, and the Hispanic population is increasing at five times the rate for the entire U.S. population. Between 1980 and 2000, Hispanics increased from 6.4% to 12.5% of the U.S. population. African Americans increased from 11.5% to 14.5% of the total population, while the number of Asian/Pacific Islanders more than doubled from 1.6% to 3.7%. The white population declined from 79.7% to 69.1% of the total population over these 2 decades. Figure 3-14 projects these trends for-

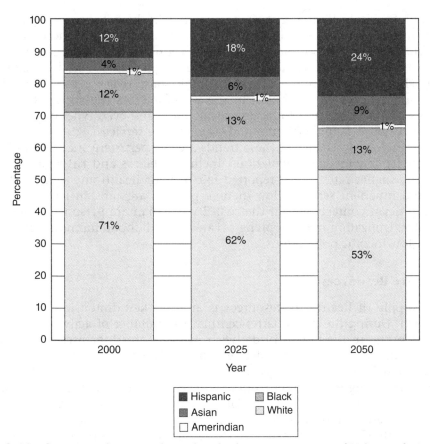

Figure 3-14 Current and projected racial and ethnic composition of U.S. population, 2000, 2025, 2050.

Data from U.S. Census Bureau, 2001.

ward through mid-century. Notably, these trends reflect differences in fertility and immigration patterns and disproportionately affect the younger age groups, suggesting that services for mothers and children will face considerable challenges in their ability to provide culturally sensitive and acceptable services. This scenario also underscores the importance of cultural competence skills for health professionals. Cultural competence is a set of behaviors and attitudes, as well as a culture within an institution or system that respects and takes into account the cultural background, cultural beliefs, and values of those served and incorporates this into the way services are delivered. At the same time, the considerably less diverse baby boom generation will be increasing its ability to affect public policy decisions and resource allocations in the early decades of the 21st century.

Changes in family structure also represent a significant demographic trend in the United States. There is only a 50% chance that married partners will reach their 25th anniversary. One in three children live part of their lives in a one-parent household; for black children, the chances are two in three. Labor force participation for women has more than doubled over the past 50 years. Even more indicative of gender changes in the labor market, the proportion of married women in the workforce with children under age 5 has been increasing in recent decades. Many American households have maintained their economic status over the recent decades with the second paycheck from women in the workforce. As the structure of families diversifies, so do their needs for access, availability, and even types of services (such as substance abuse, family violence, and child welfare services).

Intermingled with many of these trends are the persistent inequalities in access to services for low-income populations, including blacks and Hispanics. For example, despite higher rates of self-reported fair or poor health and greater utilization of hospital inpatient services, low-income persons are substantially less likely to report physician contacts within the past 2 years than are persons in high-income households. Utilization rates for prenatal care and childhood immunizations are also lower for low-income populations.

Healthcare Resources

The supply of healthcare resources is another key dimension of the healthcare system. During the past quarter-century, the number of active U.S. physicians increased by more than two-thirds, with even greater increases among women physicians and international medical graduates. The specialty composition of the physician population also changed during this period, as a result of many factors, including changing employment opportunities, advances in medical technology, and the availability of residency positions. Suffice it to say that medical and surgical subspecialties grew more rapidly than did the primary care specialties. Projections suggest that the 21st century will see a substantial shortage of primary care physicians even while there will be a surplus of physicians trained in the surgical and medical specialties. A continuing shortage of registered nurses has reached crisis proportions in many regions of the United States.

Healthcare delivery models have also experienced major changes in recent years. For example, hospital-based resources have changed dramatically. Since the mid-1970s, the number of community hospitals has decreased, and the numbers of admissions, days of care, average occupancy rates, and average length of stay have all declined, as well. On the other hand, the number of hospital employees per 100 average daily patients has continued to increase. Hospital outpatient visits have also been increasing since the mid-1970s.

The growth in the number and types of healthcare delivery systems in recent years is another reflection of a rapidly changing healthcare environment. Increasing competition, combined with cost containment initiatives, has led to the proliferation of group medical practices, health maintenance organizations, preferred provider organizations, ambulatory surgery centers, and emergency centers. Common to many of these delivery systems since the early 1990s have been managed care strategies designed to control the utilization of services. Elements of managed care strategies generally include some combination of the following:

- Risk sharing with providers to discourage the provision of unnecessary diagnostic and treatment services and, to some degree, to encourage preventive measures

- To attract specific groups, designing of tailored benefit packages that include the most important (but not necessarily all) services for that group; cost sharing for some services through deductibles and copayments can be built into these packages
- Case management, especially for high-cost conditions, to encourage seeking out of less expensive treatments or settings
- Primary care gatekeepers, generally the enrollee's primary care physician, who control referrals to specialists
- Second opinions as to the need for expensive diagnostic or elective invasive procedures
- Review and certification for hospitalizations, in general, and hospital admissions through the emergency department, in particular
- Continued-stay review for hospitalized patients as they reach the expected number of days for their illness (as determined by diagnosis-related groupings)
- Discharge planning to move patients out of hospitals to less expensive care settings as quickly as possible[11]

The growth and expansion of these delivery systems has significant implications for the cost of, access to, and quality of health services. These, in turn, have substantial impact on public health organizations and their programs and services. The majority of the U.S. population is now served through a managed care organization, and that share continues to increase.

CHANGING ROLES, THEMES, AND PARADIGMS IN THE HEALTH SYSTEM

Even a cursory review of the health sector requires an examination of the key participants or key players in the health industry. The list of major stakeholders has been expanding as the system has grown and now includes government, business, third-party payers, healthcare providers, drug companies, and labor, as well as consumers. The federal government has become the largest purchaser of health care and, along with business, has attempted to become a more prudent buyer by exerting more control over payments for services. Government seeks to reduce rising costs by altering the economic performance of the health sector through stimulation of a more competitive healthcare market. At the same time, efforts to expand access through Medicaid and state child health insurance programs and isolated state initiatives toward universal coverage require more, not less, governmental spending. Still, budget problems at all levels make it increasingly difficult for government to fulfill commitments to provide healthcare services to the poor, the disadvantaged, and the elderly. Over recent years, new and expensive medical technology, inflation, and unexpected increases in utilization forced third parties to pay out more for health care than they anticipated when premiums were determined. As a result, insurers have joined government in becoming more aggressive in efforts to contain healthcare costs. Many commercial carriers deploy methods to anticipate utilization more accurately and to control outlays through managed care strategies. Business, labor, patients, hospitals, and professional organizations are all trying to restrain costs while maintaining access to health services.

Reducing the national deficit and balancing the federal budget rely in part on controlling costs within Medicare and Medicaid, as well as in discretionary federal health programs. Except for Medicare, such efforts are likely to be politically popular, even though the public has little understanding of the federal budget. For example, a 1994 poll found that Americans believe healthcare costs comprise 5% of the federal budget, although these costs actually constituted 16% at the time.[12] At the same time, Americans believed that foreign aid and welfare comprise 27% and 19%, respectively, of the federal budget when, in fact, they constituted only 2% and 3%, respectively. When the time comes to balance the federal budget and reduce the national deficit, the American public faces difficult choices as to which programs can be reduced. Public health programs, largely discretionary spending, may not fare well in this scenario.

As these stakeholders search for methods to reduce costs and as competition intensifies, efforts to preserve the quality of health care have become increasingly important. An Institute of Medicine study concluded that medical errors account for as many deaths each year as motor vehicle crashes and breast cancer.[13] Despite the difficulty in measuring quality of medical care, it is likely that quality measurement systems will increase substantially.

Almost certainly, health policy issues will become increasingly politicized. The debate on healthcare issues will continue to expand beyond the healthcare community. Many health policy issues may no longer be determined by sound science and practice considerations, but rather by political factors. Changes in the health sector may lead to unexpected divisions and alliances on health policy issues.

The intensity of economic competition in the health sector is likely to continue to increase because of the increasing supply of healthcare personnel and because of the changes in the financing of care. Increased competition is likely to cause realignments among key participants in the healthcare sector, often depending on the particular issue involved. Dialogue and debate among the major stakeholders in the health system will be influenced by the tension between cost containment and regulation; the interdependence of access, quality, and costs; the call for greater accountability; and the slow but steady acceptance of the need for health reform.

The failure of health reform at the national policy level in 1994 did not avert the implementation of significant improvements in both the public or the private components of the health sector. With or without major changes in national health policies, the health system in the United States has been reforming itself incrementally for decades. With the persistence of cost and access as the system's twin critical problems, new approaches and models were both needed and expected. The federal, as well as state, governments have moved to control the costs of Medicaid services, primarily through attempts to enroll nondisabled Medicaid populations into capitated managed care programs. The rapid conversion of Medicaid services to managed care operations and the growth of private managed care organizations pose new issues for the delivery of clinical preventive and public health services.[11] These changes will likely result in fewer clinical preventive and treatment services being provided through public health agencies, but the extent and impact of these shifts is uncertain.

In any event, the underlying investment strategy of the U.S. health system appears to have changed little over recent decades, with more than 95% of the available resources allocated for treatment services, approximately 4% for essential public health services, and a scant 1% for population-based public health services.

Without additional investment in prevention and public health approaches, the long-term prospects for controlling costs within the U.S. health system are bleak. The health reform package enacted in 2010 was a significant step toward universal coverage and meaningful health reform, especially in terms of reducing barriers to access for the 45 million Americans on the fringes of the system and who otherwise would continue to incur excessive costs when they inappropriately accessed needed services. Universal access remains a prerequisite for eventual control of costs. Although the Affordable Care Act addressed a variety of health insurance gaps and abuses, it did relatively little to shift the balance in the U.S. health system from treatment to prevention. Table 3-3 offers a scorecard on the implementation of key Affordable Care Act (also known as Obamacare) components through 2014.

Although progress along the road to reform has been painfully slow, there is evidence that a paradigm shift is already under way. The Pew Health Professions Commission, among other authorities, argues that the American healthcare system of the 21st century will be quite different from its 1990s counterpart. The 21st century health system will be:

- More managed, with better integration of services and financing
- More accountable to those who purchase and use health services
- More aware of and responsive to the needs of enrolled populations
- More able to use fewer resources more effectively
- More innovative and diverse in how it provides for health
- More inclusive in how it defines health
- Less focused on treatment and more concerned with education, prevention, and care management
- More oriented to improving the health of the entire population
- More reliant on outcomes data and evidence[14]

These gains, however, will likely be accompanied by pain. The number of hospitals may decline by as much as 50% and the number of hospital beds by even more than that. There will be continued expansion of primary care in community and other ambulatory settings; this will foster replication of services in different settings, a development likely to confuse consumers. These forces also suggest major traumas for the health professions, with projected deficits of some professions, such as nurses and dentists, and surpluses of others, such as physicians and pharmacists.[14] An estimated 100,000–150,000 excess physicians, mainly specialists, could be joined by several hundred thousand excess nurses as the hospital sector consolidates and by as many as 40,000 excess pharmacists as drug dispensing is automated and centralized. The massive fragmentation among 200 or more allied health fields will likely cause consolidation into multiskilled professions to meet the changing needs of hospitals and other care settings. One of the few professions likely to flourish in this environment will be public health, with its focus on populations, information-driven planning, collaborative responses, and broad definition of health and health interventions.

Where these forces will move the health system is not yet known. To blend better the contributions of preventive and treatment-based approaches, several important changes are needed. There must be a new and more rational

TABLE 3-3   Timeline and Implementation Status of Selected Affordable Care Act Health Reform Provisions

Year	Affordable Care Act Provision ✓ = in effect * = delayed or not yet implemented
2010	
✓	Requires the federal government to create a process, in conjunction with states, where insurers have to justify unreasonable premium increases. Provides grants to states for reviewing premium increases.
✓	Appropriates $5 billion for fiscal years 2010 through 2014 and $2 billion for each subsequent fiscal year to support prevention and public health programs.
✓	Provides a $250 rebate to Medicare beneficiaries who reach the Part D coverage gap in 2010. Further subsidies and discounts that ultimately close the coverage gap begin in 2011.
✓	Provides tax credits to small employers with no more than 25 employees and average annual wages of less than $50,000 that provide health insurance for employees. Phase I (2010–2013): tax credit up to 35% (25% for nonprofits) of employer cost; Phase II (2014 and later): tax credit up to 50% (35% for nonprofits) of employer cost if purchased through an insurance Exchange for 2 years.
✓	Imposes additional requirements on nonprofits hospitals to conduct community needs assessments and develop a financial assistance policy and impose a tax of $50,000 per year for failure to meet these requirements.
✓	Creates a state option to provide Medicaid coverage to childless adults with incomes up to 133% of the federal poverty level. (States will be required to provide this coverage in 2014.)
✓	Creates a temporary program to provide health coverage to individuals with preexisting medical conditions who have been uninsured for at least 6 months. The plan will be operated by the states or the federal government.
✓	Creates the National Prevention, Health Promotion, and Public Health Council to develop a national prevention, health promotion, and public health strategy.
✓	Extends dependent coverage for adult children up to age 26 for all individual and group policies.
✓	Prohibits individual and group health plans from placing lifetime limits on the dollar value of coverage, rescinding coverage except in cases of fraud, and from denying children coverage based on preexisting medical conditions or from including preexisting condition exclusions for children. Restricts annual limits on the dollar value of coverage (and eliminates annual limits in 2014).
✓	Requires new health plans to provide at a minimum coverage without cost-sharing for preventive services rated A or B by the U.S. Preventive Services Task Force, recommended immunizations, preventive care for infants, children, and adolescents, and additional preventive care and screenings for women.
✓	Permanently authorizes the federally qualified health centers and NHSC programs and increases funding for FQHCs and for the NHSC for fiscal years 2010–2015.

TABLE 3-3   Timeline and Implementation Status of Selected Affordable Care Act Health Reform Provisions   (*Continued*)

Year	Affordable Care Act Provision ✓ = in effect * = delayed or not yet implemented
2011	
✓	Requires health plans to report the proportion of premium dollars spent on clinical services, quality, and other costs and provide rebates to consumers if the share of the premium spent on clinical services and quality is less than 85% for plans in the large group market and 80% for plans in the individual and small group markets.
✓	Provides a 10% Medicare bonus payment for primary care services; also, provides a 10% Medicare bonus payment to general surgeons practicing in health professional shortage areas.
✓	Eliminates cost-sharing for Medicare-covered preventive services that are recommended (rated A or B) by the U.S. Preventive Services Task Force and waives the Medicare deductible for colorectal cancer screening tests; authorizes Medicare coverage for a personalized prevention plan, including a comprehensive health risk assessment.
✓	Creates a new Medicaid state option to permit certain Medicaid enrollees to designate a provider as a health home and provides states taking up the option with 90% federal matching payments for 2 years for health home-related services.
✓	Provides 3-year grants to states to develop programs to provide Medicaid enrollees with incentives to participate in comprehensive health lifestyle programs and meet certain health behavior targets.
*	Provides grants for up to 5 years to small employers that establish wellness programs. • Funds have yet to be awarded due to budget debates related to the Prevention and Public Health Fund
✓	Requires disclosure of the nutritional content of standard menu items at chain restaurants and food sold from vending machines.
2012	
✓	Allows providers organized as accountable care organizations (ACOs) that voluntarily meet quality thresholds to share in the cost savings they achieve for the Medicare program.
✓	Requires private individual and group health plans to provide a uniform summary of benefits and coverage (SBC) to all applicants and enrollees. The intent is to help consumers compare health insurance coverage options before they enroll and understand their coverage once they enroll.
✓	Requires enhanced collection and reporting of data on race, ethnicity, sex, primary language, disability status, and for underserved rural and frontier populations.
2013	
✓	Provides a one percentage point increase in federal matching payments for preventive services in Medicaid for states that offer Medicaid coverage with no patient cost sharing for services recommended (rated A or B) by the U.S. Preventive Services Task Force and recommended immunizations.

(continues)

TABLE 3-3 Timeline and Implementation Status of Selected Affordable Care Act Health Reform Provisions (*Continued*)

Year	Affordable Care Act Provision ✓ = in effect * = delayed or not yet implemented
✓	Increases Medicaid payments for primary care services provided by primary care doctors to 100% of the Medicare payment rate for 2013 and 2014 (financed with 100% federal funding).
✓	Creates the Consumer Operated and Oriented Plan (CO-OP) to foster the creation of nonprofit, member-run health insurance companies.
✓	Extends authorization and funding for the Children's Health Insurance Program (CHIP) through 2015 (current authorization is through 2013).
2014	
✓	Expands Medicaid to all individuals not eligible for Medicare under age 65 (children, pregnant women, parents, and adults without dependent children) with incomes up to 138% FPL and provides enhanced federal matching payments for new eligibles.
✓	Allows all hospitals participating in Medicaid to make presumptive eligibility determinations for all Medicaid-eligible populations.
✓	Requires U.S. citizens and legal residents to have qualifying health coverage (there is a phased-in tax penalty for those without coverage, with certain exemptions). • States were given latitude to let people renew insurance policies that fail to meet the law's benefits standards, so that consumers may buy such policies until October 2016 and keep them for 1 year after that.
✓	Creates state-based American Health Benefit Exchanges and Small Business Health Options Program (SHOP) Exchanges, administered by a governmental agency or nonprofit organization, through which individuals and small businesses with up to 100 employees can purchase qualified coverage. Exchanges will have a single form for applying for health programs, including coverage through the Exchanges and Medicaid and CHIP programs. • Online enrollment via SHOPs delayed until November 2014 although small businesses could get coverage directly from an insurer or an insurance agent or broker before online enrollment becomes available. • Implementation of requirement that SHOPs offer two plans delayed until 2015.
✓	Provides refundable and advanceable tax credits and cost sharing subsidies to eligible individuals. Premium subsidies are available to families with incomes between 133–400% of the federal poverty level to purchase insurance through the Exchanges, while cost sharing subsidies are available to those with incomes up to 250% of the poverty level.
✓	Requires guarantee issue and renewability of health insurance regardless of health status and allows rating variation based only on age (limited to a 3 to 1 ratio), geographic area, family composition, and tobacco use (limited to 1.5 to 1 ratio) in the individual and the small group market and the Exchanges.

TABLE 3-3 Timeline and Implementation Status of Selected Affordable Care Act Health Reform Provisions (*Continued*)

Year	**Affordable Care Act Provision** ✓ = in effect * = delayed or not yet implemented
✓	Prohibits annual limits on the dollar value of coverage.
✓	Creates an essential health benefits package that provides a comprehensive set of services, limiting annual cost-sharing to the Health Savings Account limits ($5,950/individual and $11,900/family in 2010). Creates four categories of plans to be offered through the Exchanges, and in the individual and small group markets, varying based on the proportion of plan benefits they cover.
*	Permits states the option to create a Basic Health Plan for uninsured individuals with incomes between 133–200% FPL who would otherwise be eligible to receive premium subsidies in the Exchange. • Implementation delayed until 2015.
*	Assesses a fee of $2,000 per full-time employee, excluding the first 30 employees, on employers with more than 50 employees that do not offer coverage and have at least one full-time employee who receives a premium tax credit. Employers with more than 50 employees that offer coverage but have at least one full-time employee receiving a premium tax credit, will pay the lesser of $3,000 for each employee receiving a premium credit or $2,000 for each full-time employee, excluding the first 30 employees. • Implementation date moved to: January 1, 2015 for employers with 50–99 employees. • Implementation date moved to January 1, 2016 for employers with 100 or more employees.
✓	Permits employers to offer employees rewards of up to 30%, potentially increasing to 50%, of the cost of coverage for participating in a wellness program and meeting certain health-related standards; establishes 10-state pilot programs to permit participating states to apply similar rewards for participating in wellness programs in the individual market.
2016	
*	Permits states to form healthcare choice compacts and allows insurers to sell policies in any state participating in the compact. • Scheduled implementation date: January 1, 2016
2018	
*	Imposes an excise tax on insurers of employer-sponsored health plans with aggregate expenses that exceed $10,200 for individual coverage and $27,500 for family coverage. • Scheduled implementation date: January 1, 2018

Modified from Kaiser Family Foundation, Kaiser Commission on Medicaid and the Uninsured and Health Care Marketplace Project. Available at http://kff.org/interactive/implementation-timeline/. Accessed March 10, 2014.

understanding of what is meant by "health services." This understanding must include a broad view of health promotion and health protection strategies and must afford these equal standing with treatment-based strategies. Once and for all, health services must be seen to include services that focus on health, as well as those that focus on ill health. The health status of a population is determined by a complex set of considerations which include social determinants that reflect the fundamental causes of many societal ills operating within a social-ecological model of health and illness. Those considerations are very much the focus of the population-focused public health and prevention interventions. A second and companion change needed is to finance this enhanced basic benefit package from the same source, rather than funding public health and most prevention from one source (government resources) and treatment and the remaining prevention activities from private sources (business, individuals, insurance). With these changes, a gradual reallocation of resources can move the system toward a more rational and effective investment strategy.

OUTSIDE-THE-BOOK THINKING 3-5

Which problems and issues of the health system are improved by the Affordable Care Act? Which are not? What forces are most likely to fuel further movement toward major health system reform in America?

Organizations and systems that are unable to achieve their primary objectives and outcomes often justify their existence in terms of how well they do the things they are doing. Our health system is a prime example of this phenomenon. In such cases, the original outcome (here, improved health status) is displaced by a focus on how well the means to that end (the availability of complex and sophisticated services) are being executed. Processes displace outcomes as the prime purpose or mission for that entity. Instead of "doing the right things" to affect health status, the system focuses on "doing things right" (regardless of whether they actually affect population health status). This outcome displacement allows the United States to boast having the best medical care services in the world while having an inadequate health system.

CONCLUSION

Every day in America, decisions are made that influence the health status of individuals and populations. The aggregate of these decisions and the activities necessary to carry them out constitute our health system. It is important to view interventions as linked with health and illness states, as well as with the dynamic processes and multiple factors that move an individual from one state to another. Preventive interventions act at various points and through various means to prevent the development of a disease state or, if it occurs, to minimize its effects to the extent possible. These interventions differ in their linkages with public health practice, medical practice, and long-term care, as well as in their focus on individuals or groups. The framework represents a rational one, reflecting known facts concerning each of its aspects and their relationships with each other.

As this chapter has described, the U.S. health system focuses mainly on disease states and strategies for restoring, as opposed to promoting or protecting, health. It directs the vast majority of human, physical, and financial resources to tertiary prevention, particularly to acute treatment. It focuses disproportionately on individually oriented secondary and tertiary medical care. In so doing, it raises questions as to whether these policies are effective and ethical.

Characterized in the past largely by federalism, pluralism, and incrementalism, the health sector in the United States is finally undergoing fundamental change due in large part to the massive resources it consumes. We are now realizing that this investment strategy is not producing results commensurate with its costs. Health indicators, including those characterizing large disparities in outcomes and access among important minority groups, are not responding to more resources being deployed in the usual ways. How to control costs while moving toward universal access, consistent quality, and improved outcomes will challenge the U.S. healthcare system through the first quarter of the 21st century.

REFERENCES

1. National Center for Health Statistics. *Health, United States, 2013*. Hyattsville, MD: NCHS; 2014.
2. Rust G, Satcher D, Fryer GE, Levine RS, Blumenthal DS. Triangulating on success: innovation, public health, medical care, and cause-specific US mortality rates over a half century (1950–2000). *Am J Public Health*. 2010 April; *100*(Suppl 1): S95–S104. doi: 10.2105/AJPH.2009.164350
3. Leavell HR, Clark EG. *Preventive Medicine for the Doctor in His Community*. 3rd ed. New York: McGraw-Hill; 1965.
4. U.S. Preventive Services Task Force. Guide to Clinical Preventive Services. Accessible at http://www.uspreventiveservicestaskforce.org/index.html. Accessed June 13, 2014.
5. Lasker RD. *Medicine & Public Health: The Power of Collaboration*. New York: New York Academy of Medicine; 1997.
6. Weil PA, Bogue RJ. Motivating community health improvement: leading practices you can use. *Healthc Exec*. 1999; *14*: 18–24.
7. Brown RE, Elixhauser A, Corea J, Luce BR, Sheingold S. *National Expenditures for Health Promotion and Disease Prevention Activities in the United States*. Washington, DC: Medical Technology Assessment and Policy Research Center; 1991.
8. Core Functions Project, Public Health Service, Office of Disease Prevention and Health Promotion. Health Care Reform and Public Health: A Paper Based on Population-Based Core Functions. Washington, DC: PHS; 1993.
9. Frist B. Public health and national security: the critical role of increased federal support. *Health Aff* (Millwood). 2002; *21*: 117–130.
10. McGlynn EA, Asch SM, Adams J, et al. The quality of health care delivered to adults in the United States. *N Engl J Med*. 2003; *348*: 2635–2645.
11. Halvorson PK, Kaluzny AD, McLaughlin CP. *Managed Care & Public Health*. Gaithersburg, MD: Aspen Publishers; 1998.
12. Blendon RJ. *Kaiser/Harvard/KRC National Election Night Survey*. Menlo Park, CA: Henry J. Kaiser Family Foundation; 1994.
13. Institute of Medicine. *To Err Is Human*. Washington, DC: National Academy of Sciences; 1999.
14. Pew Health Professions Commission. *Critical Challenges: Revitalizing the Health Professions for the Twenty-First Century*. San Francisco: University of California Center for Health Professions; 1995

Law, Government, and Public Health

Public health is not limited to what governmental public health agencies do, although this is a widely held misperception. Still, particular aspects of public health rely on government. For example, the enforcement of laws remains one of those governmental responsibilities important to the public's health and public health practice. Yet, law and the legal system are important for public health purposes above and beyond the enforcement of laws and regulations. Laws at all levels of government bestow the basic powers of government and distribute these powers among various agencies, including public health agencies. Law represents governmental decisions and their underlying collective social values, providing the basis for actions that influence the health of the public.

Decisions and actions that take place outside the sphere of government also influence the health of the public, sometimes even more than those made by our elected officials and administrative agencies. Private sector and voluntary organizations play key roles in identifying factors important for health and advancing actions to promote and protect health for individuals and groups. Public health involves collective decisions and actions; it is often governmental forums that raise issues, make decisions, and establish priorities for action. Many governmental actions reflect the dual roles of government often portrayed on official governmental seals and vehicles of local public safety agencies—to protect and to serve. As they relate to health, the genesis of these two roles lies in separate, often conflicting, philosophies and duties of government. This chapter will examine how these roles are organized in the United States. This examination particularly emphasizes the relationships among law, government, and public health, seeking answers to the following questions:

- What are the various roles for government in serving the public's health?
- What is the legal basis for public health in the United States?
- How are public health responsibilities and roles structured at the federal, state, and local levels?

To review the organization and structure of governmental public health, this chapter will begin with federal public health roles and activities, to be followed, in turn, by those at the state and local levels. The focus is primarily on form and structure, rather than function. In most circumstances, it is logical for form to follow function. Here, however, it is necessary to understand the legal and organizational framework of governmental public health as part of the context for public health practice. The framework established through law and governmental agencies is a key element of public health's infrastructure and one of the basic building blocks of the public health system. This structure is a product of our uniquely American approach to government.

AMERICAN GOVERNMENT AND PUBLIC HEALTH

Former Speaker of the U.S. House of Representatives, Tip O'Neill, frequently observed, "all politics is local." If this is so, public health must be considered primarily a local phenomenon, as well, because politics are embedded in public health processes. After all, public health represents collective decisions as to which health outcomes are unacceptable, which factors contribute to those outcomes, which unacceptable problems will be addressed in view of resource limitations, and which participants need to be involved in addressing the problems. These are political processes, with different viewpoints and values being brought together to determine which collective decisions will be made. All too often, the term politics carries a very different connotation, one frequently associated with overtones of partisan ideologies. However, political processes are necessary and productive, and perhaps the best means devised by humans to meet our collective needs.

The public health system in the United States is a product of many forces that have shaped governmental roles in health. The framers of the U.S. Constitution did not plan for the federal government to deal directly with health or, for that matter, many other important issues. The word *health* does not even appear in that famous document, relegating health to the group of powers reserved to the states and the people. The Constitution explicitly authorized the federal government to promote and provide for the general welfare (in the Preamble and Article I, Section 8) and to regulate commerce (also in Article I, Section 8). Federal powers evolved slowly in the area of health on the basis of these explicit powers and subsequent U.S. Supreme Court decisions that broadened federal authority by determining that additional powers are implied in the explicit language of the Constitution.

The initial duties to regulate international affairs and interstate commerce led the federal government to concentrate its efforts on preventing the importation of epidemics and assisting states and localities, upon request, with their episodic needs for communicable disease control. The earliest federal health unit, the Marine Hospital Service, was established in 1798, partly to serve merchant seamen and partly to prevent importation of epidemic diseases; it evolved over time into the U.S. Public Health Service (PHS).

The power to promote health and welfare, however, did not always translate into the ability to act. The federal government acquired the ability to raise substantial financial resources through the authority to levy a federal tax on income, which was provided by the 16th Amendment in the early 20th century. The ability to raise vast sums generated the capacity to address health problems and needs through transferring resources to state and local governments in various forms of grants-in-aid. Despite its powers to provide for the general welfare and regulate commerce, the federal government could not act directly in most health matters; it could act only through states as its primary delivery system. After 1935, the power and influence of the federal government grew rapidly through its financial influence over state and local programs, such as the Hospital Services and Construction (Hill-Burton) Act of 1946 and, after 1965, through its emergence as a major purchaser of health care through Medicare and Medicaid. As for a public health presence at the federal level, the best-known and most widely respected federal public health agency, now known as the Centers for Disease Control and Prevention (CDC), was not established until 1946.[1]

The emergence of the federal government as a major influence in the health system displaced states from a position they had held since before the birth of the American republic. States were sovereign powers before agreeing to share their powers with the newly established federal government; their sovereignty included powers over matters related to health emanating from two general sources. First, they derived from the police powers of states, which provide the basis for government to limit the actions of individuals in order to control and abate hazards and nuisances. A second source for state health powers lay in the expectation for government to serve those individuals unable to provide for themselves. This expectation had its roots in the Elizabethan Poor Laws and carried over to states in the new American form of government. Despite this common heritage, states assumed these roles quite differently and at different points in time because the evolution of states themselves during the 19th century took place unevenly.

States developed structures and organizations needed to use their police powers to protect citizens from communicable diseases and environmental hazards, primarily from wastes, water, and food. State health agencies developed first in Massachusetts, then across the country, during the latter half of the 19th century. When federal grants became available, especially after 1935, states eagerly sought out their federal funding for maternal and child health services, public health laboratories, and other basic public health programs. In so doing, states surrendered some of their autonomy over health issues. Priorities were increasingly dictated by federal grants tied to specific programs and services.

Each state has the ultimate authority to create the political subunits that serve the residents of a particular jurisdiction. In this manner, counties, cities, and other forms of municipalities, townships, boroughs, parishes, and the like are established. Special-purpose districts for every conceivable purpose—from library services and mosquito control to emergency medical services and education—have also abounded. The powers delegated to or authorized for all of these local jurisdictions are established by state legislatures for health and other purposes. Although many big-city health departments were established prior to the establishment of their respective state health agencies, states are free to use a variety of approaches to structuring public health roles at the local level. Because most states use the county form of subdividing the state, counties became the primary local governmental jurisdictions with health roles after 1900.

State constitutions and statutes impart the authority for local governments to influence health. This authority comes in two forms: those responsibilities of the state specifically delegated to local governments and additional authorities allowed through home rule powers. Home rule options permit local jurisdictions to enact a local constitution or charter and to take on additional authority and powers, such as the ability to levy taxes for local public health services and activities.

Counties generally carry out duties delegated by the state. More than two-thirds of U.S. counties have a county commission form of government, with anywhere from 2 to 50 elected county commissioners (supervisors, judges, and other titles are also used).[2] These commissions carry out both legislative and executive branch functions, although they share administrative authority with other local elected officials, such as county clerks, assessors, treasurers, prosecuting attorneys, sheriffs, and coroners. Some counties—generally, the more populous ones—have a county administrator accountable to elected commissioners, and a small number of counties (less than 5%) have an elected county executive.

Local governments in U.S. cities were first on the scene in terms of public health responses, as noted in our discussion of the history of public health. Big-city health agencies remain an important force in the public health system in the United States. However, after about 1875 when states became more extensively involved, the relative role of municipal governments began to erode. Both local and state governments were enticed by the availability of federal funding, finding it preferable to take what they could get from a higher level of government rather than generating their own revenue to finance needed services.

Many forces have been at work to alter the initial relationships among the three levels of government for health roles, including:

- Gradual expansion and maturation of the federal government
- Staggered addition of new states and variability in the maturation of state governments
- Population growth and shifts over time
- Ability of the various levels of government to raise revenues commensurate with their expanding needs

- Growth of science and technology as tools for addressing public health and medical care needs
- Rapid growth of the U.S. economy
- Expectations and needs of American society for various services from their government[3,4]

The last of these factors is perhaps the most important. For the first 150 years of U.S. history, there was little expectation that the federal government should intervene in the health and welfare needs of its citizenry. The massive need and economic turmoil of the Great Depression years drastically altered this longstanding value as Americans began to turn to government to help deal with current needs and future uncertainties.

The complex public health network that exists today evolved slowly, with several shifts in relative roles and influence. Economic considerations and societal expectations, both reaching a critical point in the 1930s, set the tone for the rest of the 20th century. In general, power and influence were initially greatest at the local level, residing there until states began to develop their own machinery to carry out their police power and general welfare roles. States then served as the primary locus for these health roles until the federal government began to use its vast resource potential to meet changing public expectations in the 1930s. Federal grant programs for public health and, eventually, personal healthcare service programs soon drove state actions, especially after the 1960s. It was then that several new federal health and social service programs were targeted directly to local governments, bypassing states. At the same time, a new federal–state partnership for the medically indigent (Medicaid) was established to address the national policy concern over the plight of the medically indigent.

Political and philosophical shifts since about 1980 altered roles once again.[3] Debates over federal versus state roles continued throughout the decades that followed, initially resulting in some diminution of federal influence and enhancement of states' rights. However, the Affordable Care Act in 2010 opened the door to further expansion of the federal role in the health arena. In the end, the federal government has acquired the ability to influence the health system through its fiscal muscle power, as well as its research, regulatory, technical assistance, and training roles.

PUBLIC HEALTH LAW

One of the chief organizing forces for public health lies in the system of law. Law has many purposes in the modern world, and many of these are evident in public health laws. Unfortunately, there is no one repository where the entire body of law, even the body of public health law, can be found. This has occurred because laws are products of the legal system, which, in the United States, includes a federal system and 50 separate state-based legal systems. These developed at different times in response to somewhat different circumstances and issues. Common to each is some form of a state constitution, a considerable amount of legislation, and a substantial body of judicial decisions. If there is any road map through this maze, it lies in the federal and state constitutions, which establish the basic framework dividing governmental powers among the various branches of government in ways that allow each to create it own legal structures.

As a result, four different types of law can be distinguished by virtue of their form or authority:

- Constitutionally based law
- Legislatively based law
- Administratively based law
- Judicially based law

A brief description of each of these forms of law follows.

Types of Law

Constitutional law is ultimately derived from the U.S. Constitution, the legal foundation of the nation, in which the powers, duties, and limits of the federal government are established. States basically gave up certain powers (e.g., defense, foreign diplomacy, printing money), ceding these to the federal government while retaining all other powers and duties. Health is not one of those powers explicitly bestowed upon the federal government. States, in turn, have developed their own state constitutions, often patterned after the federal framework, although state constitutions tend to be more clear and specific in their language, leaving less room and need for judicial interpretation. State constitutions provide the broad framework from which states determine which activities will be undertaken and how those activities will be organized and funded. These decisions and actions come in the form of state statutes.

Statutory (legislatively based) law includes all of the acts and statutes enacted by Congress and the various state and local legislative bodies. This collection of law represents a wide range of governmental policy choices, including:

- Simple expressions of preferences in favor of a particular policy or service (such as the value of home visits by public health nurses)
- Authorizations for specific programs (such as the authority for local governments to license restaurants)
- Mandates or requirements for an activity to occur or, alternatively, to be prohibited (such as requiring all newborns to be screened for specific metabolic diseases or prohibiting smoking in public places)
- Providing resources for specific purposes (such as the distribution of medications to patients with acquired immune deficiency syndrome)

If the legislative intent is for something to occur, the most effective approaches are generally to require or prohibit an activity.

The basic requirement for statutory-based laws is that they must be consistent with the U.S. Constitution and, for state and local statutes, with state constitutions as well. State laws also establish the various subunits of the state and delineate their responsibilities for carrying out state mandates, as well as the limits of what they can do. At the local level, the legislative bodies of these subunits (e.g., city councils and county commissions) enact ordinances and statutes setting forth the duties and authorizations of local government and its agencies. Laws affecting public health are created at all levels in this hierarchy, but especially at the state and local levels. Among other purposes, these laws establish state and local boards of health and health departments, delineate the responsibilities of these agencies, including their programs and budgets, and establish health-related laws and requirements. Many of these laws are enforced by governmental health agencies.

Administrative law is law promulgated by administrative agencies within the executive branch of government. Rather than enact statutes that include extensive details of a professional or technical nature and to allow greater flexibility in their design and subsequent revision, administrative agencies are provided with the authority to establish law through rule-making processes. These rules, administrative law, carry the force of law and represent a unique situation in which legislative, judicial, and executive powers are carried out by one agency. Administrative agencies include cabinet-level departments, as well as other boards, commissions, and other entities that are granted this power through an enactment of the legislative body.

The fourth type of law is judicial law, also known as common law. This includes a wide range of tradition, legal custom, and previous decisions of federal and state courts. To ensure fairness and consistency, previous decisions are used to guide judgments on similar disputes. This form of law becomes especially important in areas in which laws have not been codified by legislative bodies. In public health, nuisances (unsanitary, noxious, or otherwise potentially dangerous circumstances) are one such area in which few legislative bodies have specified exactly what does and what does not constitute a public health nuisance. In this situation, the common law for nuisances is derived from previous judicial decisions. These determine under what circumstances and for what specific conditions a public health official can take action, as well as the actions that can be taken.

OUTSIDE-THE-BOOK THINKING 4-1

What is the legal basis for public health activities in the United States? What differences are there in the public health powers of federal, state, and local governments?

Purposes of Public Health Law

Two broad purposes for public health law can be described: protecting and promoting health and ensuring the protection of rights of individuals in the processes used to protect and promote health. Public health powers ultimately derive from the U.S. Constitution, which bestows the authority to regulate commerce and provide for the general welfare, and from the various state constitutions, which often provide clear but broad authorities, based largely on the police power of the state. States often have reasonably well-defined public health codes. However, there is considerable diversity in their content and scope, despite similarities in their basic sources of power and authority.

Many public health laws are enacted and enforced under what is known as the state's "police power." This is a broad concept that encompasses the functions historically undertaken by governments in protecting the health, safety, welfare, and general well-being of their citizens. A wide variety of laws derive from the police power of the state, a power that is considered one of the least limitable of all governmental powers. The police power of the state can be vested in an administrative agency, such as a state health agency, which becomes accountable for the manner in which these responsibilities are executed. In these circumstances, its use is a duty, rather than a matter of choice, although its form is left to the discretion of the user.

The courts have upheld laws that appear to limit severely or restrict the rights of individuals where these were found to be reasonable, rather than arbitrary and capricious attempts to accomplish government's ends. The state's police power is not unlimited, however. Interference with individual liberties and the taking of personal property are considerations that must be balanced on a case-by-case basis. At issue is whether the public interest in achieving a public health goal outweighs the public interest in protecting civil liberties. Public health laws requiring vaccinations or immunizations to protect the community have generally withstood legal challenges claiming that they infringed upon the rights of individuals to make their own health decisions. A precedent-setting judicial opinion upheld a Massachusetts ordinance authorizing local boards of health to require vaccinations for smallpox to be administered to residents if deemed necessary by the local boards.[5] Such decisions argue that laws that place the common good ahead of the competing rights of individuals should govern society. Similarly, courts have weighed the power of the state to appropriate an individual's property or limit the individual's use of it if the best interests of the community make such an action desirable. In some circumstances, equitable compensation must be provided. Issues of community interest and fair compensation are commonly encountered in dealing with public health nuisances in which an individual's private property can be found to be harmful to others.

OUTSIDE-THE-BOOK THINKING 4-2

What is meant by a state's police power, and how is that used in public health?

The various forms of law and the changing nature of the relationships among the three levels of government have created a patchwork of public health laws. Despite its relatively limited constitutionally based powers, the federal government can preempt state and local government action in key areas of public health regulation involving commerce and aspects of communicable disease control. States also have authority to preempt local government actions in virtually all areas of public health activity. Although this legal framework allows for a clear and rational delineation of authorities and responsibilities, a quite variable set of arrangements has arisen. Often, the higher level of government chooses not to exercise its full authority and shifts that authority to a lower level of government. This can be accomplished in some instances by delegating or requiring, and in other instances by authorizing (with incentives), the lower level of government to exercise authorities of the higher level. This has made for a complex set of relationships among the three levels of government and for 50 variations of the theme to be played in the

50 states. These relationships and their impact on the form and structure of governmental public health agencies will be evident in subsequent sections of this chapter.

There have been many critiques of the statutory basis of public health in the United States. A common one is that public health law, not unlike law affecting other areas of society, simply has not kept pace with the rapid and extensive changes in science and technology. Laws have been enacted at different points in time in response to different conditions and circumstances. These laws have often been enacted with little consideration as to their consistency with previous statutes and their overall impact on the body of public health law. For example, many states have different statutes and legal frameworks for similar risks, such as general communicable diseases, sexually transmitted diseases (STDs), and human immunodeficiency virus infections. Confidentiality and privacy provisions, which trace their origins to the vow in the Hippocratic oath not to reveal patient's secrets, are often inconsistent from law to law, and enforcement provisions vary as well. Beyond these concerns, public health laws often lack clear statements of purpose or mission and are not clearly linked to modern public health core function and essential public health services frameworks.

In view of these criticisms, recommendations have been advanced calling for a complete overhaul and recodification of public health law. Recommendations for improvement of the public health codes often call for:

- Stronger links with the overall mission and core functions of public health
- Uniform structures for similar programs and services
- Confidentiality provisions to be reviewed and made more consistent
- Clarification of police power responsibilities to deal with unusual health risks and threats
- Greater emphasis on the least restrictive means necessary to achieve the law's intent through use of intermediate sanctions and compulsive measures, based on proven effectiveness
- Fairer and more consistent enforcement and administrative practices

Although these recommendations have been advanced for several decades, little progress has been made at either the federal or state level. At times, states have sought to recodify public health statutes by relocating their placement in the statute books, rather than dealing with the more basic issues of reviewing the scope and allocation of their public health responsibilities so that these are clearly presented and assigned among the various levels of government. The intricacies of public health law often help drive the inner workings of federal, state, and local public health agencies. We will now turn to the form and structure of these agencies.

GOVERNMENTAL PUBLIC HEALTH

Federal Health Agencies

The U.S. Public Health Service (PHS) serves as the focal point for health concerns at the federal level. Although there have been frequent reorganizations affecting the structure of PHS and its placement within the massive Department of Health and Human Services (DHHS), the restructuring completed in 1996 was the most significant in recent decades. The changes were undertaken as part of the federal Reinvention of Government Initiative to bring expertise in public health and science closer to the Secretary of DHHS. In the restructuring, the line authority of the Assistant Secretary for Health over the various agencies within PHS was abolished, with those agencies now reporting directly to the Secretary of DHHS, as illustrated in Figure 4-1. The Assistant Secretary for Health became the head of the Office of Public Health and Science (OPHS), a new division reporting to the Secretary that also includes the Office of the Surgeon General. Each of the former PHS agencies became a full DHHS operating division. These eight operating agencies, the OPHS, and the regional health administrators for the 10 federal regions of the country now constitute the PHS. In effect, PHS has become a functional rather than an organizational unit of DHHS. In 2003, several activities related to emergency preparedness and response were moved into the newly established Department of Homeland Security. An Office of Public Health Emergency Preparedness and Response remained at DHHS to coordinate bioterrorism and other public health emergency activities managed by various PHS agencies. These duties were later consolidated under a new Assistant Secretary for Preparedness and Response.

PHS agencies address a wide range of public health activities, from research and training to primary care and health protection, as described in Table 4-1. The key PHS agencies are:

- Health Resources and Services Administration (HRSA)
- Indian Health Service
- Centers for Disease Control and Prevention (CDC)
- National Institutes of Health (NIH)
- Food and Drug Administration
- Substance Abuse and Mental Health Services Administration
- Agency for Toxic Substances and Disease Registry
- Agency for Healthcare Research and Quality (AHRQ)

PHS agencies comprise only a small part of DHHS. Other important operating divisions within DHHS include the Administration for Children and Families, the Administration for Community Living, and the massive Centers for Medicare and Medicaid Services (CMS). In addition, there are several administrative and support units for management and the budget.

Beyond DHHS, health responsibilities have been assigned to several other federal agencies, including the federal Environmental Protection Agency (EPA) and the Departments of Homeland Security, Education, Agriculture, Defense, Transportation, and Veterans Affairs, just to name a few. The importance of some of these other federal agencies should not be underestimated in terms of their roles and resources devoted to health purposes. Health-specific agencies at the federal level are a relatively new phenomenon. The first cabinet-level federal human services agency of any kind was the Federal Security Agency in 1939, and PHS itself remained a unit of the Treasury Department until 1944. This historical trivia demonstrates that federal engagement in public health is a relatively recent phenomenon.

The federal government is now the largest purchaser of health-related services, with spending on health representing more than one-fourth of the total federal

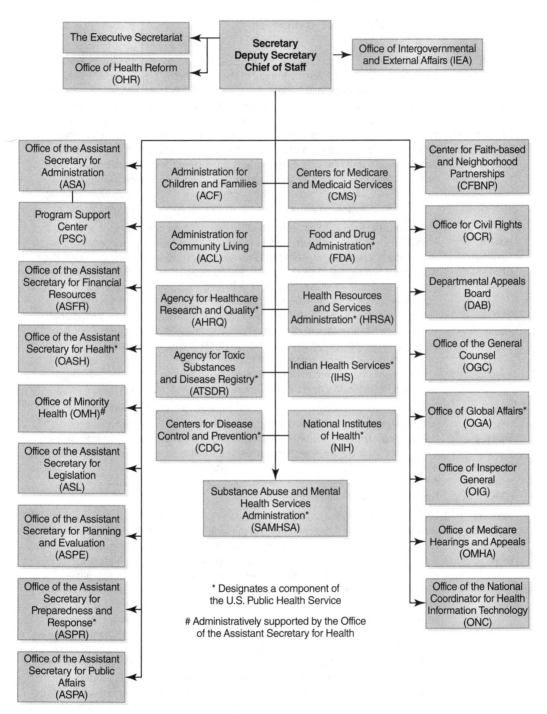

Figure 4-1   U.S. Department of Health and Human Services organization chart, 2014.

Reproduced from U.S. Department of Health and Human Services, 2014.

Table 4-1   U.S. Public Health Service Agencies

Health Resources and Services Administration (HRSA)	HRSA helps provide health resources for medically underserved populations. The main operating units of HRSA are the Bureau of Primary Health Care, Bureau of Health Professions, Maternal and Child Bureau, and the HIV/AIDS Bureau. A nationwide network of community and migrant health centers, augmented by primary care programs for the homeless and residents of public housing, serve more than 10 million Americans each year. HRSA also works to build the healthcare workforce and maintains the National Health Service Corps. The agency provides services to people with AIDS through the Ryan White Care Act programs. It oversees the organ transplantation system and works to decrease infant mortality and improve maternal and child health. HRSA was established in 1982 by bringing together several existing programs. HRSA has nearly 2,000 employees, most at its headquarters in Rockville, Maryland.
Indian Health Service (IHS)	IHS is responsible for providing federal health services to American Indians and Alaska Natives. The provision of health services to members of federally recognized tribes grew out of the special government-to-government relationship between the federal government and Indian tribes. This relationship, established in 1787, is based on Article I, Section 8 of the Constitution, and has been given form and substance by numerous treaties, laws, Supreme Court decisions, and Executive Orders. IHS is the principal federal healthcare provider and health advocate for Native Americans, and its goal is to raise their health status to the highest possible level. IHS currently provides health services to approximately 3 million American Indians and Alaska Natives who belong to more than 564 federally recognized tribes in 35 states. IHS was established in 1924; its mission was transferred from the Interior Department in 1955. Agency headquarters are in Rockville, Maryland. IHS has more than 15,000 employees.
Centers for Disease Control and Prevention (CDC)	Working with states and other partners, CDC provides a system of health surveillance to monitor and prevent disease outbreaks, including bioterrorism events and threats, and maintains national health statistics. CDC also provides for immunization services, supports research into disease and injury prevention, and guards against international disease transmission, with personnel stationed in more than 54 foreign countries. CDC was established in 1946; its headquarters are in Atlanta, Georgia. CDC has 11,000 employees.
National Institutes of Health (NIH)	Begun as a one-room Laboratory of Hygiene in 1887, NIH today is one of the world's foremost medical research centers and the federal focal point for health research. NIH is the steward of medical and behavioral research for the nation. Its mission is science in pursuit of fundamental knowledge about the nature and behavior of living systems and the application of that knowledge to extend healthy life and reduce the burdens of illness and disability. In realizing its goals, NIH provides leadership and direction to programs designed to improve the health of the nation by conducting and supporting research in the causes, diagnosis, prevention, and cure of human diseases; in the processes of human growth and development; in the biological effects of environmental contaminants; in the understanding of mental, addictive and physical disorders; and in directing programs for the collection, dissemination, and exchange of information in medicine and health, including the development and support of medical libraries and the training of medical librarians and other health information specialists. Although the majority of NIH resources sponsor external research, there is also a large in-house research program. NIH includes 27 separate health institutes and centers; its headquarters are in Bethesda, Maryland. NIH has approximately 19,000 employees.

Table 4-1   U.S. Public Health Service Agencies   (*Continued*)

Food and Drug Administration (FDA)	FDA ensures that the food we eat is safe and wholesome, that the cosmetics we use will not harm us, and that medicines, medical devices, and radiation-transmitting products such as microwave ovens are safe and effective. FDA also oversees feed and drugs for pets and farm animals. Authorized by Congress to enforce the Federal Food, Drug, and Cosmetic Act and several other public health laws, the agency monitors the manufacture, import, transport, storage, and sale of more than $1 trillion worth of goods annually. FDA has over 15,000 employees. Among its staff, FDA has chemists, microbiologists, and other scientists, as well as investigators and inspectors who visit more than 16,000 facilities a year as part of their oversight of the businesses that FDA regulates. FDA, established in 1906, has its headquarters in Silver Spring, Maryland.
Substance Abuse and Mental Health Services Administration (SAMHSA)	SAMHSA was established by Congress under Public Law 102-321 on October 1, 1992, to strengthen the nation's healthcare capacity to provide prevention, diagnosis, and treatment services for substance abuse and mental illnesses. SAMHSA works in partnership with states, communities, and private organizations to address the needs of people with substance abuse and mental illnesses as well as the community risk factors that contribute to these illnesses. SAMHSA serves as the umbrella under which substance abuse and mental health service centers are housed, including the Center for Mental Health Services (CMHS), the Center for Substance Abuse Prevention (CSAP), and the Center for Substance Abuse Treatment (CSAT). SAMHSA also houses the Office of the Administrator, the Office of Applied Studies, and the Office of Program Services. SAMHSA headquarters are in Rockville, Maryland; the agency has about 600 employees.
Agency for Toxic Substances and Disease Registry (ATSDR)	Working with states and other federal agencies, ATSDR seeks to prevent exposure to hazardous substances from waste sites. The agency conducts public health assessments, health studies, surveillance activities, and health education training in communities around waste sites on the U.S. Environmental Protection Agency's National Priorities List. ATSDR also has developed toxicity profiles of hazardous chemicals found at these sites. The agency is closely associated administratively with CDC; its headquarters are also in Atlanta, Georgia. ATSDR has more than 400 employees.
Agency for Health Care Research and Quality (AHRQ)	AHRQ supports cross-cutting research on healthcare systems, healthcare quality and cost issues, and effectiveness of medical treatments. Formerly known as the Agency for Health Care Policy and Research, AHRQ was established in 1989, assuming broadened responsibilities of its predecessor agency, the National Center for Health Services Research and Health Care Technology Assessment. The agency has about 300 employees; its headquarters are in Rockville, Maryland.

budget. Figure 4-2 compares total national health expenditures with health expenditures attributed to the federal government and to state and local governments. Escalating costs for healthcare services seriously constrain efforts to reduce the federal budget deficit, and there is little public or political support for additional taxes for health purposes.

It is no simple task to describe the federal budget development and approval process that determines funding levels for federal health programs. Although one-fourth of the federal budget supports health activities, the major share is spent on Medicare and Medicaid. These and other entitlement programs, such as Social Security, comprise two-thirds of the federal budget; this spending is mandatory and

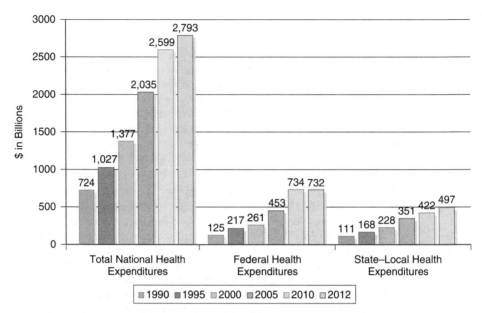

Figure 4-2 Total national health expenditures, and federal and state–local government expenditures for health-related purposes, United States, 1980–2012.

Data from Centers for Disease Control and Prevention, National Center for Health Statistics. *Health, United States, 2013.* Hyattsville, MD: NCHS; 2014.

cannot be easily controlled. The remaining one-third represents discretionary spending; half of this is related to national defense purposes. Spending for discretionary programs is more readily controlled. Nondefense discretionary spending for health purposes competes with a wide array of programs, including education, training, science, technology, housing, transportation, and foreign aid and is declining as a proportion of all federal spending.

Decisions authorizing and funding health programs are made in an annual budget approval process. The current process is a complex one that establishes ceilings for broad categories of expenditures and then reconciles individual programs and funding levels within those ceilings in omnibus budget reconciliation acts. For discretionary programs, Congress must act each year to provide spending authority. For mandatory programs, Congress may act to change the spending that current laws require. The result is a mixture of substantive decisions as to which programs will be authorized and what they will be authorized to do, together with budget decisions as to the level of resources to be made available through 13 annual appropriations bills. In recent years federal law has imposed a cap on total annual discretionary spending and requires that spending cuts must offset increased mandatory spending or new discretionary programs. This budgetary environment presents major challenges for new public health initiatives and, not infrequently, threatens continued funding for programs that have been operating for decades.

The organization of federal health responsibilities within DHHS is quite complex fiscally and operationally. In federal fiscal year 2015, the overall DHHS budget

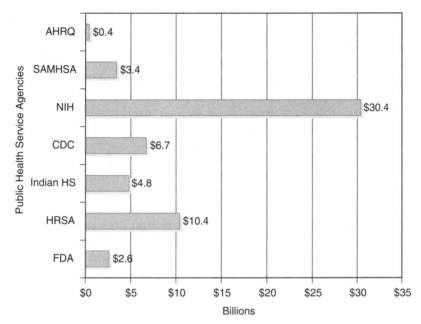

Figure 4-3 Fiscal year 2015 U.S. Public Health Service Agency program level budgets.
Data from the Fiscal Year 2015 Budget, U.S. Department of Health and Human Services, 2014.

is about $1 trillion.[6] DHHS has nearly 73,000 employees and is the largest grant-making agency in the federal government, with some 60,000 grants each year. DHHS manages more than 300 programs through its 11 operating divisions. The major share of the DHHS budget supports the Medicare and Medicaid programs within HCFA. PHS activities account for less than one-tenth of the DHHS budget.

Budgets for PHS operating divisions in federal fiscal year 2015 range from $30 billion for NIH to $400 million for AHRQ as shown in Figure 4-3. Just over 50% of all PHS funds support NIH research activities, and another $32 billion support the remaining PHS agencies with HRSA and CDC together accounting for about $18 billion, which represents only 2% of total DHHS resources and about 0.5% of all federal spending.

OUTSIDE-THE-BOX THINKING 4-3

What are the primary federal roles and responsibilities for public health in the United States? How do those roles and responsibilities comport with Public Health Service (PHS) agency budget requests for federal fiscal year 2015?

As previously described, federal grants-in-aid have long been the prime strategy and mechanism by which the federal government generates state and local action toward health priorities. A variety of approaches to grant making have been used over recent decades. These can be categorized by the extent of restrictions or flexibility imparted to grantees. The greatest flexibility and lack of requirements are associated with revenue-sharing grants. Block grants, including those initiated in the early 1980s, consolidate previously categorical grant programs into a block that generally comes with fewer restrictions than the previous collection of categorical grants. Formula grants are awarded on the basis of some predetermined formula, often based at least partly on need, which determines the level of funding for each grantee. Project grants are more limited in availability and are generally intended for a specific demonstration program or project.

In addition to being a prime strategy to influence services at the state and local level, federal grants also serve to redistribute resources to compensate for differences in the ability of states to fund and operate basic health services. They have also served as a useful approach to promoting minimum standards for specific programs and services. For example, federal grants for maternal and child health promoted personnel standards in state and local agencies that fostered the growth of civil service systems across the country. Other effects on state and local health agencies will be apparent as these are examined in the following sections.

State Health Agencies

Several factors place states at center stage when it comes to health. The U.S. Constitution gives states primacy in safeguarding the health of their citizens. From the mid-19th century until the 1930s, states largely exercised that leadership role with little competition from the federal government and only occasional conflict with the larger cities. Federal funding turned the tables on states after 1935, reaching its peak influence in the 1960s and 1970s. At that time, numerous federal health and human service initiatives (such as model cities, community health centers, and community mental health services) were funded directly to local governments and even to community-based organizations. This practice greatly concerned state officials and served to damage tenuous relationships among the three levels of government. The relative influence of states began to grow once again after 1980, with federal actions restoring some powers and resources to states and their state health agencies. Although states were finding it increasingly difficult to finance public health and medical service programs, they demanded more autonomy and control over the programs they managed, including those operated in partnership with the federal government. Ironically, local governments were making demands on state governments similar to those that states were making on the federal government. States have found themselves uncomfortably in the middle between the two other levels of government as states are one step removed from both the resources needed to address the needs of their citizens and the demands and expectations of the local citizenry.

States carry out their health responsibilities through many different state agencies, although the overall constellation of health programs and services within all of state government is roughly similar across states. In a typical state, there are often two dozen or more state agencies that carry out health responsibilities or activities. Somewhere in the maze of state agencies is an identifiable lead agency for public health. These official health agencies are often freestanding cabinet-level departments reporting to the governor of the state. In more than one-half of the states, the state health agency also reports to a state board of health or similar entity, although the prevalence of this reporting relationship is declining. Another approach to the organizational placement of state health agencies finds them within a multipurpose human service agency, often with the state's social services and substance abuse responsibilities. State health agencies are freestanding agencies in nearly 30 states and are part of multipurpose health and/or human services agencies in the others.[7]

The official with statutory authority to carry out public health laws and declare public health emergencies is generally the state health officer whose responsibilities also include serving as director of the state health department. In some states, however, this statutory authority resides with other public officials, such as the governor or director of the superagency in which the state health department is a component, or with the state board of health.

As identified in a recent profile of state public health agencies compiled by the Association of State and Territorial Health Officials (ASTHO), key activities performed by state public health agencies include:

- Running statewide prevention programs like tobacco quit lines, newborn screening programs, and disease surveillance.
- Ensuring a basic level of community public health services across the state, regardless of the level of resources or capacity of local health departments.
- Providing the services of professionals with specialized skills, such as disease outbreak specialists and restaurant and food service inspectors, who bring expertise that is otherwise hard to find, too expensive to employ at a local level, or involves overseeing local public health functions.
- Collecting and analyzing statewide vital statistics, health indicators, and morbidity data to target public health threats and diseases such as cancer.
- Directing statewide investigations of disease outbreaks, environmental hazards such as chemical spills and hurricanes, and other public health emergencies.
- Monitoring the use of funds and other resources to ensure they are used effectively and equitably throughout the state.
- Conducting statewide health planning, improvement, and evaluation.
- Licensing and regulating health care, food service, and other facilities.[7]

The range of responsibilities for the official state health agency varies considerably in terms of specific programs and services. Staffing levels and patterns also show a wide range, reflecting the diversity in agency responsibilities. The data presented on state health agencies in this chapter are derived from recent surveys of state health officials conducted by ASTHO.[7]

Figure 4-4 illustrates the variability in state health agencies' responsibilities for programs. In 2005, for example, 90% of the official state health agencies administered the Supplemental Food Program for Women, Infants, and Children, vital statistics systems, public health laboratories, and tobacco prevention and control programs. Less than one-half of the state health agencies administered the state Medicaid Program, mental health and substance abuse services, and health professional licensing. Many state health agencies administered programs for environmental health services, most frequently involving food and drinking water safety;

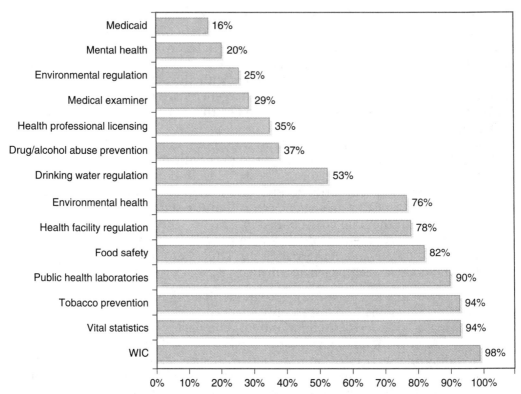

Figure 4-4   Selected organizational responsibilities of state health agencies, 2005.
Data from Association of State and Territorial Health Officials. Washington, DC: ASTHO; 2006.

however, only 20% of the state health agencies served as the environmental regulatory agency within their state, which often includes responsibility for clean air, resource conservation, clean water, superfund sites, toxic substance control, and hazardous substances. Table 4-2 and Figure 4-5 summarize a wide range of state

Table 4-2   Vital Statistics for State Health Agencies (SHAs)

Definition	• State health agency (SHA), or state department of health, is a department or agency of state government focused on public health.
Number	• 51
Jurisdiction Type	• 50 states + District of Columbia
Organizational Placement	• 58% — freestanding state agency • 42% — unit within umbrella agency
State—Local Public Health System	• 53% — decentralized or largely decentralized • 27% — centralized or largely centralized • 20% — mixed or shared

Table 4-2   Vital Statistics for State Health Agencies (SHAs) (*Continued*)

Selected Service Catego- ries Most Frequently Provided by SHAs (% of SHAs)	**Population-Based Primary Prevention Services** • 87% — tobacco • 85% — HIV • 95% — Sexually transmitted disease counseling and partner notification **Laboratory Services** • 96% — bioterrorism agent testing • 94% — foodborne illness testing • 94% — influenza typing **Maternal and Child Health Services** • 59% — children with special healthcare needs • 56% — WIC (Supplemental Food Program for Women, Infants and Children) • 44% — home visiting services **Access to Healthcare Services** • 94% — health disparities initiatives • 72% — rural health • 47% — emergency medical services
Expenditures	• Median per capita expenditures = $78 • Mean per capita expenditures = $98
Source and Use of Funds	**Sources** • 53%— federal sources • 24% — state general funds • 4% — fees • 10% — other state sources • 9% — other nonfederal and nonstate sources **Use of Funds** • 27% — consumer health • 26% — WIC • 10% — infectious diseases • 5% — environmental health • 5% — chronic diseases • 5% — quality of health services • 4% — all-hazards preparedness • 3% — administration • 2% — health laboratory • 1% — vital statistics • 1% — injury prevention • 1% — health data • 10% — other programs and services

(*continues*)

Table 4-2   Vital Statistics for State Health Agencies (SHAs)   (*Continued*)

Workforce	• Total full-time equivalent (FTE) employees = 101,000 (5,000 fewer than in 2010)
	  ○ 71% female
	  ○ 73% white
	  ○ 93% non-Hispanic
	• FTEs per 100,000 population =
	  ○ 69 for small states
	  ○ 43 for medium states
	  ○ 24 for large states
	• Median FTE employees = 1,151

Governance	• 45% of SHAs relate and/or report to a state board of health • 8% relate and/or report to a similar entity
Leadership	• 74% appointed by Governor • 71% with MD degree; 41% with MPH; 10% with DrPH or PhD degree • Mean tenure = 3.4 years

Data from Association of State and Territorial Health Officials, Profile of State Health, Volume 3. Washington, DC: ASTHO; 2014.

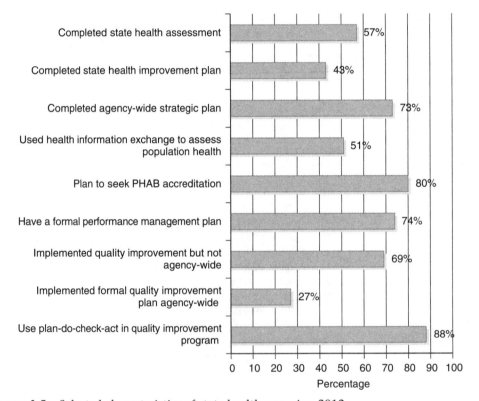

Figure 4-5   Selected characteristics of state health agencies, 2012.

Data from Association of State and Territorial Health Officials, Profile of State Health, Volume 3. Washington, DC: ASTHO; 2014.

health agency characteristics and activities. SHAs have made significant progress in completing the three prerequisites for accreditation—state health assessments, state health improvement plans, and agency-wide strategic plans—since 2010 despite budget restrictions and staff reductions.

State health agency responsibilities are anything but fixed in stone. Recent decades witnessed several changes in their public health responsibilities, including more state health agencies taking on preparedness responsibilities and expanding their health planning and development roles. On the other hand, fewer state health agencies are carrying out environmental health and institutional licensing functions and some have transferred responsibility for natural disaster preparedness. Notably, all-hazards preparedness and response is now one of the most prevalent of these emerging roles.

In some states regional or district offices carry out state responsibilities and assist local health departments (LHDs). Staff members assigned to district offices often provide consultation and technical assistance to local health agencies especially for purposes of medical oversight, budgetary management, inspectional activities and code enforcement, provision of education and training, and general planning and coordination for activities such as emergency preparedness. More than 50% of the 100,000 full-time equivalent (FTE) employees of state health departments perform their duties from regional, district, or local sites.

With public health responsibilities allocated differently across the various states, data on state public health expenditures are difficult to interpret. These data do not allow for meaningful comparison across states because of the variation in responsibilities assigned to the official state health agency. Importantly, these data often fail to differentiate between population-based public health activities and personal health services.

OUTSIDE-THE-BOOK THINKING 4-4

Access the websites of any two U.S. state health departments and compare and contrast the two state–local public health systems in terms of their structure, general functions, specific services, resources, and other important features. Your focus should be on the state–local public health systems in these two states, rather than only the state health agencies!

The organizational placement and specific responsibilities of state health agencies largely determine the size of their budgets and workforce. In order to identify state government expenditures for all public health activities, it is necessary to examine the budgets of multiple state agencies. Data on state health expenditures for fiscal year 2003 indicate that states spent about $10 billion from state sources on population-based public health activities. In addition, states expended another $9 billion of federal funding to support population-based services. Environmental protection, injury prevention, and infrastructure activities were more likely to be funded from state sources. On the other hand, funding for emergency preparedness and chronic disease prevention activity was more likely to come from federal sources. State and federal funds equally supported prevention of epidemics and spread of disease.

In most states, more than a dozen state agencies carry out environmental health roles. This pattern replicates the web of environmental responsibilities among federal agencies, creating a complex system often poorly understood by the private sector and general public. Driving the organization of state responsibilities are several key federal environmental statutes that include:

- Clean Air Act
- Clean Water Act
- Comprehensive Environmental Response, Competition, and Liability Act and Superfund Amendments and Reauthorization Act
- Federal Insecticide, Fungicide, and Rodenticide Act
- Resource Conservation and Recovery Act
- Safe Drinking Water Act
- Toxic Substance Control Act
- Food, Drug, and Cosmetic Act
- Federal Mine Safety and Health Act
- Occupational Safety and Health Act

The focus of federal statutes on specific environmental media (water, air, waste) has fostered the assignment of environmental responsibilities to a variety of state agencies other than official state health agencies. The implications of this diversification are important for public health agencies. State health agencies are becoming less involved in environmental health programs; only a handful of states utilize their state health agency as the state's lead agency for environmental concerns. This role has largely shifted to state environmental agencies, although other state agencies are also involved, resulting in state-level environmental strategies shifting from a health-oriented approach to a regulatory approach. Despite their diminished role in environmental concerns, state health agencies continue to address a very diverse set of environmental health issues and maintain epidemiologic and quantitative risk assessment capabilities not available in other state agencies. Linking this important expertise to the workings of other state agencies is a particularly challenging task.[8]

The wide variation in organization and structure of state health responsibilities suggests that there is no standard or consistent pattern to public health practice among the various states. An examination of enabling statutes and state public agency mission statements provides further support for this conclusion. One study found that only 11 of 43 state agency mission statements address the majority of the concepts related to public health purpose and mission in the Public Health in America document.[9] When state public health enabling statutes are examined for consistency with the essential public health services framework (also found in the Public Health in America document), the majority of essential public health services could be identified in only one-fifth of the states. The most frequently identified essential public health services reflected traditional public health activities, such as enforcement of laws, monitoring of health status, diagnosing and investigating health hazards, and informing and educating the public. The essential public health services least frequently referenced in these enabling statutes reflect more modern concepts of public health practice, including mobilizing community partnerships, evaluating the effects of health services, and research for innovative solutions. Only a few states were found to have both enabling statutes and state health agency mission statements highly congruent with the concepts advanced in core functions/ essential public health services framework.

State-based public health systems blend the roles of the state health agency and the LHDs in that state. In more than 40 states, all areas of the state are served by an LHD. Where there is no LHD to provide public health services, the state health agency usually provides basic public health coverage. Increasingly, states are using regional or district structures to provide oversight and support for LHDs. In more than two-thirds of states, local boards of health also provide direction and oversight of local public health activities.

In sum, states face many challenges related to the fragmentation of public health roles and responsibilities among various state agencies. Central to these are two related challenges: how to coordinate public health's core functions and essential services effectively and how to leverage changes within the health system to instill greater emphasis on population-based preventive services. These are related aims.

Local Health Departments

In the overall structuring of governmental public health responsibilities, LHDs are where the "rubber meets the road." These agencies are established to carry out the critical public health responsibilities embodied in state laws and local ordinances and to meet other needs and expectations of their communities. Although some cities had local public health boards and agencies prior to 1900, the first county health department was not established until 1911. At that time, Yakima County, Washington, created a permanent county health unit, based on the success of a county sanitation campaign to control a serious typhoid epidemic. The number of LHDs grew rapidly during the 20th century, although in recent decades, expansion has been tempered by consolidations.

LHDs should not be considered separately from the state network in which they operate. It is important to remember that states, through their state constitutions and legislatures, establish the types and powers of local governmental units that can exist in that state. In this arrangement, the state and its local subunits, however defined, share responsibilities for health and other state functions. How health duties are shared in any given state depends on a complex set of factors that include state and local statutes, history, need, and expectations.

Local health agencies relate to their state public health systems in one of three general patterns. In most states, LHDs are formed and managed by local government, reporting directly to some office of local government, such as a local Board of Health, county commission, or city or county executive officer. In this decentralized arrangement, LHDs often have considerable autonomy although they may be required to carry out specific state public health statutes.

In some states, oversight of LHDs is shared between the state health agency and local government through the power to appoint local health officers or to approve its annual budget. In other states with decentralized LHDs, some areas of the state lack coverage because the local government chooses not to form a local health agency and the state must provide services in those uncovered areas. This mixed arrangement occurs occasionally in about 20% of the states.

Another 30% of the states use a more centralized approach, in which local health agencies are directly operated by the state or there are no LHDs and the state provides all local health services. Classifying these arrangements as decentralized, centralized, or mixed is useful from the perspective of the state–local public health system. From the perspective of the LHD and the population it serves, however, the LHD is either a unit of local government or a unit of state government or both.

LHDs are established by governmental units, including counties, cities, towns, townships, and special districts, by one of two general methods. The legislative body may create an LHD through enactment of a local ordinance or a resolution, or the citizens of the jurisdiction may create a local board and agency through a referendum. Both patterns are common. Resolution health agencies are often funded from the general funds of the jurisdiction, whereas referendum health agencies often have a specific tax levy available to them. There are advantages and disadvantages to either approach. Resolution health agencies are simpler to establish and may develop close working relationships with the local legislative bodies that create them. Referendum agencies reflect the support of the local electorate and may have access to specific tax levies that preclude the need to compete with other local government funding sources.

Counties represent the most common form of subdividing states. In general, counties are geopolitical subunits of states that carry out various state responsibilities, such as law enforcement (sheriffs and state's attorneys) and public health. Counties largely function as agents of the state and carry out responsibilities delegated or assigned to them. In contrast, cities are generally not established as agents of the state. Instead, they have considerable discretion through home rule powers to take on functions that are not prohibited by state law. Cities can choose to have a health department or to rely on the state or their county for public health services. City health departments often have a wider array of programs and services because of this autonomy. As described previously, the earliest public health agencies developed in large urban centers, prior to the development of either state health agencies or county-based LHDs. This status also contributes to their sense of independence and autonomy. These considerations, as well as the increased demands and expectations to meet the needs of those who lack adequate health insurance, have made many city-based, especially big city-based, LHDs more complex than other LHDs.

Both cities and counties have resource and political bases. Both rely heavily on property and sales taxes to finance health and other services, and both struggle under the limitations of these funding sources. Political resistance to increasing taxes is the major limitation for both. Relatively few counties and cities have imposed income taxes, the form of taxation relied upon by federal and state governments.

Counties play a critical role in the public sector, the extent and importance of which is often overlooked. The overwhelming majority of LHDs are organized at the county level, serving a single county, a city–county, or several counties. As a result, counties provide a substantial portion of the community prevention and clinical preventive services offered in the United States. Counties provide care for tens of millions at a cost of tens of billions from their tax revenues through thousands of sites that include hospitals, nursing homes, clinics, health departments, and mental health facilities. Counties play an explicit role in treatment, are legally responsible for indigent health care in over 30 states, and pay a portion of the nonfederal share of Medicaid in about 20 states. In addition, counties purchase health care for several million county employees.[10]

The National Association of County and City Health Officials (NACCHO) tracks public health activities of LHDs; the most recent survey of LHDs took place in 2013.[10] Data provided in this chapter are derived from this 2013 survey, as well as from several earlier surveys.

One limitation of information on LHDs is that there is neither a clear nor a functional definition of what constitutes a LHD. The most widely used definition calls for an administrative and service unit of local government, concerned with health, employing at least one full-time person, and carrying responsibility for health of a jurisdiction smaller than the state. By this definition, more than 3,000 local health agencies operate in 3,042 U.S. counties. The number of LHDs varies widely from state to state; Rhode Island has none, whereas neighboring Connecticut and Massachusetts each report more than 100 LHDs.

More than two-thirds of LHDs are single-county health agencies, and over 80% operate out of a county base (single county, multicounty, or city–county).[10] Other LHDs function at the city, town, or township levels; some state-operated units also serve local jurisdictions. Although precise numbers are uncertain, it appears that the total number of LHDs has been increasing, from about 1,300 in 1947 to about 2,000 in the mid-1970s to somewhere near 3,000 today.

Authoritative reports going back nearly 70 years have proposed consolidation of small LHDs because of perceived lack of efficiency and coordination of services, inconsistent administration of public health laws, and the inability of small LHDs to raise adequate resources to carry out their prime functions effectively. Consolidations at the county level would appear to be the most rational approach, but only limited progress has been achieved in recent decades.

Most LHDs are relatively small organizations; as illustrated in Figure 4-6, 61% serve populations of 50,000 or fewer while 34% of LHDs serve populations of 50,000–499,999. Only 5% of LHDs serve populations of 500,000 or more residents.[10] Fully 90% of the U.S. population is served by an LHD in the medium and large population categories. Table 4-3 summarizes basic descriptive information on LHDs.

OUTSIDE-THE-BOOK THINKING 4-5

Describe the basic structure of a typical local health department (LHD) in the United States in terms of type and size of jurisdiction served, budget, staff, and agency head. (The NACCHO website may be useful here!) How does this compare with the LHD serving your community?

Some states set qualifications for local health officers or require medical supervision when the administrator is not a physician. About four-fifths of LHDs employ a full-time health officer. Health officers have a mean tenure of about 9 years.

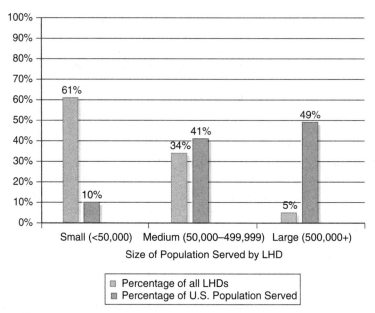

Figure 4-6   Small, medium, and large LHDs; percentage of all LHDs and percentage of population served, United States, 2013.

Data from National Association of County and City Health Officials. 2013 National Profile of Local Health Departments. Washington, DC: NACCHO; 2014.

Approximately 15% are physicians. Fewer than one-fourth of LHD directors have graduate degrees in public health.

Local boards of health are associated with most LHDs; in 2013, 70% of LHDs reported working with a local board of health. About 35 states provide for some form of local boards of health. There are an estimated 3,200 local boards of health; about 85% reported an affiliation with an LHD. However, 15% exist independently of any LHD; this pattern is most common in Massachusetts, Pennsylvania, New Hampshire, Iowa, and New Jersey.

Virtually all local boards of health establish local health policies, fees, ordinances, and regulations. Figure 4-7 indicates that most local boards of health also recommend and/or approve budgets, establish community health priorities, and hire the director of the local health agency. In recent decades, the roles of local boards of health have shifted away from policy making to more advisory duties as local governments have become more directly involved with oversight of their LHDs.

Similar to the situation with state health agencies, data on LHD expenditures lack currency and completeness. Annual LHD expenditures in 2013 ranged from less than $10,000 to over $1 billion. One-half of LHDs had budgets of $1 million or less, and 22% had budgets over $5 million. Total expenditures increase with size of population. LHDs located in metropolitan areas had substantially higher expenditures than their nonmetropolitan area counterparts. The median per capita LHD expenditure level in 2013 was $34 excluding clinical services.

Table 4-3   Vital Statistics for Local Health Departments (LHDs)

Definition	• An administrative and service unit of state or local government, concerned with health, employing at least one full-time person, and carrying responsibility for health of a jurisdiction smaller than the state
Number	• Approximately 3,200 using the above definition; 2,532 in NACCHO sampling frame • Functional definition would reduce number considerably • Ranges from zero in Rhode Island and Hawaii to more than 100 in seven states
Jurisdiction Type	• 68% — single county • 8% — multicounty • 20% — city or town • 4% — other (mostly multiple cities and towns)
Jurisdiction Population	• 61% — <50,000 • 34% — 50,000—499,999 • 5% — 500,000 and greater
Services Most Frequently Provided by LHDs	• 91% — communicable disease surveillance • 90% — adult immunizations • 90% — childhood immunizations • 83% — tuberculosis screening • 78% — environmental health surveillance • 78% — food service establishment inspection • 76% — tuberculosis testament • 72% — food safety education • 69% — population-based nutrition services • 69% — schools and daycare centers inspection
Expenditures	• Mean — $7,220,000 • 25% — <$500,000 • 22% — >$5,000,000 • Median per capita expenditures: $34 (excluding clinical revenue); $39 (all sources)
Source of Funds (from 2008 survey)	• 25% — local • 20% — state • 17% — federal funds passed through state • 2% — federal direct to local agency • 10% — Medicaid reimbursement • 5% — Medicare reimbursement • 11% — fees • 7% — other • 2% — not specified
Workforce	• Total full-time equivalent (FTE) employees = 146,000 (20,000 fewer than in 2008) • Median number of employees = 20 • Median FTE employees = 17 ○ 61% of LHDs with <25 FTE ○ 13% of LHDs with >100 FTE • Median FTEs in selected occupational categories employed by LHDs

(continued)

Table 4-3   Vital Statistics for Local Health Departments (LHDs)   (*Continued*)

Population Served								
	<10,000	10,000–24,999	25,000–49,999	50,000–99,999	100,000–249,999	250,000–499,999	500,000–999,999	1,000,000+
All LHD Staff	4	9	15	28	64	130	251	453
Manager	0.7	1	1	2	2	4	14	17
Nurse	1	2.8	4	6	12	19	34.5	44.5
Physician	0	0	0	0	0.3	1	1.7	3
Environmental Health Worker	0.1	1	1.8	3	7	14	25	34
Licensed Practical or Vocational Nurse (LPN/LVN)	0	0	0	0	0	0	2	3
Epidemiologist	0	0	0	0	0	1	2	6
Community Health Worker	0	0	0	0	0.5	2	6	20
Health Educator	0	0	0.6	1	1.7	3	5	9.9
Nutritionist	0	0	0.6	1	3	5	8.5	20.9
Information Systems Specialist	0	0	0	0	0	1	2	4.5
Public Information Specialist	0	0	0	0	0	0	1	1
Emergency Preparedness Staff	0	0.2	0.5	1	1	2	4	5
Behavioral Health Professional	0	0	0	0	0	0	1	0
Laboratory Worker	0	0	0	0	0	0	2	10
Oral Health Care Professional	0	0	0	0	0	0	0	1
Administrative/Clerical	1	2.5	4	6.8	14	28.3	48.5	101.5

Governance
- 80% of LHDs relate and/or report to a local board of health
- For 66% of local boards of health, members of the board are appointed to their positions

Leadership
- More than one-half of local health officers are women
- One-fifth of all local health officers have doctoral-level degrees
- Mean tenure = 8.7 years

Data from National Association of County and City Health Officials, 2013 National Profile of Local Health Departments. Washington, DC: NACCHO; 2014.

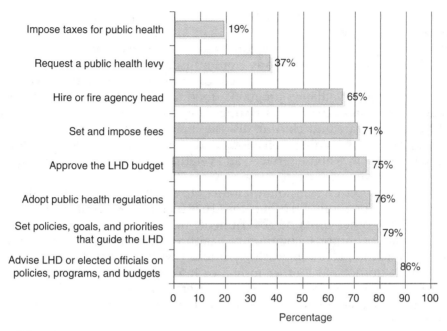

Figure 4-7   Selected functions of local boards of health

Data from 2013 National Profile of Local Health Departments, NACCHO, 2014.

LHDs derived their funding from several sources: local funds (26%), the state (37%, including 17% that were federal funds passing through the state), direct federal funds (2%), Medicaid and Medicare reimbursements (15%), fees (12%), and other sources (8%). Metropolitan LHDs and those serving smaller populations are more dependent on local sources of funding, while LHDs in nonmetropolitan areas and those serving larger populations rely more on state sources.

Revenue from virtually all sources for LHDs had been increasing until the economic recession that began in 2008. The number of FTE workers shows the same pattern. The economic downturn didn't reverse course until 2012 and 2013—well after the official end of recession.

The number of FTE employees also increases with the size of the population served. Only 11% of LHDs employ 125 or more persons, and 68% have 24 or fewer employees. The number of employees and the number of different occupations and professions are related to LHD population size. Clerical staff, nurses, sanitarians, managers, health educators, and nutritionists are the most common occupational categories.

There is considerable variability in the services provided by LHDs. Top priority areas for LHDs overall are communicable disease control, environmental health, and child health. LHDs serving both large and small populations report similar priorities, although community outreach replaces environmental health as a top priority for the largest local health jurisdictions (those over 500,000 population). Slight differences in priorities are also apparent between metropolitan and nonmetropolitan area LHDs. LHDs in metropolitan areas often include inspections as a high priority, while nonmetropolitan LHDs are more likely to include family planning and home health-care services as priorities.

Many LHDs provide a common core battery of services that generally includes adult and childhood immunizations, communicable disease control, community assessment, community outreach and education, environmental health services, epidemiology and surveillance programs, food safety and restaurant inspections, health education, and tuberculosis testing. Less commonly, LHDs provide services related to primary care and chronic disease, including cardiovascular disease, diabetes, and glaucoma screening; behavioral and mental health services; programs for the homeless; substance abuse services; and veterinary public health.

LHDs do not always provide these services themselves; increasingly, they contract for these services or contribute resources to other agencies or organizations in the community. Community partners for LHDs include state health agencies, other LHDs, hospitals, other units of government, nonprofit and voluntary organizations, academic institutions, community health centers, the faith community, and insurance companies. LHDs increasingly interact with managed care organizations, although most do not have either formal or informal agreements governing these interactions. Where agreements existed, they were more likely to be formal, to cover clinical and case management services, and to involve the provision (rather than the purchase) of services.

INTERGOVERNMENTAL RELATIONSHIPS

In terms of public health roles, no level of government predominates. The relationships between and among the three levels of government have changed considerably over time in terms of their relative importance and influence. This is especially true for the federal and local roles. The federal government had little authority and little ability to influence health priorities and interventions until after 1930. Since that time, it has exercised its influence primarily through financial leverage on both state and local governments, as well as on the private medical care system. The massive financing role of the federal government has moved it to a position of preeminence among the various levels of government in actual ability to influence health affairs. This is evident in the federal share of total national health expenditures and the federal government's role in implementing the Affordable Care Act. However federal public health spending represents only about 1% of total federal health spending, one-fourth less than in 2005 (Figure 4-8). This suggests that the relative federal commitment to public health has declined somewhat over recent decades. The federal proportion of total public health activity spending shows a similar pattern (Figure 4-9), declining from 20% in 2010 to 15% in 2012. Figure 4-10 traces public health activity spending from 1980 to 2012.

In recent decades, political initiatives have sought to diminish the powerful federal role and return some of its authority back to the states. However, little in the form of meaningful transfer of authority or resource control has taken place through 2014. It is likely that the federal government's fiscal muscle will sustain its current upper hand in its relationships with state and local government.

Local government has experienced the greatest and most disconcerting change in relative influence over the 20th century. Prior to 1900, local government was the

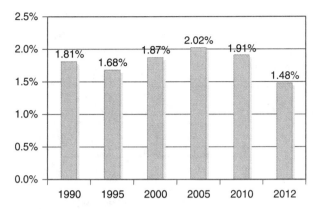

Figure 4-8 Federal public health activity spending as a percentage of total federal health spending, United States, 1990–2012.

Data from Centers for Medicare and Medicaid Services, National Health Accounts (NHA), selected years, 1990–2012.

primary locus of action, with the development of both population-based interventions for communicable disease control and environmental sanitation and locally provided charity care for the poor. However, the massive problems related to simultaneous urbanization and povertization of the big cities spawned needs that could not be met with local resources alone. States often viewed local governments in general and LHDs in particular as their delivery system for programs and services. In any event, the power of states and the growing influence of financial incentives through grant programs of both federal and state government acted to alter local priorities. Priorities were being established by higher levels of government more often than through local determinations of needs. Although the demands and expectations

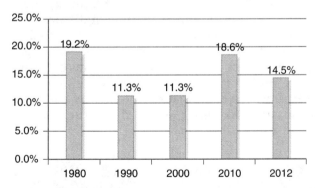

Figure 4-9 Federal public health activity spending as a percentage of total public health activity spending, United States, 1980–2012.

Data from Centers for Medicare and Medicaid Services, National Health Accounts (NHA), selected years, 1980–2012.

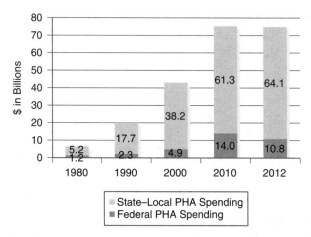

Figure 4-10 Federal and state–local public health activity spending, United States, 1980–2012.

Data from Centers for Medicare and Medicaid Services, National Health Accounts (NHA), selected years, 1980–2012.

were being directed at local governments, key decisions were being made in state capitals and in Washington, DC. Unfortunately there are signs that local governments across the country are looking for opportunities to reduce their health roles for both clinical services and population-based interventions where they can. The perception is that the responsibility for clinical services lies with federal and state government or the private sector and that even traditional public health services can be effectively outsourced. How these actions will comport with the widespread belief that services are best provided at the local level raises serious questions regarding new roles of oversight and accountability that are not easily answered. Local governments have lost control over priorities and policies; they bridle under the regulations and grant conditions imposed by state and federal funding sources. As costs increase, grant awards fail to keep pace; however, even with Obamacare wholly or partly uninsured individuals will continue to look to local government for services. These rising expectations and increasing costs are occurring at a time when local governments are unable and unwilling to seek additional tax revenues. The complexities of organizing and coordinating community-wide responses to modern public health problems and risks also push local government to look elsewhere for solutions.

OUTSIDE-THE-BOOK THINKING 4-6

What is the basis for the historic and ongoing tension between the powers of the federal government and the powers of states in public health matters?

States were slow to assume their extensive powers in the health arena but have been major players since the latter half of the 19th century. Although the growing influence of the federal government since 1930 displaced states as the most important level of government, their relative role has strengthened since about 1980. Still, states have become secondary players in the health sector. Most states lack the means, political as well as statutory, to intervene effectively in the portion of the health sector located within their jurisdictional boundaries. This is further complicated by their tradition of imitating the federal health bureaucracy whenever possible through the decentralization of health roles and responsibilities throughout dozens of administrative agencies. Coordination of programs, policies, and priorities has become exceedingly difficult within state government. Still, the widely disparate circumstances from state to state make for laboratories of opportunity in which innovative approaches can be developed and evaluated.

The relationship between state and local government in public health has traditionally been tenuous and difficult. Just as the federal government views the states, states themselves have come to view local governments as just another way to get things done. As a result, states have turned to other parties, such as community-based organizations, and have begun to deal directly with them, leaving local government on the sidelines. This undervaluing of LHDs, when coupled with competing priorities, such as education, public safety, and transportation, within local governments, presents major challenges for the future of public health services in the U.S. Instead of becoming stronger allies, these forces are working to pull apart the fabric of the national public health network.

These ever-changing and evolving relationships call into question whether the governmental public health network can be strengthened through a more centralized approach involving greater federal leadership and direction.[11] With a continued emphasis on decentralization, some states may truly be laboratories of innovation and offer creative solutions. There are many examples of creative policies and programs at the state level, but there are also many examples of state creativity being stifled by the federal government. The history of state requests for waivers of Medicaid requirements is a case in point. Many states waited several years or more for federal approval of the waivers necessary to begin innovative programs, and some of the more creative proposals were actually rejected. Still, it can be argued that state political processes are more reflective of the different political values that must be reconciled for progressive policies to develop.

CONCLUSION

Public health activities in the United States are coordinated by a network of state and local public health agencies working in partnership with the federal government. This framework is precariously balanced on a legal foundation that gives primacy for health concerns to states, a financial foundation that allows the federal government to promote consistency and minimum standards across 50 diverse states, and a practical foundation of LHDs serving as the point of contact between communities and their three-tiered government. Over time, the relative influence of these partners has shifted dramatically because of changing needs, resources, and public expectations. The challenges to this dynamic organizational structure are many. There are increasing calls for government to turn over many public programs to private interests and growing distrust of government, in general. These developments make it easy to forget that many of the public health achievements of the past century would not have been possible without a serious commitment of resources and leadership by those in the public sector. In any event, it is clear that the organizational structure of public health—its form—intimately reflects the structure of government in the United States. The extent to which public health's form facilitates or impedes its effective functioning is the focus of an upcoming chapter.

REFERENCES

1. Centers for Disease Control and Prevention. History of CDC. *MMWR*. 1996; *45*: 526–528.
2. Centers for Disease Control and Prevention. *Profile of State and Local Public Health Systems 1990.* Atlanta, GA: CDC; 1991.
3. Shonick W. *Government and Health Services: Government's Role in the Development of the U.S. Health Services 1930–1980.* New York: Oxford University Press; 1995.
4. Pickett G, Hanlon JJ. *Public Health Administration and Practice.* 9th ed. St. Louis, MO: Mosby; 1990.
5. *Jacobson v Massachusetts.* 197 US 11 (1905).
6. U.S. Department of Health and Human Services (DHHS). *The Fiscal Year 2015 Budget.* Washington, DC: DHHS; 2014.
7. Association of State and Territorial Health Officials. *Profile of State Public Health, Volume Three, 2012.* Washington, DC: ASTHO; 2014.
8. Burke TA, Shalauta NM, Tran NL, Stern BS. The environmental web: a national profile of the state infrastructure for environmental health and protection. *J Public Health Manage Pract.* 1997; *3*: 1–12.
9. Gebbie KM. State public health laws: an expression of constituency expectations. *J Public Health Manage Pract.* 2000; *6*: 46–54.
10. National Association of County and City Health Officials. *2013 National Profile of Local Health Departments.* Washington, DC; NACCHO; 2014.
11. Turnock BJ, Atchison C. Governmental public health in the United States: the implications of federalism. *Health Aff.* 2002; *6*: 68–78.

Chapter 5

Twenty-First Century Community Public Health Practice

The Institute of Medicine's (IOM) landmark report in 1988, *The Future of Public Health*, stimulated important changes in the U.S. public health system.[1] The IOM report rearticulated the mission, substance, and core functions of public health and challenged the public health community to think more strategically, plan more collectively, and perform more effectively. Exciting opportunities afforded by broader participation through engaging communities and other stakeholders, heightened public expectations for addressing threats and emergencies, and the potential for better integration of public health and medical care activities have energized these efforts. These developments brought change to the public health system while offering new hope for achieving improved health outcomes through public health practice. This chapter examines the link between public health's functions and public health practice, focusing on the organizing concepts for modern public health practice and how these have advanced new standards for public health practice. Key questions to be addressed in this chapter are as follows:

- What have been public health's main functions over the past century?
- What are the core functions of public health today?

- How are these functions translated into practice?
- What are the current standards for community public health practice?

Improvement science asserts that results reflect the systems that produce them. In other words, every system is perfectly designed to achieve the exact results it gets. This somewhat elliptical wisdom underscores a major challenge confronting efforts to enhance the results of public health practice: Improving health outcomes calls for improving the basic processes of public health practice. However, as some additional reasoning from the improvement scientists warns, to improve something, we must be able to control it; to control it, we must be able to understand it; and to understand it, we must be able to measure it. Measurement relies on operational definitions for the concepts of interest. Improving the performance of public health functions is an agenda that defines, measures, understands, and controls the processes that constitute public health practice.

For nearly 100 years, the public health community has been grappling with this agenda, with only limited success along the way.[2] For much of the 20th century, an adequate conceptual framework for defining the public health system was lacking. As a result, past efforts generally focused on measuring aspects of the public health system that only indirectly or partially characterized the functions carried out in public health practice. This limited opportunities for understanding, controlling, and improving public health practice and health outcomes. Nonetheless, these efforts paved the way for developments that were subsequently jump-started by the 1988 IOM report.

PUBLIC HEALTH FUNCTIONS AND PRACTICE BEFORE 1990

Over much of the past century, the mission and purpose of public health (what it is) and its functions (how it addresses its mission) were viewed as synonymous with the provision of public health services. In fact, public health's services were frequently characterized as its functions. Public health was known more by its deeds than its intent. As a result, early efforts to describe and measure public health practice focused primarily on measuring aspects of important public health services.

The earliest attempts to define and measure public health practice in the United States date back to 1914. Before that time, public health functions were primarily those identified in the broad statutes of state and local governments, centering on the prevention and control of infectious diseases. In 1914, however, a survey catalogued the various services of state health agencies, as well as their role in fostering the development of local health departments (LHDs). This study concluded that even though public health agencies were carrying out a wide variety of programs and services they were missing their mark. Much of what was being done through public health agencies had little effect on community health status, and there was actually much that these agencies could have been doing that would have reduced mortality and morbidity.[3] Public health practice was evaluated using a scoring system that placed greater weight on some public health activities and services than on others, allowing a basis for comparisons across agencies. Key elements of this approach were soon incorporated into local public health assessment initiatives orchestrated by the American Public Health Association (APHA).

In 1921, the first report of APHA's Committee on Municipal Health Department Practice called for the systematic collection and analysis of information on local public health practice to support the development of standards for LHDs serving the nation's largest municipalities. The committee had determined that LHDs and the communities they served would benefit from standards that would ensure a consistent level of public health services from one jurisdiction to another. The committee also sought to identify characteristics of LHD practice that produce the best results. An elaborate survey instrument and process were established; more than 80 big-city health departments were reviewed in the initial effort.

The need to examine public health practice outside the nation's large cities, especially in the growing number of county-based LHDs, was soon apparent. In 1925, the committee was reconstituted as the Committee on Administrative Practice to assess more broadly the status of public health practice in the United States. The new committee developed the first version of an "Appraisal Form" to be used as a self-assessment tool by local health officers. The intent was to measure the immediate results attained from local public health services. Examples of these immediate results follow:

- Birth and death records adequately catalogued and analyzed
- Various vaccinations provided for specific age groups
- Health problems in school-aged children identified and treated
- Tuberculosis cases hospitalized and treated
- Laboratory tests performed[4]

Successive iterations of the Appraisal Form appeared through the 1920s and 1930s; these were well received by the public health community, although there were occasional concerns that quantity was being emphasized over quality. Local health officers were able to compare their ratings with those of other public health agencies. The basis for comparison was a numerical rating score, based on aggregated points awarded across key administrative and service areas. Comparative ratings were used to improve health programs, advocate for resources, summarize health agency activities in annual reports, and engage other health interests in the community. Agency ratings often attracted considerable public interest, resulting in both good and bad publicity for local agencies. Despite the initial intent to emphasize immediate results, however, the major focus of the ratings remained on measuring the more concrete aspects of public health practice, such as staff, clinic sites, patient visits, and the number of services rendered.

In 1943, a new instrument, the "Evaluation Schedule," which was scored centrally by the APHA Committee on Administrative Practice, replaced the self-assessment approach used in the Appraisal Form. The scores for health agencies of varying size and type were widely disseminated so that individual LHDs could directly compare their performance in meeting community needs with that of their peers. Table 5-1 lists some of the key performance measures included in the 1947 version of the Evaluation Schedule.

To develop a blueprint for a national network of LHDs that would provide every American with public health coverage, the Committee on Administrative Practice established a Subcommittee on Local Health Units. The subcommittee's major report (widely known as the Emerson Report) in 1945 was a landmark for

Table 5-1   Public Health Practice Performance Measures from 1947 Evaluation Schedule

1. Hospital beds: percentage in approved hospitals
2. Practicing physicians: population per physician
3. Practicing dentists: population per dentist
4. Water: percentage of population in communities over 2,500 served with approved water
5. Sewerage: percentage of population in communities over 2,500 served with approved sewerage systems
6. Water: percentage of rural schoolchildren served with approved water supplies
7. Excreta disposal: percentage of rural schoolchildren served with approved means of excreta disposal
8. Food: percentage of food handlers reached by group instruction program
9. Food: percentage of restaurants and lunch counters with satisfactory facilities
10. Milk: percentage of bottled milk pasteurized
11. Diphtheria: percentage of children under 2 years given immunizing agent
12. Smallpox: percentage of children under 2 years given immunizing agent
13. Whooping cough: percentage of children under 2 years given immunizing agent
14. Tuberculosis: newly reported cases per death, 5-year period
15. Tuberculosis: deaths per 100,000 population, 5-year period
16. Tuberculosis: percentage of cases reported by death certificate
17. Syphilis: percentage of cases reported in primary, secondary, and early latent stage
18. Syphilis: percentage of reported contacts examined
19. Maternal: puerperal deaths per 1,000 total births, 5-year rate
20. Maternal: percentage of antepartum cases under medical supervision seen before the sixth month
21. Maternal: percentage of women delivered at home under postpartum nursing supervision
22. Maternal: percentage of births in hospital
23. Infant: deaths under 1 year of age per 1,000 live births, 5-year rate
24. Infant: deaths from diarrhea and enteritis under 1 year per 1,000 live births, 2-year rate
25. Infant: percentage of infants under nursing supervision before 1 month
26. School: percentage of elementary children with dental work neglected
27. Accidents: deaths from motor accidents per 100,000 population, 5-year rate
28. Health department budget: cents per capita spent by health department

Data from American Public Health Association, Committee on Administrative Practice. *Evaluation Schedule for Use in Study and Appraisal of Community Health Programs*. New York, NY:APHA; 1947.

recommendations regarding local public health practice. The Emerson Report became the postwar plan for public health in the United States. The report's far-reaching recommendations called for a minimum population base of 50,000 people for each LHD and included state-by-state proposals for networks of LHDs that would cover all Americans while reducing the number of LHDs by about 50% through consolidation of smaller units.[5]

The Emerson Report gave increased prominence to six basic services believed to represent local government's public health responsibilities to its citizens: vital statistics, environmental sanitation, communicable disease control, maternal and child health services, public health education, and public health laboratory services.[5,6] This was not a new formulation for local public health services. Rather,

Table 5-2   Basic Six Services of Local Public Health

1. Vital statistics—collection and interpretation.
2. Sanitation.
3. Communicable disease control, including immunization, quarantine, and other measures such as identifying communicable disease carriers and distributing vaccines to physicians as well as doing immunizations directly.
4. Maternal and child health (MCH), consisting of prenatal and postpartum care for mothers and babies and supervision of the health of schoolchildren. In some places, immunization of children was handled by the MCH program.
5. Health education, including instruction in personal and family hygiene, sanitation and nutrition, given in schools, at neighborhood health center classes, and in home visits.
6. Laboratory services to physicians, sanitarians, and other interested parties.

Data from Shonick W. *Government and Health Services: Government's Role in the Development of U.S. Health Services 1930–1980*. New York: Oxford University Press; 1995.

it was essentially the same package of services that had been considered the standard of practice among LHDs for several decades. Over time, these services had become widely known as the six basic functions of public health ("Basic Six"); Table 5-2 describes the Basic Six. With the added impetus of the Emerson Report, these six activities became the cornerstone for structuring local public health practice. Although the report's extensive recommendations never became national public policy, they promoted positive changes in many states.

The Committee on Administrative Practice stimulated considerable interest in local public health practice. After about 1950 and continuing into the 1980s, there were repeated efforts to reexamine and redefine the boundaries of local public health practice. This search for mission redefinition is evident in a series of APHA policy statements from 1950 to 1970.[6] In a 1950 APHA statement on LHD services and responsibilities, the Basic Six were presented as desirable minimal services, and several new "optimal" responsibilities were identified: recording and analysis of health data, health education and information, supervision and regulation, provision of direct environmental health services, administration of personal health services, and coordination of activities and services within the community. Another APHA policy statement in 1963 added seventh and eighth services to the Basic Six: operation of health facilities and area-wide planning and coordination. Then, in 1970, APHA adopted another policy statement, expanding on these concepts and calling for increased involvement of state and LHDs in coordinating, monitoring, and assessing the adequacy of health services in their jurisdictions. The evolution of these various characterizations of public health practice is traced in Table 5-3.

In the closing decades of the 20th century, important new expectations for local public health practice emerged. Inadequate access to medical care was increasingly identified as a significant impediment to promoting and improving community health. This resulted in local health departments increasingly serving a safety net function. This expanded direct service provision role moved LHDs into new territory, beyond the boundaries of the expanded six functions that characterized public health

Table 5-3   Expansion of the Basic Six Public Health Services, 1920–1980

Initial "Basic Six"
- Vital statistics
- Sanitation
- Communicable disease control
- Maternal and child health
- Health education
- Laboratory services

"Optimal" Services in 1950s
- Basic Six as minimal level
- Analysis and recording of health data
- Health education and information
- Supervision and regulation
- Provision of direct environmental health services
- Administration of personal health services
- Coordination of activities and services within the community

Added in 1960s
- Operation of health facilities
- Area-wide planning and coordination

Added in the 1970s
- Coordinating, monitoring, and assessing the adequacy of health services

Data from Shonick W. *Government and Health Services: Government's Role in the Development of U.S. Health Services 1930–1980.* New York: Oxford University Press; 1995.

practice throughout the first half of the 20th century. There was considerable debate as to whether this new role was appropriate, as well as whether LHDs should play leadership roles within their communities in integrating medical and community health services. The movement into medical care was controversial from its inception. Hanlon, in examining the future of LHDs in 1973, urged official public health agencies to withdraw from the business of providing personal health services (whether preventive or therapeutic) and instead to "concentrate upon [their] important and unique potential as community health conscience and leader"[7(p901)] in promoting the establishment of sound social policy. Despite these admonitions, direct medical care services increased among LHDs throughout the 1960s, 1970s, and 1980s, largely as a result of new federal and state grant programs. LHDs were becoming significant providers of safety-net medical services, joining public hospitals and community health centers in this important role.

Quietly emerging through these developments was a unique concept that began to shift the emphasis from the services of public health to its mission and functions. This concept, often characterized as *a governmental presence at the local level* (AGPALL), emerged in the 1970s in the process of fashioning model standards for communities to participate in establishment of the 1990 national health objectives.[8] As described in Table 5-4, AGPALL asserts that local government, acting through various means, is ultimately responsible and accountable for ensuring that

Table 5-4   Governmental Presence at the Local Level

The concept of governmental presence at the local level is based upon a multifaceted, multi-tiered governmental responsibility for ensuring that standards are met—a responsibility that often involves agencies in addition to the public health agency at any particular level. Regardless of the structure, every community must be served by a governmental entity charged with that responsibility, and general-purpose government must assign and coordinate responsibility for providing and ensuring public health and safety services. Where services in any area covered by standards are readily available, government may also (but need not also) be involved in delivery of such services. Conversely, where there is a gap in service availability, it is the responsibility of government to have, or to develop, the capacity to deliver such services. Where county and municipal responsibilities overlap, agreements on division of responsibility are necessary.

In summary, government at the local level has the responsibility for ensuring that a health problem is monitored and that services to correct that problem are available. The state government must monitor the effectiveness of local efforts to control health problems and act as a residual guarantor of services where community resources are inadequate, recognizing of course that state resources are also limited.

Reproduced from the U.S. Conference of City Health Officials, National Association of County Health Officials, Association of State and Territorial Health Officials, American Public Health Association, and U.S. Department of Health, Education and Welfare, Public Health Service, Centers for Disease Control. Model Standards for Community Preventive Health Services [Preamble to original model standards]. Public Health Service: Atlanta, GA; 1978.

minimum standards are met in the community. Every locality is served by a unit of government that has responsibility for the health of that locality and population. This responsibility can be executed through an organization other than the official public health agency, but government, through its presence and interest in health, is responsible to see that necessary, agreed-on services are available, accessible, acceptable, and of good quality.

The AGPALL concept emphasizes the leadership and change agent dimensions of community public health practice; however, exercising leadership to serve the community's health is neither simple nor straightforward. The complexities of 20th century health problems and their contributing factors often called for collaborative, rather than command-and-control solutions. Key to identifying and solving important community health problems is the ability to engage diverse interests and build constituencies. The AGPALL concept suggests that modern public health practice involves more than the provision of services. This broader view of public health's functions was powerfully reinforced by the IOM report.

PUBLIC HEALTH FUNCTIONS AND PRACTICE AFTER 1990

The forecast for the public health system provided in the 1988 IOM report (appropriately titled *The Future of Public Health*) was more dismal than many had expected. After all, the infrastructure of the national public health system had grown substantially throughout the century, especially in terms of LHD coverage of the population. There was widespread acceptance that appropriate community services should include chronic disease prevention and medical care, in addition to the basic six services. Also, importantly, health status had never been better. Nevertheless, the HIV/AIDS epidemic had emerged, and there was no shortage of intractable health and social issues being placed on the public health agenda. Resources to meet these challenges were greatly limited, in part because of the insatiable appetite of the medical care delivery system for every available health dollar. These forces acted together to dissipate public appreciation and support for public health, and the IOM feared that public health would not be able to overcome these challenges without a new vision that would engender the support of the public, policy makers, the media, the medical establishment, and other key stakeholders.

The vision articulated in the IOM report was grounded in a broader view of public health functions than had existed in the past. Throughout earlier decades, the services provided by public health agencies had come to be viewed by many as public health's functions. In identifying three core functions, the IOM report suggested that the function to serve—whether described in terms of specific services or as the more abstract concept of assurance—incompletely characterizes the unique role of public health in our society. Public health interventions represent the products of carrying out public health's core functions, rather than the functions themselves. The IOM examination explicated three public health core functions: assessment, policy development, and assurance.[1]

> Assessment calls for public health to regularly and systematically collect, assemble, analyze, and make available information on the health of the community, including statistics on health status, community health needs, and epidemiologic and other studies of health problems. Not every agency is large enough to conduct these activities directly; intergovernmental and interagency cooperation is essential. Nevertheless, each agency bears the responsibility for seeing that the assessment function is fulfilled. This basic function of public health cannot be delegated.[1(p7)]
>
> Policy development calls for public health to serve the public interest in the development of comprehensive public health policies by promoting the use of the scientific knowledge base in decision making about public health and by leading in developing public health policy. Agencies must take a strategic approach, developed on the basis of a positive appreciation for the democratic political process.[1(p8)]
>
> Assurance calls for public health to ensure their constituents that services necessary to achieve agreed on goals are provided, either by encouraging actions by other entities (private or public), by requiring such action through regulation or by providing services directly. Each public health agency is to involve key policy makers and the general public in determining a set of high-priority personal and community-wide health services that government will guarantee to every member of the community. This guarantee should include subsidization or direct provision of high-priority personal health services for those unable to afford them.[1(p8)]

This new core function framework resonated widely within the public health community; its broader characterization of the important functions of public health led to the definition and measurement of their operational aspects, facilitating assessment of their performance. Several key aspects of the assessment, policy development, and assurance functions are processes that identify and address health problems; others are processes (e.g., services and other interventions) generated to ensure that these problems are addressed. To explicate the core functions and provide a framework for characterizing modern public health practice, a work group representing the national public health organizations developed the essential public health services framework.[9] Since 1995, virtually all national and state public health initiatives have adopted the essential public health services framework as the foundation for efforts to characterize, measure, and improve the performance of public health practice. Unfortunately, the use of the term services in the essential public health services framework can be a source of confusion. Although they are not services in the same sense that most people view clinical services (e.g., immunizations) or community preventive services (e.g., fluoridating water), the essential public health services are important processes that operationalize the core functions—assessment, policy development, and assurance—into actionable elements of public health practice.

OUTSIDE-THE-BOOK THINKING 5-1

Review the organization of health responsibilities in the state of your choice and describe how public health's core functions and essential services are distributed among various offices and agencies of state government beyond the state health department.

Public health strives to identify health problems and their causative factors, develop strategies to address these problems, and see that these strategies are implemented in a way that achieves the desired goals. Whereas a comprehensive description for public health practice is yet to be agreed on, the best depiction of what contemporary public health practice is all about can be found in the mission, vision, and functions outlined in the Public Health in America statement.[10] This one-page document articulates a vision (healthy people in healthy communities), a mission (promoting physical and mental health and preventing disease, injury, and disability), and statements of what public health practice does and how it accomplishes these ends. As presented in Table 5-5, these statements offer a framework for establishing and measuring practice standards for public health systems, organizations, and workers. The processes embodied in the essential public health services and their links to the three core functions are critical to an understanding of modern public health practice.

Assessment in Public Health

Two important processes (or essential public health services) characterize the assessment function of public health: (1) monitoring health status to identify community health problems and (2) diagnosing and investigating health problems and health hazards in the community.

Table 5-5   Relationship of Public Health in America Statement to Public Health Practice

Public Health in America Elements	Relationship to Public Health Practice
Vision: Healthy people in healthy communities **Mission:** Promote physical and mental health and prevent disease, injury, and disability	Vision and mission statements for public health practice
Public Health	
• Prevents epidemics and the spread of disease • Protects against environmental hazards • Prevents injuries • Promotes and encourages healthy behaviors • Responds to disasters and assists communities in recovery • Ensures the quality and accessibility of health services	Statements of the broad categories of outcomes affected by public health practice; sometimes viewed as what public health does
Essential Public Health Services	
1. Monitor health status to identify community health problems 2. Diagnose and investigate health problems and health hazards in the community 3. Inform, educate, and empower people about health issues 4. Mobilize community partnerships to identify and solve health problems 5. Develop policies and plans that support individual and community health efforts 6. Enforce laws and regulations that protect health and ensure safety 7. Link people with needed personal health services and ensure the provision of health care when otherwise unavailable 8. Ensure a competent public health and personal healthcare workforce 9. Evaluate effectiveness, accessibility, and quality of personal and population-based health services 10. Research for new insights and innovative solutions to health problems	Statements of the processes of public health practice that affect public health outcomes; sometimes viewed as how public health does what it does

Data from Public Health Functions Steering Committee. Public Health in America. Washington, DC: PHS; 1994.

Monitoring health status to identify community health problems encompasses:

- Accurate, ongoing assessment of the community's health status
- Identification of threats to health
- Determination of health service needs
- Attention to the health needs of groups that are at higher risk than the total population

- Identification of community assets and resources that support the public health system in promoting health and improving quality of life
- Use of appropriate methods and technology to interpret and communicate data to diverse audiences
- Collaboration with other stakeholders, including private providers and health benefit plans, to manage multisectoral integrated information systems

Diagnosing and investigating health problems and health hazards in the community encompass:

- Access to a public health laboratory capable of conducting rapid screening and high-volume testing
- Active infectious disease epidemiology programs
- Technical capacity for epidemiologic investigation of disease outbreaks and patterns of infectious and chronic diseases and injuries and other adverse health behaviors and conditions

Policy Development for Public Health

The assessment function and its related processes provide a foundation for policy development and its key processes, including (1) informing, educating, and empowering people about health issues; (2) mobilizing community partnerships to identify and solve health problems; and (3) developing policies and plans that support individual and community health efforts.

Informing, educating, and empowering people about health issues encompass:

- Community development activities
- Social marketing and targeted media public communication
- Provision of accessible health information resources at community levels
- Active collaboration with personal healthcare providers to reinforce health promotion messages and programs
- Joint health education programs with schools, churches, work sites, and others

Mobilizing community partnerships to identify and solve health problems encompasses:

- Convening and facilitating partnerships among groups and associations (including those not typically considered to be health related)
- Undertaking defined health improvement planning process and health projects, including preventive, screening, rehabilitation, and support programs
- Building a coalition to draw on the full range of potential human and material resources to improve community health

Developing policies and plans that support individual and community health efforts encompasses:

- Leadership development at all levels of public health
- Systematic community-level and state-level planning for health improvement in all jurisdictions

- Development and tracking of measurable health objectives from the community health plan as a part of a continuous quality improvement strategy
- Joint evaluation with the medical healthcare system to define consistent policy regarding prevention and treatment services
- Development of policy and legislation to guide the practice of public health

OUTSIDE-THE-BOOK THINKING 5-2

How are the essential public health services related to public health's three core functions? How are these operationalized in public health practice?

Assurance of the Public's Health

Whereas assessment and policy development set interventions into motion, the assurance function keeps them on track through five important processes: (1) enforcing laws and regulations that protect health and ensure safety; (2) linking people to needed personal health services and ensuring the provision of health care when otherwise unavailable; (3) ensuring a competent public health and personal healthcare workforce; (4) evaluating effectiveness, accessibility, and quality of personal and population-based health services; and (5) researching for new insights and innovative solutions to health problems.

Enforcing laws and regulations that protect health and ensure safety encompasses:

- Enforcement of sanitary codes, especially in the food industry
- Protection of drinking water supplies
- Enforcement of clean air standards
- Animal control activities
- Follow-up of hazards, preventable injuries, and exposure-related diseases identified in occupational and community settings
- Monitoring quality of medical services (e.g., laboratories, nursing homes, and home healthcare providers)
- Review of new drug, biologic, and medical device applications

Linking people to needed personal health services and ensuring the provision of health care when otherwise unavailable (sometimes referred to as outreach or enabling services) encompass:

- Assurance of effective entry for socially disadvantaged people into a coordinated system of clinical care
- Culturally and linguistically appropriate materials and staff to ensure linkage to services for special population groups
- Ongoing care management
- Transportation services
- Targeted health education/promotion/disease prevention to high-risk population groups

Ensuring a competent public and personal healthcare workforce encompasses:

- Education, training, and assessment of personnel (including volunteers and other lay community health workers) to meet community needs for public and personal health services
- Efficient processes for licensure of professionals
- Adoption of continuous quality improvement and lifelong learning programs
- Active partnerships with professional training programs to ensure community-relevant learning experiences for all students
- Continuing education in management and leadership development programs for those charged with administrative/executive roles

Evaluating effectiveness, accessibility, and quality of personal and population-based health services encompasses:

- Assessing program effectiveness
- Providing information necessary for allocating resources and reshaping programs

Researching for new insights and innovative solutions to health problems encompasses:

- Full continuum of innovation, ranging from practical, field-based efforts to fostering change in public health practice to more academic efforts to encourage new directions in scientific research
- Continuous linkage with institutions of higher learning and research
- Internal capacity to mount timely epidemiologic and economic analyses and conduct health services research

The important processes embodied in the essential public health services framework underscore the complexities of public health practice. The essential public health services framework is relevant to both programs and organizations and is evident in virtually any public health intervention (although to different degrees), constituting what might be considered generic public health practice. The core functions and essential services framework demonstrate that public health practice is more than a collection of programs and services; it embodies the AGPALL concept and the tools to carry out that role.

COMMUNITY HEALTH ASSESSMENT AND IMPROVEMENT TOOLS

The delineation of core functions and essential public health services fortified the foundation for public health practice.[11] Over the 2 decades after the appearance of the IOM report, several important new tools for public health practice came onto the scene to build on this foundation.

Mobilizing for Action through Planning and Partnerships

Among the early post-IOM report initiatives, the Assessment Protocol for Excellence in Public Health (APEXPH), developed by the National Association of County and City Health Officials (NACCHO), in collaboration with other national public health organizations, had an extensive and positive influence on public health practice.[12] Even greater reach and impact are expected from the second generation of this tool, *Mobilizing for Action through Planning and Partnerships* (MAPP).[13]

OUTSIDE-THE-BOOK THINKING 5-3

Determine whether your LHD has completed a community health assessment and/or improvement process. If it has, what approaches and tools were used? What were the products and results? If it has not, why?

The original APEXPH was a tool for organizational self-assessment and improvement for LHDs, as well as a simple and effective community needs assessment process. APEXPH provided a means for LHDs to enhance their organizational capacity and strengthen their leadership role in their communities. APEXPH guided health department officials in two principal areas of activity: (1) assessing and improving the organizational capacity of the agency, and (2) working with the local community to improve the health status of its citizens. There were three principal parts to this process:[12]

1. An organizational capacity assessment—self-assessed key aspects of operations, including authority to operate, community relations, community health assessment, public policy development, assurance of public health services, financial management, personnel management, and program management, resulting in an organizational action plan that set priorities for correcting perceived weaknesses.
2. A community health assessment process—guided formation of a community advisory committee that identified health problems requiring priority attention and then set health status goals and programmatic objectives. The aim was to mobilize community resources in pursuit of locally relevant public health objectives consistent with the Healthy People objectives.
3. Completing the cycle—ensured that the activities from the organizational and community processes were effectively carried out and that they accomplished the desired results through policy development, assurance, monitoring, and evaluation activities.

After its appearance in 1991, APEXPH steadily gained acceptance with the majority of all LHDs using all or part of APEXPH during the 1990s. Although the decade's experience with APEXPH was highly positive, opportunities for strengthening the tool became apparent. Heightened interest in community health improvement efforts, widespread acceptance of the essential public health services as the framework for public health practice, the need to strategically engage a wider range of community interests, and the opportunity to formalize and activate local public health systems converged to suggest that an even more strategic approach to community health improvement was needed.

The development of MAPP addressed these needs in the form of a robust tool of public health practice that could be used by communities with effective LHD leadership to create a local system that ensures the delivery of health services essential to protecting the health of the public.[13] Distinguishing features of MAPP include:

- Incorporation of strategic planning concepts—to assist LHDs in more effectively engaging their communities, securing resources, and managing the process of change. Visioning, contextual environment assessment, strategic issue identification, and strategy formulation principles are among the strategic planning concepts embedded in MAPP.
- Grounding in local public health practice—to ensure that the process is practical, flexible, and user friendly. The instruments rely heavily on the previous experiences and successes of typical communities through vignettes, case studies, and other examples.
- A focus on the local public health system—to broaden community health improvement efforts by recognizing and including all public and private organizations contributing to public health at the local level.

Because public health involves more than what public health agencies do, MAPP provides a framework for actualizing this assertion through:

- A common approach for assessing local public health systems—to promote consistent quality of public health practice from community to community and state to state. The essential public health services framework provides the measures used to assess local public health systems consistent with other national and state efforts to promote a basic set of public health performance standards.
- Expansion of the basic indicators for health status—to reflect better the demographic and socioeconomic determinants of health, community assets, environmental and behavioral risks, and quality of life. MAPP includes a core set of measures for all communities and an extended menu of additional measures for use, where appropriate.
- Recognition that community themes and strengths play an important role in community health improvement efforts—to balance overreliance on data and expert opinion, provide new insights into factors affecting community health, and increase buy-in and active participation as stakeholders feel their concerns and opinions are important to the process.

The model developed for MAPP incorporates interrelated and interactive components. To be practical for use in widely diverse communities and to meld basic strategic planning concepts with public health and community health improvement concepts, MAPP is both simple and complex, as illustrated in Figure 5-1. There is no fixed or even preferred sequencing of its components. The boundaries of the model identify the four assessments that comprise the MAPP process; these are usually completed after visioning has taken place but before strategic issues are identified in the steps indicated in the center of the model. Each element of the model is briefly described here:

- Organizing for success/partnership development—involves establishing values and outcomes for the process and determining the scope, form, and timing for planning process, as well as its participants.

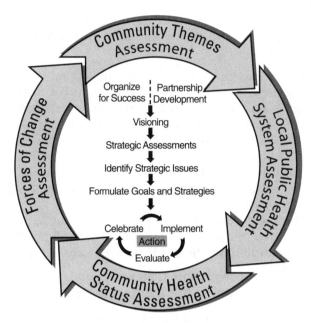

Figure 5-1   MAPP model.
Reproduced from National Association of County and City Health Officials; 2000.

- Visioning—involves developing a shared vision of the ideal future for the community, which serves to provide the process with focus, purpose, direction, and buy-in.
- Four MAPP assessments—these inform the planning process and drive the identification of strategic issues. All are critical to the success of the process, although there is no prescribed order in which they need to be undertaken. The four strategic assessments are described below:
  1. Community themes and strengths assessment—involves the collection of inputs and insights from throughout the community in order to understand issues that residents feel are important.
  2. Local public health assessment—involves an analysis of mission, vision, and goals through the use of performance measures for the essential public health services. Both strengths and areas for improvement are identified.
  3. Community health status assessment—involves an extensive assessment of indicators in 11 domains, including asset mapping and quality of life; environmental health; socioeconomic, demographic, and behavioral risk factors; infectious diseases; sentinel events; social and mental health; maternal and child health; health resource availability; and health status indicators.
  4. Forces of change assessment—identifies broader forces affecting the community, such as technology and legislation.

- Identify strategic issues—involves fundamental policy questions for achieving the shared vision, arising from the information developed in the previous phases. Some are more important than others and require action.
- Formulate goals and strategies—involves developing and examining options for addressing strategic issues, including questions of feasibility and barriers to implementation. Preferred strategies are selected.
- The action cycle—involves implementation, evaluation, and celebration of achievements after LHD leaders have selected and agreed-upon strategies.

As depicted in Figure 5-2, MAPP offers a virtual road map for community public health systems. Widespread use of MAPP began in 2001, and after only a few years, its impact was apparent in an evaluation of early adopters.[14] LHDs, other local government agencies, hospitals, and social service providers were the most frequent community participants in the MAPP process, as shown in Figure 5-3. Educational institutions, nonprofit organizations, community residents, local businesses and employers, and civic interest groups were the most frequently identified new partners. Managed care organizations, health professional organizations, environmental agencies, and neighborhood organizations were substantially less likely to be engaged in the MAPP process. LHDs reported that the most frequent results from MAPP were the strengthened existing partnerships, an increased understanding of community health problems, and greater community engagement.

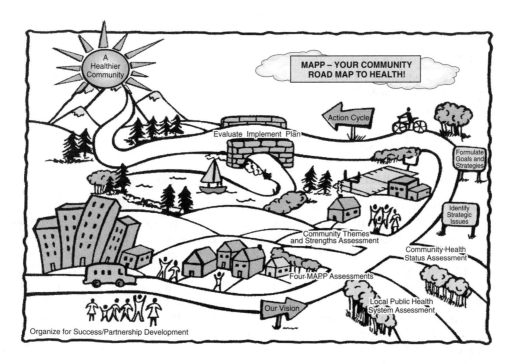

Figure 5-2 MAPP as a road map for community public health systems.
Reproduced from National Association of County and City Health Officials, 2000

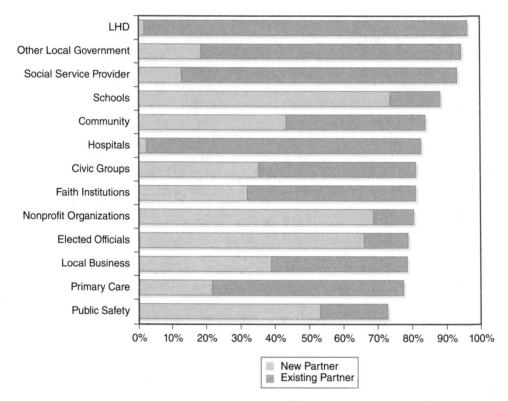

Figure 5-3   Top participant categories for communities using MAPP.

Data from Lenihan DP, Landrum LB, Turnock BJ. *An Evaluation of MAPP and NPHPS in Local Health Jurisdictions.* Chicago, IL: Illinois Public Health Institute; 2006.

Other Community Health Assessment and Improvement Tools

In addition to the essential public health services framework and the APEXPH/MAPP processes, the IOM report stimulated several other important initiatives to promote core function-related performance, especially for the assessment and policy development functions. One of the first community health planning tools to be widely used was the Planned Approach to Community Health (PATCH), a process for community organization and community needs assessment that emphasizes community mobilization and constituency building. PATCH focuses on orienting and training community leaders and other community participants in all aspects of the community needs assessment process and includes excellent documentation and resource materials. Although originally developed by the Centers for Disease Control and Prevention (CDC) to focus on chronic health conditions and stimulate health promotion and disease prevention interventions, PATCH is flexible enough to be used in a wide variety of community health needs assessment applications.

Yet another important tool for addressing public health core functions and their associated processes is the Model Standards framework.[8] The steps outlined for community implementation of the Model Standards process link many of the various core function-related tools; these steps represent, in effect, a pathway for organizations to participate in community health improvement activities. The steps include:

1. Assessment of organizational role. Communities are organized and structured differently. As a result, the specific roles of local public health organizations will vary from community to community. This essential first step is to reexamine organizational purpose and mission and develop a long-range vision through strategic planning involving its internal and external constituencies. The resulting mission statement and long-range vision serve to guide the organization (leadership and board, as well as employees) and to define it for its community partners. This critical step should be completed before the remaining steps can be successfully addressed. Part 1 of APEXPH and the expanded strategic planning elements of MAPP are useful in accomplishing this task.

2. Assessment of organizational capacity. After a mission and role have been defined, it is necessary to examine an organization's capacity to carry out its role in the community. This calls for an assessment of the major operational elements of the organization, including its structure and performance for specific tasks. This type of organizational and local public health system self-assessment is best carried out through broad participation from all levels. Both APEXPH and MAPP include hundreds of indicators that can be used in this capacity assessment. These indicators can be modified or eliminated if they are deemed inappropriate, and additional indicators can also be used. This step serves to identify strengths and weaknesses relative to the mission and role.

3. Development of a capacity-building plan. The development of a capacity-building plan incorporates the organization's strengths and prioritizes its weaknesses so that the most important are addressed first. As in any plan, specific objectives for addressing these weaknesses are developed, responsibilities are assigned, and a process for tracking progress over time is established. Again, APEXPH and MAPP are valuable tools for accomplishing this task.

4. Assessment of community organizational structure. Having looked internally at its capacity and ability to exercise its leadership role for identifying and addressing priority health needs in the community, the public health organization must assess the key stakeholders and necessary participants for a community-wide needs assessment and intervention initiative. This is often a long-term and continuous process in which the relationship of all important community stakeholders and partners (e.g., the health agency, community providers of health-related services, community organizations, community leaders, interest groups, the media, and the general public) is assessed. This step determines how and under whose auspices community health planning will take place within the community. Both APEXPH/MAPP and PATCH processes support the successful completion of this step.

5. Organization of community. This step calls for organizing the community so that it represents a strong constituency for public health and will participate collaboratively in partnership with the health agency. Specific strategies and activities will vary from community to community but will generally include

hearings, dialogues, discussion forums, meetings, and collaborative planning sessions. The specific roles and authority of community participants should be clarified so that the process is not perceived as one driven largely by the health agency and so-called experts. Both APEXPH/MAPP and PATCH are useful for completing this step.

6. Assessment of community health needs. The actual process of identifying health problems of importance to the community is one that must carefully balance information derived from data sets with information derived from the community's perceptions of which problems are most important. Often, community readiness to mitigate specific problems greatly increases the chances for success, as well as support for the overall process within the community. In addition to generating information on possible health problems, this step gathers information on resources available within the community. This step serves to provide the information necessary for the community's most important health problems to be identified. The community needs assessment tools provided in both APEXPH/MAPP and PATCH are useful in accomplishing this step.

7. Determination of local priorities and community health resources. After important health problems are identified, decisions must be made as to which are most important for community action. This step requires broad participation from community participants in the process so that priorities will be viewed as community rather than agency-specific priorities. Debate and negotiation are essential for this step, and there are many approaches to coming to consensus around specific priorities. Both APEXPH/MAPP and PATCH support this step.

8. Selection of outcome objectives. After priorities are determined, the process must establish a target level to be achieved for each priority problem. For this step, the Model Standards process is especially useful in linking community priorities to national health objectives and establishing targets that are appropriate for the current status and improvement possible from a community intervention. This step also calls for negotiation within the community because deployment and reallocation of resources may be needed to achieve the agreed-upon target outcomes. In addition to Model Standards, both APEXPH/MAPP and PATCH can be useful in accomplishing this step.

9. Development of intervention strategies. This step is one of determining strategies and methods of achieving the outcome objectives established for each priority health problem. This can be quite difficult and, at times, contentious. For some problems, there may be few or even no effective interventions. For others, there may be widely divergent strategies available, some of which may be deemed unacceptable or not feasible. After agreement is reached as to strategies and methods, responsibilities for implementing and evaluating interventions will be assigned. With community-wide interventions, overall coordination of efforts may also need to be addressed as part of the intervention strategy.

10. Implementation of intervention strategies. After the establishment of goals, objectives, strategies, and methods, specific plans of action for the intervention are developed, and specific tasks and work plans are developed. Clear delineation of responsibilities and time lines is essential for this step.

11. Continuous monitoring and evaluation of effort. The evaluation strategy for the intervention will track performance related to outcome objectives, as well

as process objectives and activity measures over time. If activity measures and process objectives are being accomplished, there should be progress toward achieving the desired outcome objectives. If this does not occur, the selected intervention strategy needs to be reconsidered and revised.

OUTSIDE-THE-BOOK THINKING 5-4

What features are similar among MAPP, PATCH, CHIP, and Model Standards? What features differ? What role do these tools play in carrying out public health's core functions at the local level?

In 1996, and again in 2002, the IOM revisited issues addressed in its 1988 report, concluding that different organizations, leadership, and political and economic realities were transforming how public health carried out its core functions and essential services.[15,16] On one hand, market-driven health care was forcing public health to clarify and strengthen its public role in a predominantly private health system. On the other, public health was increasingly identifying and working with a variety of entities within the community that shape community health and well-being. Another important IOM report in 1997 advanced an expanded community health improvement planning (CHIP) model that extended the tools developed earlier in the decade and the steps described previously here.[17] Its main features are its expanded perspective on the wide variety of factors that influence health, its support for broad participation by community stakeholders, and its emphasis on the use of performance measures to ensure accountability of partners and track progress over time.

Community health assessments leading toward community health improvement plans increased in quantity as well as quality during the 25 years between 1988 and 2013. A survey conducted by NACCHO in 2013 found that more than two-thirds of local health jurisdictions (LHJs) nationwide had conducted a community health assessment in the past 5 years (58% within the past 3 years) and only 11% either had not completed one or were not planning one in the near future. Similar results were reported for community health improvement plans and organizational strategic plans, although at somewhat lower levels.[18] Those LHDs not planning to conduct assessments, CHIPs, and strategic plans were primarily the smallest local health jurisdictions with few full-time employees. State health agencies have also been active in completing state health assessments, statewide health improvement plans, and agency-wide strategic plans, as demonstrated in Figure 5-4. State agency commitment to these planning activities provides an additional impetus for LHDs.

In most communities, LHDs serve as the primary instigators of community health assessments or serve as the lead agency or full partner in a community-wide coalition that assumes responsibility for the assessment. A provision of the Affordable Care Act health reform legislation requires nonprofit hospitals to engage in community health assessments at least every 3 years and encourages hospitals to collaborate with public health agencies where possible. Figure 5-5 documents that two-thirds of LHDs either had already been collaborating with their local hospitals

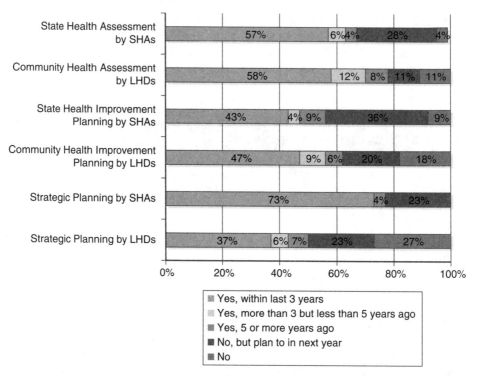

Figure 5-4 State health agency (SHA) and local health department (LHD) participation in health assessment, health improvement planning, and strategic planning activities, United States, 2012 and 2013.

Adapted from National Association of County and City Health Officials. 2013 *National Profile of Local Health Departments*. Washington, DC: NACCHO; 2014 and Association of State and Territorial Health Officials. *Profile of State Health, Volume Three, 2012*. Washington, DC: ASTHO; 2014.

by 2013 or were in discussions to incorporate hospitals into their existing community health assessment efforts.

Community Engagement

Communities remain the battlefields on which public health threats are met and public health challenges are addressed in the 21st century. There was steady growth in the armamentarium of community public health practice during the late 20th century in the form of community health assessment and improvement tools based on the core functions and essential public health services framework. Community health improvement is grounded in the realization that more doctors, more clinics, and more sophisticated diagnostic and treatment advances will not alleviate the major health problems facing Americans. Instead, the greatest gains will come from what people do or do not do for themselves, individually and collectively. Acting collectively can take place at many levels; at the community level, it often works best.

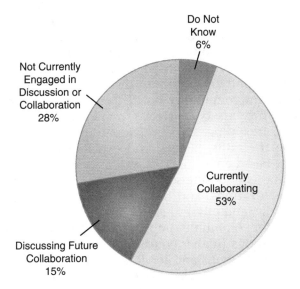

Figure 5-5 Collaboration between LHDs and nonprofit hospitals on community health assessments, United States, 2013.

Data from National Association of County and City Health Officials. *2013 National Profile of Local Health Departments*. Washington, DC: NACCHO; 2014.

The notion of community is an elusive concept. Generally, communities are aggregates of individuals who share common characteristics or other bonds. One person can be part of many different communities. One definition views community as the associative, self-generated gathering of common people who have sufficient resources in their lives to cope with life's demands and not suffer ill health. This definition of community focuses on the capacity of communities to achieve their health goals through the effective use of their own assets. It differs considerably from the view of communities as locations in which health problems reside and health services are delivered. Rather than focusing on the level of individual actions and behaviors, it recognizes the importance of social determinants of health and of the environmental and policy levels for public health responses. Community public health practice revolves around engaging communities to work collectively on their own behalf. Community engagement is the process of working collaboratively with groups of people who are affiliated by geographic proximity, special interests, or similar situations, with respect to issues affecting their well-being. Although community engagement is a relatively recent phenomenon for many governmental public health organizations, health education specialists have been using these principles for decades, based on the simple guiding principle of starting where the people are.[19]

This positive approach emphasizes that all communities have assets. All too often, communities have been viewed solely in terms of their needs and problems. The implication of these different perspectives is important. If communities are viewed from their needs, the policies and interventions will be based on needs. If they are to be viewed from their assets, the policies and interventions will be based on the community's capacities, skills, and assets. Community health improvement seldom occurs from the actions of outside interests; the most successful community development efforts are driven by the commitment of those investing themselves and their resources in the effort. Identifying community assets is possible through approaches that catalog and actually map the basic building blocks that will be used to address important community health problems.[20] Primary building blocks include those community assets that are most readily available for community health improvement, including both individual and organizational assets. Individual assets include the skills, talents, and experiences of residents, individual businesses, and home-based enterprises, as well as personal income. Organizational assets include associations of businesses, citizen associations, cultural organizations, communications organizations, and religious organizations. Secondary building blocks are private, public, and physical assets, which can be brought under community control and used for community improvement purposes. These include private and nonprofit organizations (higher educational institutions, hospitals, social service agencies), public institutions and services (public schools, police, libraries, fire departments, parks), and physical resources (vacant land, commercial and industrial structures, housing, energy, and waste resources).

In addition to community engagement and asset-mapping strategies, performance measurement offers another tool for community health improvement activities. Performance measures are also not new to public health practice. The use of performance measures to track progress toward community or national health objectives and to monitor programs has long been standard practice. The CHIP proposed by the IOM in its report on performance monitoring, however, takes performance measurement to a new level. In these processes, performance measures serve to hold communities (acting through stakeholders and partnerships) accountable for actions for which they have accepted responsibility.[17] This supports the development of a shared vision and a collaborative and integrative approach to community problem solving for the purpose of improving health status. It offers a pathway for stakeholders and partners to assume responsibility collectively and to marshal their resources and assets in pursuit of agreed-upon objectives.

The CHIP model incorporates a problem identification and prioritization cycle, followed by an analysis and implementation cycle. This second cycle develops, implements, and evaluates health intervention strategies that address priority community health problems. The distinguishing feature of this approach is the emphasis on measurement to link performance and accountability on a community-wide basis, rather than solely on the LHD or another public entity. Several recommendations were developed to operationalize the community health improvement concept, including:

- Communities should base a health improvement process on a broad definition of health and a comprehensive conceptual model of how health is produced within the community.
- A CHIP should develop its own set of specific, quantitative performance measures, linking accountable entities to the performance of specific activities expected to lead to the production of desired health outcomes in the community.

- A CHIP should seek a balance between strategic opportunities for long-term health improvement and goals that are achievable in the short term.
- Community conditions guiding CHIPs should strive for strategic inclusiveness, incorporating individuals, groups, and organizations that have an interest in health outcomes; can take actions necessary to improve community health; or can contribute data and analytic capabilities needed for performance monitoring.
- A CHIP should be centered in a community health coalition or similar entity.[17]

Numerous useful tools and guides are available via the Internet to support the expanded community health improvement efforts in models such as CHIP, MAPP, and similar initiatives. Prominent among these tools are CDC's Principles of Community Engagement, the Community Tool Box (developed by the University of Kansas), and the *Healthy People 2020* Tool Kit (produced by the Public Health Foundation).[21-23]

The maturation of community-driven models of public health practice was fostered in part by the National Turning Point Initiative.[24] Funded jointly by the Kellogg Foundation and Robert Wood Johnson Foundation, Turning Point sought to transform and strengthen the public health infrastructure at the state and local levels, in effect, reforming public health practice. More than 20 states participated in Turning Point through statewide and local partnerships that brought together a broad spectrum of health interests to develop a shared vision and strategic plans to improve statewide public health systems. The collaborations in the various Turning Point sites varied significantly, nurturing and developing many different models for systems change.

The Healthy Communities framework represents another successful model for community health improvement, using health as a metaphor for a broader approach to building community.[25] Because health cuts across lines of race, ethnicity, class, culture, and sector, the focus on a healthy community enables the entire community to collaborate in community renewal. Healthy Communities is based on the belief that change in public policies and actions will occur only when people act together to participate directly in the public work of our society and problems occur. A key to success involves community institutions using their organizational skills, relationships, in-kind resources, and credibility to engage the rest of the community in mobilizing the creativity and resources of the community to improve health and well-being. Focusing on systems change, Healthy Communities seeks to build broad citizen participation that encourages new players and honors diversity. It looks to build true collaborations between business, government, nonprofit organizations, and citizens stimulating the community and political will to act together.

Community-based health policy development is also receiving greater attention in these collaborations and partnerships. Public policy serves as a guide to influence governmental decisions and action at any jurisdictional level, thereby affecting what would otherwise occur.[26] For the health and well-being of communities, policies indicate broad directions toward important goals, cutting across many different stakeholders and affecting large populations. Policies focus on both goals and the means to achieve those goals, often affecting the decisions and actions of individual organizations. At the community level, health policy has many options, such as more and better health services to address unmet needs in the community or advocacy for broader support to improve the conditions influencing health in the community. Increasingly, community-driven public health initiatives are tackling the broader social and community factors, even as they seek to ensure that gaps in services are somehow met.

Little research is available to elucidate the value of community-driven health policy development initiatives. There is some evidence that widespread initiation of CHIPs increases the frequency with which key policy development components take place. Policy development may be the public health core function most heavily impacted by CHIPs. The increase in performance of specific practices related to the core functions has been greatest for those related to policy development, and generally, the baseline level of measures of policy development lags behind that of assessment and assurance where CHIPs have not been implemented.

Together, these strategies, initiatives, and tools can make substantial contributions to improving public health practice in the United States. In addition, there is reason to believe that improvement is needed in view of assessments of performance that were completed over recent decades.

OUTSIDE-THE-BOOK THINKING 5-5

You are the administrator of a typical county-based LHD in a largely rural state. Your newly elected county board chairman has ordered you to come up with new health-related initiatives that will improve the health of the county's residents. How would you approach this charge?

STRATEGIC PLANNING, STANDARDS, AND ACCREDITATION

Community health assessments, and community health improvement plans offer public health organizations an opportunity to reexamine their mission, vision, and goals and to better align their strategic direction with community needs and priorities. Strategic planning has become a third pillar of modern public health practice that is now institutionalized in a process that accredits state and local public health agencies through the Public Health Accreditation Board.

Strategic planning has long been recognized as an effective management practice and tool among private sector organizations. More recently, the practice has become widely established among nonprofit and public sector organizations. Strategic planning encompasses a series of key steps from laying the groundwork through implementing, evaluating, and revising the plan. Preplanning calls for identifying key stakeholders, assessing the availability of necessary information, and developing a plan, process, and timeline for the strategic planning project. These preparatory activities provide a foundation for the critically important step of developing clear statements of mission, vision, and values.

Many strategic planning processes begin with the identification of core values for the organization with the input of key stakeholders and after careful consideration

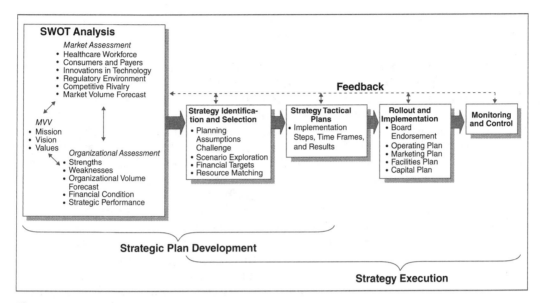

Figure 5-6   Strategic planning process.

Reproduced from Buchbinder SP and Shanks NH. *Introduction to Health Care Management, Second Edition*, 2012.

of both formal and informal mandates for the organization. An initial mission statement is then developed as well as a vision statement that articulates where the organization wants to be in the future. The vision statement is critical here, as it characterizes the difference between where an organization is and where it wants to be. This sets the stage for the identification of strategic issues that must be addressed for the vision to be achieved. Figure 5-6 illustrates the key components of an organizational strategic planning process.

Examination of strategic issues depends in part on the availability of relevant information. Existing reports and data may or may not be useful. Additional data and information are often needed, as are appropriate methods of summarizing data and information for the analysis step that follows.

Many methods are used to analyze data for strategic planning purposes, although one commonly used approach is the SWOT/SWOC Analysis. In this method, strengths, weaknesses, opportunities, and threats (or challenges) are identified as quadrants of an analysis matrix. Making these dimensions explicit facilitates the identification of emerging trends, cross-cutting themes, and ultimately, key strategic issues and priorities.

It is these key strategic issues and priorities that drive the strategic plan in the form of its strategies, goals and objectives, timelines, accountabilities, and evaluation framework. These are captured in a strategic planning document that is widely communicated to staff and stakeholders.

As the plan is implemented, activities and objectives are monitored closely using quality improvement practices that emphasize outcomes, yet foster flexibility to shift strategies when results dictate the need to do so. Revisions and updates for the original strategic plan should be viewed as the rule, rather than the exception. It is equally important that results be shared widely among staff and stakeholders.

Strategic plans for public health organizations benefit greatly from preexisting community health assessments and community health improvement plans. Together, these three tools define the minimal requirements for an effective public health organization. It should not be surprising that these three elements comprise the basic prerequisites for PHAB accreditation. Public health organizations without a community health assessment, community health improvement plan, and strategic plan simply aren't living up to the standards and expectations of 21st century community public health practice.

Accreditation of state and local public health organizations has been a controversial idea for decades. For many years, the public health community did not view the observation, "If you've seen one health department, you've seen one health department" as disparaging. For some, it was a badge of honor in that health departments should differ from each other due to their unique populations, political structures, and community health needs. As discussed earlier in this chapter, public health was long viewed as the programs and services provided, which understandably differed from one community or state to another. After the IOM report in 1988, however, a view that core functions rather than programs and community services defined a public health organization promoted a view that health departments should in fact be more alike than different. These commonalities offered a template for common standards to be developed and applied through national or state strategies to promote their widespread adoption.

Standards are basically explicit performance expectations. Progress toward the development of public health practice standards came quickly after 1990. At the national level, CDC collaborating with the major national public health practice organizations developed the National Public Health Performance Standards Program.[27] These standards were based on the 10 essential public health services framework and designed so that they could be used in several applications that would synergize their adoption. These national standards could be used by health departments for self-assessment and improvement. The standards or a subset of the standards could also be used for national surveillance purposes to determine how many health departments or what proportion of the population were being served by a health department meeting some level of these standards. The standards framework could also be adopted or adapted by states, which would then require or incentivize their LHDs to meet the standards. Finally, some external entity could apply the standards through a national voluntary accreditation program.

NACCHO extended and focused the content of the national public health performance standards in the development of a panel of standards, again based largely on the essential public health services framework, that constituted an operational definition of a functional local health department.[28] Relatively soon thereafter with substantial financial support from the Robert Wood Johnson Foundation, NACCHO and the other national public health practice organizations collaborated to explore the feasibility and ultimately established a national voluntary program for public health agency accreditation.

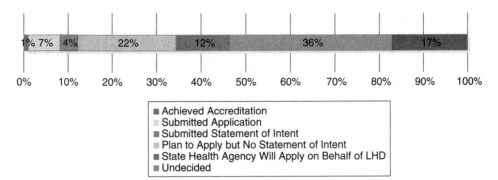

Figure 5-7 Level of local health department engagement with PHAB accreditation, 2014 (n = 609).

Reproduced from National Association of County and City Health Officials. *Local Health Department Accreditation: Findings from the 2014 Forces of Change Study*. Washington, DC: NACCHO; 2014.

The standards and process for the national program were developed by the Public Health Accreditation Board over several years.[29] The PHAB standards focused on the same catalog of concepts captured in the NPHPS program and the operational definition of a functional local health department. Once again the 10 essential public health services served as organizing domains. The accreditation process calls for an extensive self-assessment activity before an on-site verification and review by a site visit team. Notably, public health agencies must demonstrate completion of a CHA, CHIP, and strategic plan in order to even submit an application for accreditation.

In 2013, PHAB announced the initial cohort of accredited public health agencies. Additional approvals steadily followed as many agencies sought to be early adopters. Surveys of local and state health agencies, document that demand for accreditation is already substantial. As indicated in Figure 5-7, by early 2014, nearly one-half of LHDs had either been accredited or entered the pipeline for accreditation by submitting an application or letter of intent, or by indicating that they planned to submit a letter of intent or apply through their state health agency.[30] Only 17% of LHDs indicated that they did not intend to seek accreditation, virtually guaranteeing that PHAB will be busy reviewing applicants for years to come. Interest among state health agencies was even higher with 80% either already applying or planning to apply as of later 2012.[31]

CONCLUSION

For more than a century, public health has sought to measure its efforts through standards that reflected its mission to promote and protect population health and well-being. The 1988 IOM report emphasized the need for stronger assessment and policy development functions to complement the long-standing view that public health's role is one of assurance. The essential public health services framework operationalizes the core functions and serves as the organizing construct for modern public health practice standards. For public health organizations, those standards are achieved in part through community health assessments, community health improvement plans, and organizational strategic plans. These activities are now recognized by the Public Health Accreditation Board as prerequisites for recognition by that body, further establishing the core functions and essential public health services framework as the bedrock of modern public health practice.

REFERENCES

1. Institute of Medicine, Committee on the Future of Public Health. *The Future of Public Health.* Washington, DC: National Academy Press; 1988.

2. Turnock BJ, Handler AS. From measuring to improving public health practice. *Annu Rev Public Health.* 1997; *18*: 261–282.

3. Vaughan HF. Local health services in the United States: the story of CAP. *Am J Public Health.* 1972; *62*: 95–108.

4. American Public Health Association, Committee on Administrative Practice. Appraisal form for city health work. *Am J Public Health.* 1926; *16*(Suppl): 1–65.

5. Emerson H, Luginbuhl M. *Local Health Units for the Nation.* New York: Commonwealth Fund; 1945.

6. Shonick W. *Government and Health Services: Government's Role in the Development of U.S. Health Services 1930-1980.* New York: Oxford University Press; 1995.

7. Hanlon JJ. Is there a future for local health departments? *Health Serv Rep.* 1973; *88*: 898–901.

8. American Public Health Association. *Healthy Communities 2000: Model Standards.* Washington, DC: American Public Health Association; 1991.

9. Harrell JA, Baker EL. The essential services of public health. *Leadership Public Health.* 1994; *3*: 27–31.

10. Public Health Functions Steering Committee. *Public Health in America.* Washington, DC: U.S. Public Health Service; 1994.

11. Corso LC, Wiesner PJ, Halverson PK, Brown CK. Using the essential services as a foundation for performance measurement and assessment of local public health systems. *J Public Health Manage Pract.* 2000; *6*: 1–18.

12. National Association of County and City Health Officials. *Assessment Protocol for Excellence in Public Health.* Washington, DC: National Association of County and City Health Officials; 1991.

13. National Association of County and City Health Officials. *Mobilizing for Action through Planning and Partnerships.* Washington, DC: National Association of County and City Health Officials; 2000.

14. Lenihan DP, Landrum LB, Turnock BJ. *An Evaluation of MAPP and NPHPS in Local Public Health Jurisdictions.* Chicago, IL: Illinois Public Health Institute; 2006.

15. Institute of Medicine. *Healthy Communities: New Partnerships for the Future of Public Health.* Washington, DC: National Academy Press; 1996.

16. Committee on the Future of the Public's Health in the 21st Century, Institute of Medicine. *The Future of the Public's Health in the 21st Century.* Washington, DC: National Academy Press; 2003.

17. Institute of Medicine. *Improving Health in the Community: A Role for Performance Monitoring.* Washington, DC: National Academy Press; 1997.

18. National Association of County and City Health Officials. *2013 National Profile of Local Health Departments.* Washington, DC: National Association of County and City Health Officials; 2014.

19. Minkler M. Ten commitments for community health education. *Health Educ Res Theory Pract.* 1994; *9*: 527–534.

20. McKnight JL, Kretzmann J. Mapping community capacity. *New Designs.* 1992; Winter: 9–15.

21. Centers for Disease Control/ATSDR Committee on Community Engagement. *Principles of Community Engagement.* Atlanta, GA: Centers for Disease Control; 1997.

22. University of Kansas. Community Tool Box. http://ctb.ku.edu/en. Accessed September 27, 2014.

23. Public Health Foundation. *Healthy People 2010 Tool Kit.* Washington, DC: American Public Health Foundation; 1999.

24. Berkowitz B. Collaboration for health improvement: models for state, community, and academic partnerships. *J Public Health Manage Pract.* 2000; *6*: 67–72.

25. Norris T. Healthy communities. *Natl Civic Rev.* 1997; *86*: 3–10.

26. Milio N. Priorities and strategies for promoting community-based prevention policies. *J Public Health Manage Pract.* 1998; *4*: 14–28.

27. Centers for Disease Control and Prevention, Public Health Practice Program Office. Available at www.cdc.gov/nphpsp/.

28. National Association of County and City Health Officials. *Operational Definition of a Functional Local Health Department.* Washington, DC: NACCHO; 2005.

29. Public Health Accreditation Board. Available at www.phaboard.org. Accessed June 14, 2014.

30. National Association of County and City Health Officials. *Local Health Department Accreditation: Findings from the 2014 Forces of Change Study.* Washington, DC: NACCHO; 2014.

31. Association of State and Territorial Health Officials. *Profile of State Health, Volume Three, 2012.* Washington, DC: ASTHO; 2014.

Chapter 6

Public Health Workforce

LEARNING OBJECTIVES

Given the current status of public health activities in the United States, identify and explain how various occupations, positions, and roles in the public health work-force contribute to carrying out public health's core functions and essential services. Key aspects of this competency expectation include being able to:

- Describe the size, composition, and distribution of the current public health workforce.

- Identify and discuss competency frameworks for routine and emergency public health practice.

- Identify information sources for examining key dimensions of the current and future public health workforce.

- Identify three or more issues that will impact the future public health workforce in terms of its size, composition, and distribution.

Public health is important work, and the people who carry out that work contribute substantially to the health status and quality of life of the individuals, families, and communities they serve. Yet public health is not among the best known or most highly respected careers, in part because when public health efforts are successful, nothing happens. Events that don't occur don't attract attention. For example, the remarkable record of declining mortality rates and ever increasing spans of healthy life, due in large part to public health efforts, draws little public attention. Indeed, the vast majority of those who will ultimately benefit from the efforts of past and present public health workers are yet to be born. With the work of public health not widely recognized and valued for its accomplishments and contributions, it is not surprising that careers in public health are among the least understood and appreciated in the health sector.

Nonetheless, even if the public views public health as poorly defined and abstract, public health workers are real and tangible. These workers make up a public health workforce that can be defined and described in several important dimensions, including its size, distribution, composition, skills, and career pathways. Unfortunately, there is less information on these vital statistics of the public health workforce than for many other professional and occupational categories working in the health sector today.

For too long, too little attention has been directed to the public health workforce and its needs. Despite ample warnings in the 1988 Institute of Medicine (IOM) report, there were few efforts between 1980, when the Health Resources and Services Administration (HRSA) produced crude estimates of the size and composition for the United States Congress and 2000, when Kristine Gebbie and colleagues completed their landmark enumeration report on the public health workforce at the turn of the century.[1-3] Two decades of inattention provide eloquent testimony to the low priority given to the public health system's most important asset—its workforce.

Beginning in the year 2002, funding for public health workforce preparedness and training increased dramatically. This influx of funding also brought increased expectations for positive change and greater accountability for results. As a result, the public health system is now under the microscope, with federal, state, and local governments needing to show that the vital signs of the public health infrastructure, including its workforce, are improving. Unfortunately, decades of inattention left little information to serve as a basis for comparison.

A central challenge for public health workforce development efforts today is to provide more and better information about key dimensions of the public health workforce in terms of its size, distribution, composition, and competency, as well as its impact on public health goals and community health. This chapter, like the *Public Health Workforce Enumeration 2000* report, seeks to advance this important agenda by highlighting what public health workers do and how they contribute to societal well-being in the 21st century. The following questions guide this investigation:

- What is the public health workforce?
- How large is this workforce and how is it distributed?
- What professions and occupations are included?
- How does the public health workforce impact the health of populations?
- Will the public health workforce continue to grow? What trends in the overall economy, the health sector, or the public sector will impact public health jobs and career opportunities in the future?

PUBLIC HEALTH WORK AND PUBLIC HEALTH WORKERS

From a functional perspective, it is the individuals involved in carrying out the core functions and essential services of public health who constitute the public health workforce. Critical to an understanding of this characterization of the public health workforce are the terms *core functions* and *essential public health services*. These terms are examined in depth in other chapters with a useful summary of these concepts provided in the "Public Health in America" statement.[4] In it, the practice of public health is described in terms of both its ends (vision, mission, and six broad responsibilities) and how it accomplishes those ends (essential public health services). These essential public health services constitute an aggregate job description for the entire public health workforce, with the workload divided among the many different professional and occupational categories comprising the total public health workforce.

This functional perspective clearly links public health workers to public health practice. Unfortunately, this does not simplify the practical task of determining who is, and who is not, part of the public health workforce. There has never been any specific academic degree, even the master's of public health (MPH) degree, or unique set of experiences that distinguish public health's workers from those in other fields. Many public health workers have a primary professional discipline in addition to their attachment to public health. Physicians, nurses, dentists, social workers, nutritionists, health educators, anthropologists, psychologists, architects, sanitarians, economists, political scientists, engineers, epidemiologists, biostatisticians, managers, lawyers, and dozens of other professions and disciplines carry out the work of public health. This multidisciplinary workforce, with somewhat divided loyalties to multiple professions, blurs the distinctiveness of public health as a unified profession. At the same time, however, it facilitates interdisciplinary approaches to community problem identification and problem solving, which are hallmarks of modern public health practice.

OUTSIDE-THE-BOOK THINKING 6-1

What distinguishes a public health professional from a clinical professional working for a public health organization?

SIZE AND DISTRIBUTION OF THE PUBLIC HEALTH WORKFORCE

There is little agreement as to the size of the public health workforce in the United States except that it is only a small subset of the more than 15 million persons employed in the health sector of the American economy. Enumerations and estimates of public health workers suffer from one central limitation—the definition of a public health worker is unclear. An influential 2003 IOM report on public health education offered a seemingly straightforward definition of a public health professional as "a person educated in public health or a related discipline who is employed to improve health through a population focus."[5] Yet even this definition lacks precision and impedes enumeration; many public health professionals were not educated in public health or related disciplines; many others are not employed in organizations seeking to improve health through a population focus. Public health workers employed outside governmental public health agencies are especially difficult to identify; and not all employees of public health organizations and agencies have population health responsibilities associated with their jobs. Identifying specific types of public health workers is also difficult, since many have other professional affiliations.

Because of these limitations, a precise picture of the public health workforce is not available. But it is clear that efforts to identify and categorize public health workers must take into account three important aspects of public health practice:[6]

- Work setting: Public health workers work for organizations actively engaged in promoting, protecting, and preserving the health of a defined population group. The organization may be public or private, and its public health objectives may be secondary or subsidiary to its principal objectives. In addition to governmental public health agencies, other public and private organizations employ public health workers. For example, school health nurses working for the local school district and health educators employed by the local Red Cross chapter are part of the public health workforce.
- Work content: Public health workers perform work addressing one or more of the essential public health services. Relatively few job descriptions for public health workers are tailored from the essential public health services, and even when they are, the scope of tasks can be very broad. A focus on populations, as opposed to individuals, is often a distinguishing characteristic of these job descriptions. For example, an individual trained as a health educator who works for a community-based teen pregnancy prevention program is clearly a public health worker. But the same can't be said of a health educator working for a commercial advertising firm promoting cosmetics.
- Worker: The individual must occupy a position that conventionally requires at least 1 year of postsecondary specialized public health training and that is (or can be) assigned a professional, administrative, or technical occupational title (to be defined later in this chapter). This distinction may seem artificial but rests on the notion that public health practice relies on a foundation of knowledge, skills, and attitudes that, in most circumstances, cannot be completely acquired through work experiences alone.[6]

The relationships among these three aspects are illustrated in Figure 6-1, although there is no attempt to draw this modified Venn diagram to scale. Nonetheless, the total area captured with this composite represents all workers who might meet one or more of the definitions established for the individual workers, work content, and work settings using these three dimensions. For example, workers could be defined at some level of educational attainment and/or work experience. Perhaps an undergraduate or graduate level degree in public health and/or 5 years of experience could be elements of this definition.

Similarly, the definition of the work setting could call for working in an organization or entity whose mission focused on achieving public health goals. A more restrictive definition might focus on public or voluntary sector organizations or perhaps only on governmental health agencies. A definition for the content of the work could require consistency with the public health core functions/essential public health services framework. For example, if more than 50% of the work effort encompassed core functions or essential public health services, this could meet the definition.

Once definitions for the worker, work setting, and work content are established, the universe of public health workers would be established and cover different

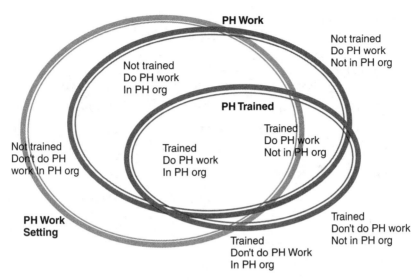

Figure 6-1   Relationships of key aspects of the public health workforce based on worker skills, work setting, and content of work.

sectors within that universe could be identified. Whether everyone meeting any of the three definitions would be considered a public health worker, or whether some combination of categories (e.g., trained, doing public health work, within a governmental health agency) would be used to establish a conceptual definition of the public health workforce requires discussion and eventual consensus. With a rational definition of who is and who is not a public health worker, strategies to enumerate and capture key information on public health workers can be devised and implemented. Without a common frame of reference, widely varying estimates of the current and past public health workforce will proliferate. This has in fact occurred as will be discussed later in this chapter.

Despite these uncertainties as to the size of the public health workforce, there is information documenting general trends over recent decades. For example, the number of workers in the health sector of the U.S. economy has been steadily increasing while the proportion of total national health expenditures attributed to public health activity has remained fairly constant.[1] This evidence suggests the number of public health workers has grown at a rate generally consistent with that of all health workers and that the public health workforce likely includes 500,000–750,000 workers (and perhaps even more if public health workers in industries outside the governmental and health industry sectors are included).

This range is consistent with the crude enumeration of the public health workforce conducted for the year 2000, which identified 450,000 public health workers.[3] The year 2000 enumeration did not include most public health workers employed by nongovernmental agencies as well as many public health workers employed by government agencies other than official public health agencies. As a result the actual total exceeded the 450,000 number reported in the enumeration.

Table 6-1 Full-Time Equivalent (FTE) Workers of Federal, State, and Local Governmental Health* Agencies, Selected Years, 1995–2012, United States

Year	Federal Health Full Time	State Health FTE	Local Health FTE	State + Local FTE	Total (F+S+L) FTE
1995	125,048	160,061	208,558	368,619	493,667
2000	120,362	172,678	236,496	409,174	529,536
2005	125,163	178,465	246,300	424,765	549,918
2008	140,026	185,667	260,416	446,083	586,109
2009	141,713	184,539	254,005	438,544	580,257
2010	147,165	193,456	254,463	447,919	595,084
2011	152,347	196,424	249,242	445,666	598,013
2012	153,578	199,508	243,319	442,827	596,405

*Health: public health services, emergency medical services, mental health, alcohol and drug abuse, outpatient clinics, visiting nurses, food and sanitary inspections, animal control, other environmental health activities (e.g., pollution control), etc.

Data from U.S. Bureau of the Census, Federal, State, and Local Governments, Public Employment and Payroll Data. Available at www.census.gov/govs/apes/. Accessed June 10, 2014.

Another indication that the public health workforce has been increasing over recent decades comes from data collected in the ongoing employment and payroll census of federal, state, and local governments by the U.S. Bureau of the Census.[7] Data from this source indicated that there were 103,000 more full-time equivalent (FTE) workers of federal, state, and local health agencies in 2012 than in 1995 (see Table 6-1).

Between 1995 and 2008 the number of workers employed in federal, state, and local government health agencies increased steadily, with the greatest gains at the local government level. The economic recession of 2008/2009 temporarily slowed the increase for workers in federal and state health agencies, but the pattern of steady increases reappeared when the recession ended. The number of workers in health agencies of local government fell both during and after the recession through 2012. It is likely that the influx of financial support for state and local governments associated with the American Recovery and Reinvestment Act of 2009 minimized the loss of local government employees through 2010, when this funding was discontinued. Fiscal and political pressures on local governments persisted after 2010 accounting for continuing losses of local government workers. This downward trend persisted through 2012, after which stabilization and small increases reappeared. Figure 6-2 traces the ratio of state and local government health agency workers to population between 1995 and 2012 further illustrating these trends. By 2012 the ratio of state and local government health agency workers to population had reverted to levels not seen since the late 1990s.

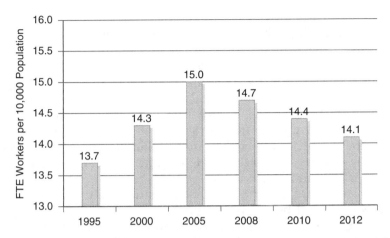

Figure 6-2 Full-time equivalent (FTE) workers for state and local health* agencies per 10,000 population, selected years 1995–2012, United States

*Health: public health services, emergency medical services, mental health, alcohol and drug abuse, outpatient clinics, visiting nurses, food and sanitary inspections, animal control, other environmental health activities (e.g., pollution control), etc.

Data from U.S. Bureau of the Census. Federal, state, and local governments, and public employment and payroll data. www.census.gov/govs/www/apes. Accessed June 15, 2014.

OUTSIDE-THE-BOOK THINKING 6-2

Choose a recent (within the last 3 years) outbreak or other public health emergency situation that has drawn significant media attention. Describe how specific occupational categories in the public health infrastructure contributed to either the emergency situation or its solution. The *Morbidity and Mortality Weekly Report* contents for recent weeks would be a good place to look for recent outbreaks; various print and electronic media may also be useful sources of information.

Similar to other health sector workers, public health workers are more likely to be found in urban and suburban settings rather than rural communities. The public health worker to population ratio, however, is often higher in rural areas than in urban areas. States show significant variation as well, with higher ratios in many of the smaller and less urban states in the East and West and lower ratios in the Central states.

The national public health workforce enumeration study completed in 2000 found that one-third of the public health workforce were employed by state agencies and another one-third by local governmental agencies.[3] This enumeration also reported that 20% worked for federal agencies and 14% worked for nongovernmental organizations in the voluntary and private sectors. Government employment census data, which excludes nongovernmental workers, also classify one-third as state workers but 44% as employees of local government and 24% as working for federal agencies. Some of these differences can be attributed to state public health systems in which state employees work at the local level but are counted as state employees in the employment census data and as local health department (LHD) employees in the public health enumeration study. These differences may also be partly attributed to the inclusion of workers in state and local governmental agencies other than the local public health agency in the government employment census data; these were not captured in the year 2000 public health enumeration study. For example, substance abuse and mental health prevention services, school health services, or restaurant inspections may operate from local mental health agencies, school districts, or consumer affairs agencies rather than from the LHD. The National Association of County and City Health Officials (NACCHO) estimated that LHDs employed 162,000 workers (146,000 FTEs) in 2013.[8]

Although recent decades have witnessed an increase in the number of public health workers employed by nongovernmental agencies because of expanded partnerships for public health priorities, governmental public health workers are often considered the primary public health workforce. Their number, composition, distribution, and competence are issues of public concern.

Government employment census data provide useful insights into overall trends at the national level and among the various levels of government. The year 2000 public health enumeration study, together with periodic surveys of state and local public health agencies, provide richer information on the composition of the public health workforce, such as the proportion and types of professional occupational categories within that workforce. Together these sources enrich our understanding of the size and composition of the public health workforce today.

COMPOSITION OF THE PUBLIC HEALTH WORKFORCE

Public health is multidisciplinary, with many different professions and occupations involved in its work. The Bureau of Labor Statistics (BLS) tracks workers in hundreds of standard occupational classifications (SOCs) regardless of the industry (such as government, health care, etc.) in which they are employed. In recent years, there has been an effort to link standard occupational classifications for public health worker titles and positions, although this effort has been challenging. Because the overall universe of public health workers is poorly defined, the precise proportion of the various occupational categories within it cannot be determined. It is clear that nurses and environmental health practitioners constitute the largest subgroups of public health workers. Managers, epidemiologists, health educators, nutritionists, and laboratory workers are also significant subgroups. Figure 6-3 provides general information on occupational categories and titles from the public health workforce enumeration completed in 2000. Specific categories and titles were not reported for one-fourth of the workers in this study.

Despite the lack of precise information, it appears that professional occupational categories comprise more than one-half of the estimated 500,000–800,000 workers in the public health workforce. For comparison purposes, there were 2.7 million nurses, 900,000 physicians, 200,000 pharmacists, 170,000 dentists, and 90,000 dietitians/nutritionists employed in the United States in 2012.[9]

Ongoing surveys of local health departments (LHDs) document that three positions are found in more than 80% of all LHDs—public health nurse, administrator,

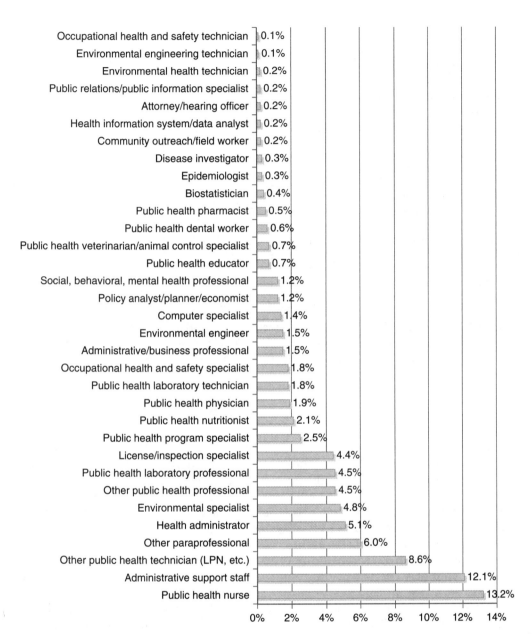

Figure 6-3 Percentage of public health workers in selected occupational categories and titles, United States, 2000.

Data from Health Resources and Services Administration, Bureau of Health Professions, National Center for Health Workforce Information and Analysis and Center for Health Policy, Columbia School of Nursing. *The Public Health Workforce Enumeration 2000.* Washington, DC: HRSA; 2000.

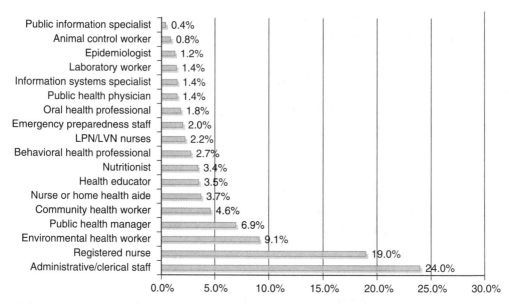

Figure 6-4 Percentage of local health department (LHD) workforce for selected occupations, United States, 2013. Estimated total employees = 162,000. Estimated total FTEs = 146,000.

Data from National Association of County and City Health Officials. *2013 National Profile of Local Health Departments.* Washington, DC: NACCHO; 2014.

and sanitarian/environmental health specialist.[8,10] These positions are present in large and small agencies alike. The next most frequent positions (emergency preparedness coordinator, health educator, dietitian/nutritionist, and physician) are found in only 40–60% of LHDs. There is considerable variation in the median FTEs in these positions, largely associated with agency size. Figure 6-4 presents a breakdown of occupational categories in the LHD workforce.

Two general patterns of LHD staffing exist around a core set of employees. One pattern focuses on clinical services, the other on more population-based programs.[11] The core employees consist of dietitian/nutritionists, sanitarians/environmental specialists, administrators, lab specialists, and health educators. The clinical pattern adds physicians, nurses, and dental health workers. The population-based pattern includes epidemiologists, public health nurses, social workers, and program specialists.

The availability of information on public health workers at the state and local level varies from state to state and is often inconsistent and incomplete. Detailed information from the official state health departments has only recently become available, although this does not include public health workers employed by state agencies other than the official state health department. The periodic profiles of LHDs completed by NACCHO before 2005 provide only general data on the proportion of responding agencies that employ specific public health job titles, either directly or through contracted services. The national profiles of LHDs completed after 2005 provide national estimates on the total number of full-time equivalent (FTE) workers as well as FTEs for 10–15 specific titles.

Gaps in information on the public health workforce extend to some of the most basic and important characteristics of that workforce. For example, there is very little information available on the racial and ethnic characteristics of the overall public health workforce. Although important, information on cultural competency is virtually nonexistent.

PUBLIC HEALTH WORKER ETHICS AND EDUCATION

Public health workers may come from different academic, professional, and experiential backgrounds, but they share a common bond. All are committed to a common mission and share common ethical principles, as exemplified by the following list advanced by the American Public Health Association:

- Public health should address principally the fundamental causes of disease and requirements for health, aiming to prevent adverse health outcomes.
- Public health should achieve community health in a way that respects the rights of individuals in the community.
- Public health policies, programs, and priorities should be developed and evaluated through processes that ensure an opportunity for input from community members.
- Public health should advocate and work for the empowerment of disenfranchised community members, aiming to ensure that the basic resources and conditions necessary for health are accessible to all.
- Public health should seek the information needed to implement effective policies and programs that protect and promote health.
- Public health institutions should provide communities with the information they have that is needed for decisions on policies or programs and should obtain the community's consent for their implementation.
- Public health institutions should act in a timely manner on the information they have within the resources and the mandate given to them by the public.
- Public health programs and policies should incorporate a variety of approaches that anticipate and respect diverse values, beliefs, and cultures in the community.
- Public health programs and policies should be implemented in a manner that most enhances the physical and social environment.
- Public health institutions should protect the confidentiality of information that can bring harm to an individual or community if made public. Exceptions must be justified on the basis of the high likelihood of significant harm to the individual or others.
- Public health institutions should ensure the professional competence of their employees.
- Public health institutions and their employees should engage in collaborations and affiliations in ways that build the public's trust and the institution's effectiveness.[12]

Information from national and state surveys indicates that the majority of public health workers lack formal education and training in public health. In 1980, HRSA determined that only 20% of the 250,000 professionals in the primary public health workforce had formal training in public health.[2] More than 3 decades later, there is little evidence that this situation has improved. While the proportion of those who have formal training varies by category of worker, the lack of formal training is striking in even some of the most critical categories. For example, NACCHO surveys from the early 1990s through 2013 found that only 20–25% of local health department leaders had formal public health education or training.[13]

This is not surprising in view of the small number of undergraduate, graduate, and doctoral degrees in public health that are awarded each year. Public health degrees at the undergraduate level represent only 0.2% of all undergraduate degrees, and public health doctoral degrees comprise the same percentage of all doctoral degrees. Master's degrees in public health, however, comprise about 1.3% of all master's-level degrees.[14]

Formal training for many public health workers focuses only on a specific aspect of public health practice, such as environmental health or community or school health nursing. Environmental health practitioners, nurses, administrators, and health educators account for the majority of public health workers with formal training in public health. Even among those with formal training in public health, public health workers with graduate degrees from schools of public health or other graduate public health programs represent only a small fraction of the total. The total number of master's-level graduates of schools of public health and other graduate-level public health degree programs was about 12,000 in 2010.

OUTSIDE-THE-BOOK THINKING 6-3

Are public health professionals viewed as change agents in their communities today? Why or why not? Do you hold the same opinion for public health organizations? Why or why not?

Evidence of the lack of formal training within this workforce, however, does not necessarily lead to the conclusion that public health workers are unprepared.[15] Instead, public health workers enter the field having earned a wide variety of degrees and professional training credentials from academic programs and institutions unrelated to public health. Often overlooked, these institutions produce the bulk of the public health workforce and represent major assets for addressing unmet needs.

On-the-job training and work experience contribute substantially to the overall competency and preparedness of the public health workforce. For example, public health workers are frequently involved in responses to earthquakes, floods, and other disasters and have increasingly acquired and demonstrated skills in assessing community health needs and devising community health improvement plans. These are skills that most public health workers acquired through real-world work experience rather than through their formal training.

Continuing education and career development for public health workers has long been a cottage industry involving many different parties. Academic institutions certainly are contributors, but public health agencies at the state and local level, public health associations and institutes (national, state, and local), and other voluntary-sector health organizations participate as well. Many different entities offer credits for continuing education, including professional organizations, academic institutions, and hospitals, among others. Public health workers value continuing education credits as a means to satisfy requirements of their core disciplines in order to maintain some level of credentialing status (such as licensed physicians and nurses, certified health education specialists, and so on). Very few states enforce continuing education requirements for the public health disciplines licensed by that state. There is no formal system of public health-specific continuing education units (CEUs) and only fledgling efforts toward credentialing public health workers. The notable development in this area is the Certified in Public Health (CPH) credential offered since 2008 by the National Board of Public Health Examiners for graduates of master's degree programs accredited by the Council on Education in Public Health. As of 2014, more than 3,000 public health workers had earned the CPH credential.[16]

CHARACTERISTICS OF PUBLIC HEALTH OCCUPATIONS

The remaining sections of this chapter define and describe several key dimensions of public health occupations and organizations that provide a framework for examining specific positions and careers for public health workers. Information on the full spectrum of occupations in the public health workforce is available from a variety of sources, including federal health and labor agencies and national public health organizations. Table 6-2 summarizes selected public health titles, occupational categories, and careers. The first column identifies the public health job titles and careers; the second column lists specific BLS standard occupational categories (SOCs). SOCs are explained more fully later in this chapter.

There are many aspects of an occupation or career that are important to current and prospective public health workers, including:

- Occupational classification: These are based on job titles and whether the duties of the job are primarily administrative, professional, technical, or supportive in nature. Many positions in public health practice have a variety of job titles associated with them. Similarly, the same job title can have a variety of regular duties and day-to-day responsibilities.
- Public health practice profile: The public health functions and essential public health services addressed by each occupational grouping can be presented in a public health practice profile.
- Important and essential duties: These are the defining characteristics of any position describing what the worker does on a daily basis.
- Minimum qualifications: Some positions require a specific academic degree or credential; many do not. Some require previous experience, while others do not. All require some particular minimum level of knowledge, skills, and abilities. Many also require specific physical capabilities.

Table 6-2 Selected Public Health Occupations and Careers

Career Category with Examples of Titles Used in Public Health Organizations	*Bureau of Labor Statistics Standard Occupational Categories Related to Public Health*
Public Health Administration • Health Services Manager • Public Health Agency Director • Health Officer • Emergency Preparedness and Response Director	Professional Occupations • Emergency Management Directors • Medical and Health Services Managers • Social and Community Services Managers
Environmental and Occupational Health • Environmental Engineer • Environmental Health Specialist (entry level) • Environmental Health Specialist (midlevel) • Environmental Health Specialist (senior level) • Occupational Health and Safety Specialist	Professional Occupations • Environmental Engineers • Environmental Scientists and Specialists (including Health) • Health and Safety Engineers (except Mining Safety Engineers and Inspectors) • Occupational Health and Safety Specialists Technical Occupations • Environmental Engineering Technicians • Environmental Science and Protection Technicians (including Health) • Occupational Health and Safety Technicians
Public Health Nursing • Public Health Nurse (entry level) • Public Health Nurse (senior level) • Licensed Practical/Vocational Nurse	Professional Occupations • Nurse Practitioners • Registered Nurses Technical Occupations • Home Health Aides • Licensed Practical and Licensed Vocational Nurses • Nursing Assistants
Epidemiology and Disease Control • Disease Investigator • Epidemiologist (entry level) • Epidemiologist (senior level)	Professional Occupations • Epidemiologists • Statisticians

Table 6-2 Selected Public Health Occupations and Careers (*Continued*)

Career Category with Examples of Titles Used in Public Health Organizations	*Bureau of Labor Statistics Standard Occupational Categories Related to Public Health*
Public Health Education and Information	
• Public Health Educator (entry level)	Professional Occupations
• Public Health Educator (senior level)	• Health Educators
• Public Information Officer	• Public Relations Specialists
• Community Health Workers (and other Outreach Occupations)	Technical Occupations
	• Community Health Workers
Other Public Health Professional and Technical Personnel	
• Public Health Nutritionist/Dietician	Professional Occupations
• Public Health Social, Behavioral and Mental Health Worker	• Audiologists
• Public Health Laboratory Worker	• Administrative Law Judges, Adjudicators, and Hearing Officers
• Public Health Physician	• Dental Hygienists
• Public Health Veterinarian	• Dentists (General Dentist)
• Public Health Pharmacist	• Dieticians and Nutritionists
• Public Health Oral Health Professional	• Healthcare Social Workers
• Administrative Law Judge/Hearing Officer	• Medical and Clinical Laboratory Technologists
• Public Health Program Specialist/Coordinator	• Mental Health Counselors
• Public Health Policy Analyst	• Mental Health and Substance Abuse Social Workers
• Public Health Information Specialist	• Microbiologists
	• Optometrists
	• Pharmacists
	• Physician Assistants
	• Physicians (Family or General Practitioners)
	• Substance Abuse and Behavioral Disorder Counselors
	• Veterinarians
	Technical Occupations
	• Animal Control Workers
	• Emergency Medical Technicians and Paramedics
	• Medical and Clinical Laboratory Technicians

- Workplace considerations: This description will identify levels of government that employ significant numbers of workers in each occupational category as well as important nongovernmental work settings for public health workers. This section will also highlight considerations related to physical demands, work schedules, travel, and general working conditions.
- Salary estimates: Salary levels for public health workers can be estimated based on information from current job postings and the most recent survey of employment and wages coordinated by the Labor Department's BLS.
- Career prospects: Estimates as to current need and future demand for specific public health occupations and career paths are provided, based on the analyses performed by public health organizations and the BLS' projections for various occupations.
- Additional information: Sources of additional information for each occupation or career are identified, including education and training opportunities.

The following sections briefly describe the type and source of information included for each of these characteristics.

Occupational Classifications

Throughout the economy, including the health sector, occupations are broadly classified as either white collar or blue collar, depending on the degree of education and experience normally required. White collar occupations include five major occupational categories (professional, administrative, technical, clerical, and other), based on the subject matter of work, the level of difficulty or responsibility involved, and the educational requirements established for each occupation. Blue collar occupations are composed of the trades, crafts, and manual labor (unskilled, semiskilled, skilled), including foreman and supervisory positions entailing trade, craft, or laboring experience and knowledge as the paramount requirement.

The U.S. Office of Personnel Management tracks occupations in various industries using four general categories—professional, administrative, technical, and support.

- Professional occupations are those that require knowledge in a field of science or learning characteristically acquired through education or training equivalent to a bachelor's or higher degree with major study in or pertinent to the specialized field, as distinguished from general education. The work of a professional occupation requires the exercise of discretion, judgment, and personal responsibility for the application of an organized body of knowledge that is continuously studied to make new discoveries and interpretations, and to improve the data, materials, and methods. Professionals require specialized and theoretical knowledge. Well-known examples of professional job titles include physicians, registered nurses (RNs), dietitians, health educators, social workers, psychologists, lawyers, accountants, economists, system analysts, and personnel and labor relations workers. Professionals comprise the majority of public health workers.
- Administrative occupations are those that involve the exercise of analytical ability, judgment, discretion, personal responsibility, and the application of a substantial body of knowledge of principles, concepts, and practices

applicable to one or more fields of administration or management. Although these positions do not require specialized educational majors, they do involve the type of skills (analytical, research, writing, judgment) typically gained through a college-level general education, or through progressively responsible experience. Administrators set broad policies, oversee overall responsibility for the execution of these policies, direct individual departments or special phases of the agency's operations, or provide specialized consultation on a regional, district, or area basis. Common job titles for administrators include department heads, bureau chiefs, division chiefs, directors, deputy directors, and similar titles. Administrators and managers comprise 5% of all public health workers.

- Technical occupations are those that involve work that is not routine in nature and is typically associated with, and supportive of, a professional or administrative field. Such occupations involve extensive practical knowledge gained through on-the-job experience, or specific training less than that represented by college graduation. Work in these occupations may involve substantial elements of the work of the professional or administrative field but requires less than full competence in the field involved. Technical occupations require a combination of basic scientific or technical knowledge and manual skills. Titles include computer specialists, licensed practical nurses (LPNs), inspectors, programmers, and a variety of technicians (environmental, laboratory, medical, nursing, dental, and so on). The technical occupations category also includes paraprofessionals who perform some of the duties of a professional or technician in a supportive role usually requiring less formal training and experience than that normally required for professional status. Included are community health workers, outreach workers, research assistants, medical aides, child support workers, home health aides, emergency medical technicians, among others. Workers in technical occupations account for 20% of all public health workers.

- Administrative support occupations are those that involve structured work in support of office, business, or fiscal operations; duties are performed according to established policies or techniques and require training, experience, or working knowledge related to the tasks to be performed. Clerical titles are often responsible for internal and external communication as well as recording and retrieval of data, information, and other paperwork required in an office. This category includes bookkeepers, messengers, clerk typists, stenographers, court transcribers, hearing reporters, statistical clerks, dispatchers, license distributors, payroll clerks, office machine and computer operators, telephone operators, legal assistants, and so on. In addition, workers in any of the blue-collar occupational categories are considered support workers within the public health workforce. About 19% of public health workers are in the administrative support category.

As documented in Figure 6-5, 81% of public health workers fall into the professional, administrative, and technical categories. More than one half (56%) are classified as professionals, similar to the proportion of professionals among all 15 million health workers. Nursing and environmental health activities account for the largest number of public health workers when both professional and technical

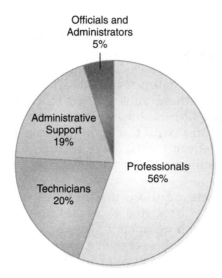

Figure 6-5 Percentage of public health workers in selected occupational categories, United States, 2000.

Data from Health Resources and Services Administration, Bureau of Health Professions, National Center for Health Workforce Information and Analysis and Center for Health Policy, Columbia School of Nursing. *The Public Health Workforce Enumeration 2000*. Washington, DC: HRSA; 2000.

occupations are considered. RNs represent the largest professional category within the public health workforce.

The U.S. Department of Labor collects information on occupations throughout the economy, including the public sector. An official taxonomy for occupations allows the Department of Labor's BLS to track information on hundreds of SOCs in terms of the number and location of jobs, salaries, and duties performed. BLS also develops projections for the number of future positions for these occupational categories based on economic and employment trends. Occupations generally can be found in a variety of industries, making it difficult to pinpoint trends and needs specific to the public health system. For example, RNs are the largest occupational category in the overall health workforce, with 2.7 million workers, but only a small percentage of all RNs (about 75,000) work in public health agencies. Many more work in hospitals and other healthcare organizations. This is also true for physicians, health services administrators, health educators, nutritionists, and many other occupations. Public health agencies, however, are the largest employers of several SOCs, such as environmental health specialists and epidemiologists. For those occupational categories, BLS information is especially useful.

SOCs relevant for public health are identified in the second column of Table 6-2, with nearly 40 specific categories listed.[17] These occupational categories clearly do not cover all titles found in public health organizations. Nor do they capture the entire scope of work undertaken by public health workers.

A second important source of estimates for public health workers in relevant SOCs is the *Public Health Workforce Enumeration 2000* study commissioned by HRSA.[3] This enumeration collected information on workers of federal, state, and local public health agencies in the year 2000 based on existing data, reports, and surveys. As such, it was as much a qualitative and descriptive enumeration as a quantitative one. The year 2000 public health workforce enumeration identified a total of 450,000 public health workers, including 15,000 workers in voluntary sector organizations and 15,000 public health students. Occupational categories could not be established for 112,000 public health workers, making it difficult to project the actual number of workers in specific categories, such as public health nurses or epidemiologists. Both sources provide insights useful for estimating the number of existing positions for each occupational category and title.

Public Health Practice Profile

Individual workers, as well as occupational categories, produce work important to achieving public health goals and objectives. As described in previous chapters, key public health goals and objectives address preventing disease and injury, promoting healthy behaviors, protecting against health risks and threats, responding to emergencies, and ensuring the quality of health services.[4] This overall public health practice framework provides the basis for channeling contributions both by individuals and organizations toward common goals. The specific public health practice tasks of different occupations and individuals generally fall into one or more of the 10 essential public health services. Earlier chapters characterized the essential public health services as how the work of public health is accomplished and its ends are achieved. It is useful to view these functions and essential public health services as an aggregate job description for the entire public health workforce, with the workload then shared among the many different professional and occupational categories composing the total public health workforce.

For each occupational category, several purposes and essential public health services that form the core of the duties and job descriptions can be identified. An example of this format is provided in Table 6-3.

In this example, the public health occupational category is primarily involved in addressing three public health goals: preventing epidemics, preventing injuries, and promoting healthy behaviors. This public health occupational category works to address these goals largely through performing five essential public health services—monitoring health status, investigating health problems, educating people about health, evaluating effectiveness, and researching new solutions to health problems.

For this example, the assignment of specific public health purposes and essential public health services may appear somewhat arbitrary. In this case, however, judgments are made as to which purposes and essential services are most closely associated with this occupational category. Some occupational categories may appear to have a relatively limited focus (e.g., public health laboratory workers) in comparison with others (e.g., public health nurses) that may have very broad roles that could conceivably cover all purposes and services. For each occupational category and title, however, the number of purposes and essential services identified for each

Table 6-3   Public Health Profile Example

(Example) *Public Health Practitioners* *Make a Difference by:*
Public Health Purposes ✓ Preventing epidemics and the spread of disease • Protecting against environmental hazards ✓ Preventing injuries ✓ Promoting and encouraging healthy behaviors • Responding to disasters and assisting communities in recovery • Ensuring the quality and accessibility of health services *Essential Public Health Services* ✓ Monitoring health status to identify community health problems ✓ Diagnosing and investigating health problems and health hazards in the community ✓ Informing, educating, and empowering people about health issues • Mobilizing community partnerships to identify and solve health problems • Developing policies and plans that support individual and community health efforts • Enforcing laws and regulations that protect health and ensure safety • Linking people with needed personal health services and ensuring the provision of health care when otherwise unavailable • Ensuring a competent public health and personal healthcare workforce ✓ Evaluating effectiveness, accessibility, and quality of personal and population-based health services ✓ Researching new insights and innovative solutions to health problems

occupational category is limited to no more than one half the number possible (3 of 6 purposes, 5 of 10 essential public health services). Table 6-4 provides a composite profile that aggregates information from selected public health occupations.

Characterizing the work of an occupational category in this manner provides a functional view of the work performed. It also facilitates an understanding of how the work of one occupational category relates to the work of other categories and how the overall workload is distributed across the various public health occupational categories.

Important and Essential Duties

The most important aspect of any job or career is what workers do day in and day out. It is those basic and routine duties that best define positions in public health or any other field of endeavor. This list varies considerably from one position to another and often from one level of the same position to a higher level (e.g., from an entry-level environmental health specialist to a midlevel environmental health specialist). Important and essential duties for various titles within subsequent chapters are based on information from a sampling of job and position descriptions from a variety of public health organizations.

Table 6-4 Composite Public Health Practice Profile for Selected Public Health Occupations and Titles

Selected Public Health Professional Occupations Make a Difference by:	Adm	EH	PHN	Epi	HE	Nutr	BH	Lab	Docs	Oral	Law	Prog	Pol
Public Health Purposes													
Preventing epidemics and the spread of disease	✓	✓	✓	✓	✓	✓		✓	✓	✓	✓		✓
Protecting against environmental hazards		✓		✓				✓			✓	✓	✓
Preventing injuries		✓		✓	✓							✓	
Promoting and encouraging healthy behaviors		✓			✓	✓	✓		✓	✓		✓	
Responding to disasters and assisting communities in recovery	✓						✓						
Assuring the quality and accessibility of health services	✓		✓			✓	✓	✓	✓	✓	✓		✓
Essential Public Health Services													
Monitoring health status to identify community health problems		✓		✓		✓		✓	✓	✓		✓	
Diagnosing and investigating health problems and health hazards in the community		✓	✓	✓				✓	✓			✓	
Informing, educating, and empowering people about health issues		✓			✓	✓	✓			✓			✓
Mobilizing community partnerships to identify and solve health problems	✓				✓		✓						✓
Developing policies and plans that support individual and community health efforts	✓				✓		✓				✓	✓	✓
Enforcing laws and regulations that protect health and ensure safety	✓	✓						✓			✓	✓	

(continues)

Table 6-4 Composite Public Health Practice Profile for Selected Public Health Occupations and Titles (*Continued*)

Selected Public Health Professional Occupations Make a Difference by:	Adm	EH	PHN	Epi	HE	Nutr	BH	Lab	Docs	Oral	Law	Prog	Pol
Linking people with needed personal health services and assuring the provision of health care when otherwise unavailable			✓		✓	✓	✓		✓	✓			
Assuring a competent public health and personal healthcare workforce	✓				✓						✓		
Evaluating effectiveness, accessibility, and quality of personal and population-based health services	✓	✓	✓	✓		✓	✓	✓	✓	✓	✓	✓	✓
Researching new insights and innovative solutions to health problems			✓	✓		✓		✓	✓		✓		✓

Notes: Adm: public health managers; EH: environmental health workers; PHN: public health nurses; Epi: epidemiologists; HE: health educators; Nutr: nutritionists and dieticians; BH: behavioral health professionals; Lab: public health laboratory workers; Docs: physicians, veterinarians, optometrists, pharmacists; Oral: oral health professionals; Law: administrative judges and hearing officers: Spec; public health program specialists/coordinators; Pol: policy analysts.

Minimum Qualifications

Another key dimension of a position is a statement of the minimum qualifications necessary for that job. Often these minimum qualifications must be met in order for a worker to apply for a particular position. Minimum qualifications may emphasize experience or education or both. In any event, there is a battery of skills or competencies that are expected of those applying for and those working in public health positions. Minimum levels of knowledge, skills, and abilities are presented for public health job titles addressed in the subsequent occupation-specific chapters. Additional qualifications, such as physical capabilities appropriate for specific jobs or job locations, are also presented. These qualifications can be synthesized from a sampling of current position descriptions.

The range of public health occupations and careers extends from those requiring considerable education and training to those that require relatively little. For example, some state and local health officials may hold several degrees, such as a bachelor's degree in science, an MPH, and a doctoral degree in medicine. At the same time, key staff performing investigations of communicable disease or environmental threats may have only an associate or bachelor's degree at the under-graduate level. It is not uncommon for some technical and clerical staff to have attained no more than a high school diploma with on-the-job training.

Workplace Considerations

Public health work takes place in many organizations and settings other than governmental public health agencies such as state health agencies or local public health departments. Many community and voluntary organizations collaborate with governmental public health agencies and employ staff whose work parallels that of workers in governmental public health agencies. This is true both for nongovernmental public health efforts here in the United States and those on the international level.

Another important workplace consideration relates to special physical capabilities, travel requirements, and other unique aspects of specific jobs. For example, some positions may require the ability to lift and move items weighing up to 50 pounds. Other jobs may require the ability to walk great distances or to have normal vision or hearing. Others may require the ability to work outside in cold and inclement weather, or to work unusual hours.

Salary Estimates

Detailed and specific salary information is not widely available. Information will be provided based on limited sources, including BLS data and current job postings. This information should not be considered to be definitive, timely, or completely accurate. Salary scales vary widely from agency to agency depending on a variety of circumstances and conditions. Figure 6-6 indicates that the overall average salary of a full-time workers employed by a state or local health agency increased by 50% to more than $50,000 between 1998 and 2012.

Career Prospects

Current and future opportunities for public health careers, as do careers in all fields, are a function of relationships among the population, the labor force, the overall economy, and the demand for public health programs and services.[17] The size and composition of the population strongly influence both the size of the workforce and the types of services needed by the population.

The U.S. population continues to increase, although at a slower rate than in recent decades. The average age of the population continues to increase as well, and the proportion of the population in the older age categories will continue to increase. As older workers near retirement, replacement of workers will create job opportunities and career advancement possibilities in addition to those created by the continued growth of the overall population.

Among the various sectors of the U.S. economy, the health sector is projected to grow faster and add more jobs than other sectors. About one in every four new jobs will be in the health sector, with professional and technical occupational categories exhibiting the greatest growth and offering the greatest opportunities for new jobs and career advancement. In sum, the overall outlook for professional and technical occupations in public health is very bright for those now in or about to enter the job market.

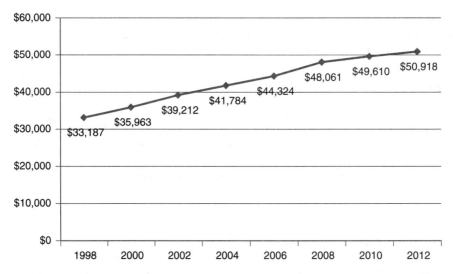

Figure 6-6   Mean salary for full-time equivalent workers of state and local health* agencies, selected years, 1998–2012, United States.

*Health: public health services, emergency medical services, mental health, alcohol and drug abuse, outpatient clinics, visiting nurses, food and sanitary inspections, animal control, other environmental health activities (e.g., pollution control), etc.

Data from U.S. Bureau of the Census. Federal, state, and local governments, and public employment and payroll data. www.census.gov/govs/apes. Accessed June 15, 2014.

The optimal number of public health workers is controversial and uncertain. There is widespread concern within the public health community that there will soon be a shortage of public health workers. Several key public health occupational categories are currently in short supply, such as public health nurses and epidemiologists. The information provided in the career prospect section will identify specific occupational categories that are projected to be in greatest need. Despite the uncertainties, the BLS provides projections for the number of positions likely to be needed in 10 years and the number of job openings that will occur through new positions and retirements.

Careers in public health, like those in many fields, are not always straightforward. Individual workers can begin in one career pathway and then shift into another. For example, administrators of public health agencies could come up through the ranks of program and agency management or from one of the public health professional categories, such as environmental health, nursing, or health education.

OUTSIDE-THE-BOOK THINKING 6-4

How have the needs for different public health occupations changed over the past century? How will the need for various public health occupations change over the next 2 decades?

PUBLIC HEALTH WORKFORCE GROWTH PROSPECTS

Will the public health workforce increase or decrease in size over the next several decades? There should be little debate over this question, but there is. One reason for controversy derives from the general lack of information on the public health workforce between 1980 and 2000. Another relates to the many complex forces within public health and the broader economy that influence the number of public health workers needed.

In hindsight, it is clear that HRSA's estimate as to the size of the public health workforce in 1980 lacked precision. This is unfortunate, because the 500,000 figure from 1980 is frequently cited as documentation that the public health workforce must be shrinking because only 450,000 public health workers were enumerated in 2000. On closer examination, however, the HRSA 1980 estimate actually indicated that only 250,000 of the 500,000 public health workers were in the primary public health workforce consisting of federal, state, and local public health agency workers and selected others who devoted most of their work efforts to public health activities.[2] Even within this 250,000 figure were faculty and researchers at academic institutions; occupational health physicians and nurses working for various private companies; health educators teaching in schools; and administrators working in hospitals, nursing homes, and other medical care settings. The actual number of public health professionals working for federal, state, and local public health agencies in 1980, after adjusting for these inclusions, was closer to 140,000. The total for the comparable categories from the *Public Health Workforce Enumeration 2000* was 260,000, a figure that indicates the public health workforce grew rather than shrank between 1980 and 2000. Data from the employment census of governmental agencies support this conclusion, showing there has been a steady increase in FTE workers of governmental health agencies over the past several decades.

Together this evidence suggests that the public health workforce has been increasing throughout the 1990s, and into the first and second decades of the new century. This is consistent with the documented expansion of the health sector within the overall economy, which continues to grow at a more rapid rate than the rest of the economy. If public health activities continue to maintain even their current small share of total health spending, funding for public health activities and public health workers will grow commensurately. It is conceivable that public health activities could even increase their share of overall health spending, fostering even more rapid growth of employment opportunities. Several prevention and public health provisions of the Affordable Care Act suggest that this is possible.

There are mounting concerns, however, that the growth of the public health workforce may be slowing, at least in the public sector. It was somewhat surprising that the infusion of bioterrorism preparedness funding after 2001 didn't result in even greater numbers of state and local public health workers than are reflected in Table 6-1. It appears that state and local governments initially shifted some workers onto federal bioterrorism grant payrolls, thereby saving state and local resources or possibly shifting resources from public health to other priorities such as education. The severe national economic downturn in 2008/2009 forced many states and localities to suspend hiring and subject workers to furloughs and layoffs. The massive infusion of funding to state and local governments through the American Recovery and Reinvestment Act of 2009 also served to temporarily support positions in public health agencies until this funding ended in 2010. The long-term impact of the recession on the national public health workforce remains uncertain, although surveys conducted by the Association of State and Territorial Health Officials and NACCHO suggest that state and local health departments suffered significant staff reductions between 2008 and 2012.[18]

Recent history indicates that federal funding to states and localities for bioterrorism preparedness served as a temptation to replace or supplant state and local support for public health with federal money. The funding of epidemiologists further illustrates this phenomenon. In 2004, federal bioterrorism funds paid the salaries of 460 epidemiologists; among 390 epidemiologists working on bioterrorism and emergency response activities, 62% were funded by the federal government. Infectious disease epidemiologists did not increase between 2001 and 2004, but in 2004 nearly 20% were paid through federal bioterrorism funds.[19] This scenario likely affected several other public health occupational categories, such as laboratory workers and emergency response coordinators. It underscores the important role of the underlying fiscal environment of state and local governments in determining the size of the public health workforce.

OUTSIDE-THE-BOOK THINKING 6-5

What factors determine the optimum size of the public health workforce in a community? Are these the same factors that would determine the optimum size of the public health workforce at the state or national level?

Two additional modern forces affect public health workforce size. These are the expansion of information technology and the resulting increase in worker productivity. Public health practice, by its very nature, is information dependent and information driven. Enhanced information technology tools and increased individual worker productivity mean fewer workers are needed to support the work of administrators, professionals, and technical staff. This trend would tend to increase the proportion of professionals within the public health workforce; however, these trends also mean fewer professionals are needed to perform the same volume of work. The net effect is therefore difficult to forecast in terms of the number and type of workers needed.

Trends within the health sector will also continue to affect public health workers. Health is highly valued both as a personal and societal goal. The economic value placed on health exceeds $3 trillion annually, or nearly $10,000 per person in the United States.[9] There is no indication that health will assume a lower priority within the American social value system. In recent years, for example, expenditures for health purposes have grown faster than the rate for the overall economy. In effect, health is becoming an even greater priority. Between the two general strategies to achieve health—preventive and therapeutic approaches—the balance may be slowly shifting toward more prevention. There is still a notable imbalance, with a 20 to 1 ratio; however, this shift is likely to continue. Taken together with an increased priority on health itself, public health activities, including those carried out by public health agencies and workers, should continue to increase in size, importance, and value to society.

The value placed on public health activities can be measured in economic terms, such as funding levels for programs, services, and the workers who implement public health programs and services. To sustain or even enhance public health funding, national leadership is necessary. Federal health agencies such as CDC and HRSA are especially important in the area of public health workforce development. Complementing sustained national leadership, state and local governments must remain committed to and invested in public health objectives. However, states and local governments across the United States face difficult economic circumstances and tough choices as they look to cut back services that are either low priority or that have other funding sources.

Beyond funding, administrative and bureaucratic obstacles challenge public health workforce development efforts in the public sector. State and local agencies are often the locus of some of the most significant recruitment and retention problems facing the public health workforce. These include slow hiring by governmental agencies, civil service systems, hiring freezes, budget crises affecting state and local government, and the lack of career ladders, competitive salary structures, and other forms of recognition that value workers for their skill and performance.

Despite the uncertainties inherent in these influences, past trends and current forces suggest that professional and administrative jobs and careers in public health are likely to grow over the next decade. Unfortunately, it will be difficult to measure progress without deployment of a standard taxonomy for public health occupations and more comprehensive enumeration strategies and tools that provide better information on the key dimensions of the public health workforce.[20,21]

Job opportunities generally track with population density and demographic shifts. Within the health sector, job opportunities cluster around metropolitan areas. Public health positions also follow this pattern. There are more positions, and therefore more opportunities, in metropolitan areas than there are in rural areas. General demographic trends indicate a continuing shift of population from the Northeast and Midwest regions of the United States to the South, Southwest, and West Coast. It is likely that health sector jobs and public health positions will also follow this pattern.

The ratio of positions to population, however, is higher in rural areas (and states that have higher proportions of their population living in nonmetropolitan areas). This occurs because there is a basic core staffing that must be present regardless of the size of the population and because rural and remote communities often lack other public health resources and assets. Higher public health worker to population ratios in rural areas raise questions as to whether scarce resources, in the form of public health professionals, are used efficiently in state–local public health systems. Given limited resources, this finding argues in favor of further consolidation of small local public health agencies into larger ones.

The demand for many public health professional occupations is growing steadily. In recent decades, an increasing number of LHDs employed epidemiologists, health educators, health information specialists, emergency response coordinators, and public health information officers. The aftermath of terrorist events of 2001, including the series of anthrax spore attacks through the postal system, spotlighted the need for two professional positions in particular. The first, emergency response coordinators, is new to the list of public health occupations; the second, epidemiologists, is one of the oldest public health professional occupations. State and local public health agencies are rapidly hiring emergency response coordinators. These people come to these new positions with a wide range of academic and experiential qualifications. Epidemiologists, on the other hand, have more restrictive qualifications in terms of academic preparation such as master's and doctoral degrees. Concerns over the past few decades that epidemiologists were in short supply and great demand are now heightened as agencies seek to hire more of these specialists. The number of epidemiologists coming out of graduate programs does not appear to be keeping pace with the need, despite an increase in interest as measured by the number of applications for epidemiology training programs.

Prior to 2001, health educators and community health planners were steadily growing professional categories in the public health workforce. Expansion of health education and promotion programs, and an increase in community health planning and community health improvement activities account for this trend. More recently, the Affordable Care Act has focused increased attention on the potential roles for community health workers. If the U.S. health system shifts even slightly toward a greater emphasis on public health and prevention activities, other public health occupations may benefit as well.

PUBLIC HEALTH PRACTITIONER COMPETENCIES

Beyond workforce size, distribution, and composition are issues related to the essential competencies and skills that will be most important in public health practice and how these skills are best acquired. Establishing and promoting competencies for public health workers is tricky business. For one thing, public health workers come from a variety of professional backgrounds, many of which have their own core competencies. For example, public health nursing has a set of core competencies and health educators use a sophisticated competency framework for purposes of certification. The same is true for public health physicians, administrators, epidemiologists, and several other public health professional occupations. Identifying a common core for these various professional categories generally leads to a framework with very general and nonspecific competencies that are difficult to relate to a specific situation or problem. The Council on Linkages between Academia and Public Health Practice spent 2 decades grappling with this problem before arriving at the set of core competencies for public health professionals summarized in Table 6-5 for entry-level workers.

CONCLUSION

Recent decades witnessed an increase in the number of public health workers employed by both governmental and nongovernmental agencies. This expansion of the workforce, however, leaves many questions unanswered as to the appropriate number, distribution, training, and preparedness of the public health workforce, making these issues of public concern. Some of these concerns have persisted since the late 1800s, as suggested by an editorial appearing in the *Journal of the American Medical Association* more than a century ago:

> It is unfortunate that in the absence of epidemics or pestilence, too little attention is paid to the protection of the public health, and as a necessary consequence, to the selection of those whose duties require them to guard the public health.[22(p189)]

Table 6-5   Core Competencies for Tier 1 (Entry-Level) Public Health Workers

Analytical/Assessment Skills

1. Describes factors affecting the health of a community (e.g., equity, income, education, environment)
2. Identifies quantitative and qualitative data and information (e.g., vital statistics, electronic health records, transportation patterns, unemployment rates, community input, health equity impact assessments) that can be used for assessing the health of a community
3. Applies ethical principles in accessing, collecting, analyzing, using, maintaining, and disseminating data and information
4. Uses information technology in accessing, collecting, analyzing, using, maintaining, and disseminating data and information
5. Selects valid and reliable data
6. Selects comparable data (e.g., data being age-adjusted to the same year, data variables across datasets having similar definitions)
7. Identifies gaps in data
8. Collects valid and reliable quantitative and qualitative data
9. Describes public health applications of quantitative and qualitative data
10. Uses quantitative and qualitative data
11. Describes assets and resources that can be used for improving the health of a community (e.g., Boys & Girls Clubs, public libraries, hospitals, faith-based organizations, academic institutions, federal grants, fellowship programs)
12. Contributes to assessments of community health status and factors influencing health in a community (e.g., quality, availability, accessibility, and use of health services; access to affordable housing)
13. Explains how community health assessments use information about health status, factors influencing health, and assets and resources
14. Describes how evidence (e.g., data, findings reported in peer-reviewed literature) is used in decision making

Policy Development/Program Planning Skills

1. Contributes to state/Tribal/community health improvement planning (e.g., providing data to supplement community health assessments, communicating observations from work in the field)
2. Contributes to development of program goals and objectives
3. Describes organizational strategic plan (e.g., includes measurable objectives and targets; relationship to community health improvement plan, workforce development plan, quality improvement plan, and other plans)
4. Contributes to implementation of organizational strategic plan
5. Identifies current trends (e.g., health, fiscal, social, political, environmental) affecting the health of a community
6. Gathers information that can inform options for policies, programs, and services (e.g., secondhand smoking policies, data use policies, HR policies, immunization programs, food safety programs)
7. Describes implications of policies, programs, and services
8. Implements policies, programs, and services
9. Explains the importance of evaluations for improving policies, programs, and services
10. Gathers information for evaluating policies, programs, and services (e.g., outputs, outcomes, processes, procedures, return on investment)
11. Applies strategies for continuous quality improvement
12. Describes how public health informatics is used in developing, implementing, evaluating, and improving policies, programs, and services (e.g., integrated data systems, electronic reporting, knowledge management systems, geographic information systems)

(continues)

Table 6-5   Core Competencies for Tier 1 (Entry-Level) Public Health Workers

Communication Skills

1. Identifies the literacy of populations served (e.g., ability to obtain, interpret, and use health and other information; social media literacy)
2. Communicates in writing and orally with linguistic and cultural proficiency (e.g., using age-appropriate materials, incorporating images)
3. Solicits input from individuals and organizations (e.g., chambers of commerce, religious organizations, schools, social service organizations, hospitals, government, community-based organizations, various populations served) for improving the health of a community
4. Suggests approaches for disseminating public health data and information (e.g., social media, newspapers, newsletters, journals, town hall meetings, libraries, neighborhood gatherings)
5. Conveys data and information to professionals and the public using a variety of approaches (e.g., reports, presentations, email, letters)
6. Communicates information to influence behavior and improve health (e.g., uses social marketing methods, considers behavioral theories such as the Health Belief Model or Stages of Change Model)
7. Facilitates communication among individuals, groups, and organizations
8. Describes the roles of governmental public health, health care, and other partners in improving the health of a community

Cultural Competency Skills

1. Describes the concept of diversity as it applies to individuals and populations (e.g., language, culture, values, socioeconomic status, geography, education, race, gender, age, ethnicity, sexual orientation, profession, religious affiliation, mental and physical abilities, historical experiences)
2. Describes the diversity of individuals and populations in a community
3. Describes the ways diversity may influence policies, programs, services, and the health of a community
4. Recognizes the contribution of diverse perspectives in developing, implementing, and evaluating policies, programs, and services that affect the health of a community
5. Recognizes the contribution of diverse perspectives in developing, implementing, and evaluating policies, programs, and services that affect the health of a community
6. Describes the effects of policies, programs, and services on different populations in a community
7. Describes the value of a diverse public health workforce

Community Dimensions of Practice Skills

1. Describes the programs and services provided by governmental and nongovernmental organizations to improve the health of a community
2. Recognizes relationships that are affecting health in a community (e.g., relationships among health departments, hospitals, community health centers, primary care providers, schools, community-based organizations, and other types of organizations)
3. Suggests relationships that may be needed to improve health in a community
4. Supports relationships that improve health in a community
5. Collaborates with community partners to improve health in a community (e.g., participates in committees, shares data and information, connects people to resources)
6. Engages community members (e.g., focus groups, talking circles, formal meetings, key informant interviews) to improve health in a community
7. Provides input for developing, implementing, evaluating, and improving policies, programs, and services
8. Uses assets and resources (e.g., Boys & Girls Clubs, public libraries, hospitals, faith-based organizations, academic institutions, federal grants, fellowship programs) to improve health in a community
9. Informs the public about policies, programs, and resources that improve health in a community
10. Describes the importance of community-based participatory research

Table 6-5 Core Competencies for Tier 1 (Entry-Level) Public Health Workers (*Continued*)

Public Health Sciences Skills

1. Describes the scientific foundation of the field of public health
2. Identifies prominent events in the history of public health (e.g., smallpox eradication, development of vaccinations, infectious disease control, safe drinking water, emphasis on hygiene and hand washing, access to health care for people with disabilities)
3. Describes how public health sciences (e.g., biostatistics, epidemiology, environmental health sciences, health services administration, social and behavioral sciences, and public health informatics) are used in the delivery of the 10 Essential Public Health Services
4. Retrieves evidence (e.g., research findings, case reports, community surveys) from print and electronic sources (e.g., PubMed, *Journal of Public Health Management and Practice*, *Morbidity and Mortality Weekly Report*, *The World Health Report*) to support decision making
5. Recognizes limitations of evidence (e.g., validity, reliability, sample size, bias, generalizability)
6. Describes evidence used in developing, implementing, evaluating, and improving policies, programs, and services
7. Describes the laws, regulations, policies, and procedures for the ethical conduct of research (e.g., patient confidentiality, protection of human subjects, Americans with Disabilities Act)
8. Contributes to the public health evidence base (e.g., participating in Public Health Practice-Based Research Networks, community-based participatory research, and academic health departments; authoring articles; making data available to researchers)
9. Suggests partnerships that may increase use of evidence in public health practice (e.g., between practice and academic organizations, with health sciences libraries)

Financial Planning and Management Skills

1. Describes the structures, functions, and authorizations of governmental public health programs and organizations
2. Describes government agencies with authority to impact the health of a community
3. Adheres to organizational policies and procedures
4. Describes public health funding mechanisms (e.g., categorical grants, fees, third-party reimbursement, tobacco taxes)
5. Contributes to development of program budgets
6. Provides information for proposals for funding (e.g., foundations, government agencies, corporations)
7. Provides information for development of contracts and other agreements for programs and services
8. Describes financial analysis methods used in making decisions about policies, programs, and services (e.g., cost-effectiveness, cost-benefit, cost-utility analysis, return on investment)
9. Operates programs within budget
10. Describes how teams help achieve program and organizational goals (e.g., the value of different disciplines, sectors, skills, experiences, and perspectives; scope of work and timeline)
11. Motivates colleagues for the purpose of achieving program and organizational goals (e.g., participating in teams, encouraging sharing of ideas, respecting different points of view)
12. Uses evaluation results to improve program and organizational performance
13. Describes program performance standards and measures
14. Uses performance management systems for program and organizational improvement (e.g., achieving performance objectives and targets, increasing efficiency, refining processes, meeting *Healthy People* objectives, sustaining accreditation)

(*continues*)

Table 6-5   Core Competencies for Tier 1 (Entry-Level) Public Health Workers (*Continued*)

Leadership and Systems Thinking Skills

1. Incorporates ethical standards of practice (e.g., Public Health Code of Ethics) into all interactions with individuals, organizations, and communities
2. Describes public health as part of a larger interrelated system of organizations that influence the health of populations at local, national, and global levels
3. Describes the ways public health, health care, and other organizations can work together or individually to impact the health of a community
4. Contributes to development of a vision for a healthy community (e.g., emphasis on prevention, health equity for all, excellence and innovation)
5. Identifies internal and external facilitators and barriers that may affect the delivery of the 10 Essential Public Health Services (e.g., using root cause analysis and other quality improvement methods and tools, problem solving)
6. Describes needs for professional development (e.g., training, mentoring, peer advising, coaching)
7. Participates in professional development opportunities
8. Describes the impact of changes (e.g., social, political, economic, scientific) on organizational practices
9. Describes ways to improve individual and program performance

Note: Tier 1 competencies apply to public health professionals who carry out the day-to-day tasks of public health organizations and are not in management positions. Responsibilities of these professionals may include data collection and analysis, fieldwork, program planning, outreach, communications, customer service, and program support.

Reproduced from Council on Linkages between Academia and Public Health Practice; 2010.

Other concerns are of more recent vintage. The economic recession of 2008/2009 displaced millions of workers in both the public and private sectors of the economy. State and local governments were especially hard hit, and are recovering slowly. Sources point to the aging of the public health workforce, current shortages of public health nurses and epidemiologists, and the imminent retirement of many public health professionals. On the other hand, national health reform legislation enacted in 2010 included several provisions for stabilizing and strengthening the public health workforce and an increased emphasis on population-focused prevention.

The public health workforce is growing and will continue to grow for years to come. Many public health occupational categories will see a steady increase; others will grow even more rapidly. Core public health practice competencies will increasingly influence education and training programs and hopefully find their way into the human resource activities and personnel systems of governmental public health agencies. Worker recognition initiatives based on relevant competencies, such as credentialing and certification programs, will also grow in order to address the need for both heightened accountability and expanded career pathways.

Although strategies that focus on the pipeline are necessary and useful, they will never be sufficient to ensure an effective public health workforce over the long term. Comprehensive workforce development strategies must focus not only on current and future workers, but also on the organizations in which the work of public health is performed. In the decades that lie ahead, the most important resource and asset of the public health system—its workforce—faces as many challenges as opportunities.

REFERENCES

1. Institute of Medicine, National Academy of Sciences. *The Future of Public Health.* Washington, DC: National Academy Press; 1988.

2. Health Resources and Services Administration, U.S. Department of Health and Human Services. *Public Health Personnel in the United States, 1980: Second Report to Congress.* Washington, DC: U.S. Public Health Service; 1982.

3. Health Resources and Services Administration, U.S. Department of Health and Human Services. *Public Health Workforce Enumeration 2000.* Washington, DC: Government Printing Office; December 2000.

4. Public Health Functions Steering Committee. *Public Health America.* I. Washington, DC: U.S. Public Health Service; 1995.

5. Institute of Medicine, National Academy of Sciences. *Who Will Keep the Public Healthy? Education Public Health Professionals for the 21st Century.* Washington, DC: National Academy Press; 2003.

6. Kennedy VC, Moore FI. A systems approach to public health workforce development. *J Public Health Manage Pract.* 2001; *7:* 17–22.

7. U.S. Bureau of the Census. *Federal, State, and Local Governments, Public Employment and Payroll Data.* Available at www.census.gov/govs/apes/. Accessed June 16, 2014.

8. National Association of County and City Health Officials. *2013 National Profile of Local Health Departments.* Washington, DC: National Association of County and City Health Officials; 2014.

9. Centers for Disease Control and Prevention, National Center for *Health Statistics. Health United States, 2013.* Hyattsville, MD: National Center for Health Statistics; 2014.

10. National Association of County and City Health Officials. *2008 National Profile of Local Health Departments.* Washington, DC: National Association of County and City Health Officials; 2009.

11. Gerzoff RB, Baker EL. The use of scaling techniques to analyze U.S. local health department staffing structures, 1992–1993. *Proceedings of the Section on Government Statistics and Section on Social Statistics of the American Statistical Association.* 1998: 209–213.

12. Thomas JC, Sage M, Dillenberg J, Guillory VJ. A code of ethics for public health. *Am J Public Health.* 2002; *92:* 1057–1059.

13. Gerzoff RB, Richards TB. The education of local health department top executives. *J Public Health Manage Pract.* 1997; *3:* 50–56.

14. U.S. Department of Education, National Center for Education Statistics, Integrated Postsecondary Education Data System (IPEDS), Fall 2010, Completions component. 2011.

15. Turnock BJ. Roadmap for public health workforce preparedness. *J Public Health Manage Pract.* 2003; *9:* 471–480.

16. National Board of Public Health Examiners. Available at http://www.nbphe.org. Accessed June 9, 2014.

17. Bureau of Labor Statistics, U.S. Department of Labor. Available at www.bls.gov. Accessed June 15, 2014.

18. National Association of County and City Health Officials. Local health department job looses and program cuts: Findings from the 2013 Profile study. Washington, DC: NACCHO; 2013.

19. Council of State and Territorial Epidemiologists. *2004 National Assessment of Epidemiologic Capacity: Findings and Recommendations.* Washington, DC: Council of State and Territorial Epidemiologists; 2004. Available at http://www.cste.org/Assessment/ECA/pdffiles/ECAfinal05.pdf. Accessed October 8, 2014.

20. Tilson H, Gebbie KM. The public health workforce. *Ann Rev Public Health.* 2004; *25:* 341–356.

21. Gebbie KM, Turnock BJ. The public health workforce, 2006: new challenges. *Health Aff (Millwood).* 2006, *25:* 923 933.

22. American Medical Association. Editorial. *JAMA.* 1893; *20:* 189.

Managing Public Health Infrastructure

After the violin virtuoso had finished her concert performance and was attempting to slip out of the orchestra hall through the delivery entrance, several adoring fans mobbed her. One particularly aggressive young man pushed his way to the front of the throng and grabbed the musician's hand, shaking it furiously. "Maestro, you played those notes just brilliantly tonight." Taken aback a little by this adulation, the virtuoso replied, "Young man, anyone can play the notes correctly. It's the intervals between the notes that create truly great music." Similar to the maestro's music, public health derives its effectiveness from both its components and how they are blended together. This chapter examines the basic ingredients of public health practice that are integrated and managed to carry out its work.

This ground-level view of public health focuses on infrastructure, a concept that is more readily understood in our everyday lives. When we think of infrastructure, we commonly envision roads, bridges, sewers, power lines, and water supplies. The similarities between these concrete and visible structures in our communities and their counterparts in public health are not so easily appreciated. An analogy might picture the public health infrastructure as a bridge over which trucks delivering public health services must pass, as illustrated in Figure 7-1. Community needs and

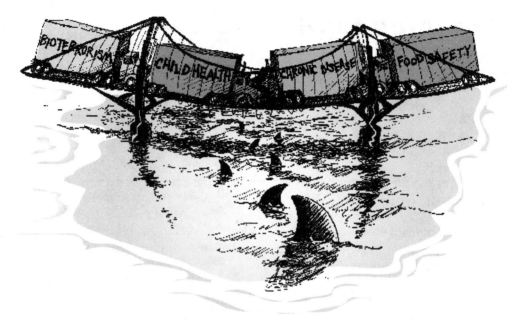

Figure 7-1   Public health infrastructure.

Reproduced from Centers for Disease Control and Prevention, Public Health Practice Program Office, 1999.

expectations are met by using more and bigger trucks to deliver more and better public health services. Yet this example suggests that the infrastructure has limits in terms of its ability to accommodate those trucks, just as the state of the nation's roads, bridges, and tunnels limits the effectiveness of the national transportation system. Attention to the infrastructure is essential for public health services to be delivered effectively.[1] However, there are different views as to what the concept of public health infrastructure actually represents.

Infrastructure has both static and dynamic attributes. In a static representation, such as the bridge described previously, public health infrastructure is the foundation for public health activities; this foundation consists of building blocks and other basic materials. In a more dynamic representation, infrastructure is the capacity or capability of that foundation to serve its purpose. As the virtual nerve center of the public health system, and representing the capacity necessary to carry out public health's core functions and essential services, public health infrastructure is a composite that can be dismantled to reveal its basic building blocks. Both of these views—what the infrastructure is and what the infrastructure does—offer insights into modern public health practice. Importantly, both also portray infrastructure as absolutely necessary in order to effectively carry out public health's mission and purpose.

This chapter examines several important components of the public health infrastructure, focusing on the following questions:

- What are the critical components of public health infrastructure?

- What is the current status of these components?
- How can these components be managed and enhanced to improve the performance of public health organizations and systems?

PUBLIC HEALTH INFRASTRUCTURE COMPONENTS

In simple terms, the public health infrastructure consists of the resources and relationships necessary to carry out the core functions and essential services of public health. Contributing to the system's capacity are human, informational, financial, and organizational resources, including aspects of organizational relationships (such as statutes, leadership, and partnerships) that delineate how these building blocks relate to one another—similar to the intervals between the notes in the virtuoso's music.

Separating the elements of the public health infrastructure into discrete categories is a challenging task. For example, distinguishing between the knowledge and skills of public health workers and the information resources available to them seems arbitrary and may be a distinction without a difference in real-world public health practice. Similarly, financial resources can be considered as system resources or as a metric for measuring the other resources in economic terms or the value society places on its results. Still, it is useful to delineate different dimensions of the public health infrastructure, realizing that they can be lumped, split, or conceptualized in different ways.

Human resources include the workforce of public health and the knowledge, skills, and abilities of public health workers. Key dimensions of this critical resource were examined in the public health workforce chapter. This chapter will focus on the workforce development and workplace management aspects of this infrastructure component. Organizational resources include the relationships among the various system participants—public and private—and the mechanisms that manage and coordinate collective action. These mechanisms include leadership and collaborative components, as well as statutory and governance elements examined in the chapter on governmental public health roles. Information resources include various data, information, and communication systems. Fiscal resources are the funding levels and financial management skills that support the work of public health. Each of these elements contributes to the system's capacity to perform, and each will be examined in the sections that follow. Physical resources, such as equipment and physical facilities, also contribute to the work of public health; however, these are not discussed here.

HUMAN RESOURCES MANAGEMENT IN PUBLIC HEALTH

The people who do the actual work of public health are the most important component—and the most valuable asset—of public health's infrastructure. The size, distribution, composition, skills, practice profiles, growth prospects, and competency frameworks discussed in a previous chapter underscore the value of education and training as an important public health workforce development strategy. Yet, as illustrated in Figure 7-7, education and training are not by themselves sufficient. A complementary set of strategies that promote workforce development through

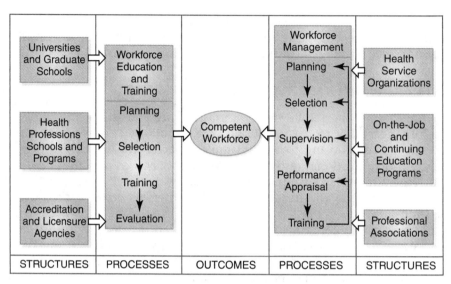

Figure 7-2   Conceptual model for workforce development.

Reproduced from Kennedy VC, Moore FI. A systems approach to public health workforce development. *J Public Health Manage Pract.* 2001;7:17–22. Data from FI Moore, Functional Job Analysis: Guidelines for Task Analysis and Job Design. World Health Organization, Geneva, 1999.

human resources and workplace management activities is also necessary.[2] Workplace management strategies continuously assess and promote competent performance in the context of the organization's mission and objectives. Figure 7-2 suggests that separate workforce development subsystems contribute to workforce development— one focusing on education and training strategies and the other emphasizing workplace management strategies. Yet each subsystem plans and manages its activities separately. One produces potential workers identified by occupational and professional labels; the other places workers into job titles and positions that serve the needs of the organization. But occupational categories and job titles are imprecise vehicles for achieving their intended ends. Ultimately, the common denominator for public health workers and the public health workforce is the job and work performed to accomplish public health goals. A common conceptual framework for work-doing that links the worker, work, and work setting can effectively merge the strategies across these subsystems to achieve their common goals. This merger offers a common conceptual basis and language organized around critical skills and core competencies that drive both training and workplace management activities. The work to be done, consistent with the public heath core functions and essential services framework, the expected level of performance, and the technologies employed must all contribute to this common culture and language.[3]

In this scenario, critical skills and core competencies are the organizing principles for education and training interventions while, at the same time, they are promoted in the workplace through job descriptions with performance standards and performance appraisals. Managers and supervisors help to guide the professional development of workers and build skills that are necessary for career advancement.

These administrative and personnel policies promote a culture that values competent performance and the mastery of new skills.

A complementary strategy to promote workforce competency relies on external bodies to validate and recognize skill levels through professional credentialing programs. Credentials distinguish someone who is recognized for a particular status from others who are not. Identifying individuals who have demonstrated practice-relevant competencies at a specified level (such as frontline workers, senior professionals, specialists, and leaders) provides an incentive for individuals to enhance their skills. Health professions take various approaches to credentialing that include licensing, certification, and registration. For example, physicians and nurses are licensed, paramedics and laboratory workers are certified, and dieticians are registered. Public health disciplines and occupations also seek various forms of credentialing. For example, public health nutritionists may earn the registered dietitian credential, public health nurses can earn certification in community health nursing, public health educators may become certified health education specialists, public health physicians may achieve board certification in preventive medicine and public health, and several different credentials are available to environmental health practitioners. With discipline-specific credentials available to many public health worker occupational categories, it is not surprising that a more general, common credential would emerge to serve those who do not qualify for these profession-specific credentials. A common public health credential would also establish a basic level of general expertise across multiple professional and occupational categories in the public health workforce. Such a credentialing process was initiated in 2008 by the Board of Public Health Examiners, which offers a credential (CPH: Certified in Public Health) for graduates of master's in public health degree programs based on a national test.[4] By 2015, several thousand public health professionals had attained the CPH credential.

For workers to value credentials and the competencies on which they are based, employers and health agencies must value them and base decisions about hiring, promotion, salaries, and the like on an individual worker's acquisition and demonstration of those competencies. In sum, improving workers' ability to perform their job functions competently relies on both worker training and work-management strategies.[2,3] As performance standards for public health organizations and public health systems gain headway through initiatives such as the Public Health Accreditation Board, competency-based performance standards for workers will increasingly be viewed as key ingredients of both workforce development and organizational performance.

ORGANIZATIONAL MANAGEMENT IN PUBLIC HEALTH

Organizational resources in public health include the complex web of federal, state, local, and tribal health agencies and their public, private, and voluntary sector partners and collaborators. Before collaboration patterns are addressed, several organizational aspects of public health organizations merit discussion.

Organizational Aspects of Public Health Systems

Organizations are groups of individuals linked by common goals and objectives. Each organization has a specific mission or purpose, resources appropriate to work toward that purpose, the ability to determine progress toward its goals and objectives, and a defined process for making decisions that change the direction or speed of the organization in pursuit of its goals. Each organization takes on a structure to delegate its activities to specific units or individuals and to coordinate the tasks among them. Communication pathways facilitate the accomplishment of the organization's goals and objectives. In one respect, communication channels define the organization, even as the organizational structure defines the communication pathways. A variety of forces shape an organization's ability to survive and thrive in a changing environment. These include the organization's vision, mission, and leadership, as well as key aspects of its operations, such as planning, collaboration, and communications. The specifics of these organizational arrangements are best left to texts in health administration and organizational behavior; only selected issues are addressed in this section.

Public sector organizations differ in many important respects from their private and voluntary sector counterparts. The most obvious, and perhaps most important, difference is apparent in their bottom lines. The bottom line of public health organizations is measured in health and quality of life outcomes, with efficiency valued but not nearly as highly. For the private sector, the bottom line is often profits and customer satisfaction, with efficiency and effectiveness viewed as means to those ends. Many community and voluntary organizations address missions that resemble those of public organizations; however, public sector organizations often have political and bureaucratic environments that are unique among organizations.

The presence of a civil service-based workforce in many public health agencies is often cited as an impediment to getting things done, although the real problem may be more related to inadequate management practices than to institutionalized inertia. Civil service personnel systems were established in state and local governments, in large part through personnel standards fostered by Maternal and Child Health funding associated with the enactment of Title V of the Social Security Act in 1935. Although the initial intent was to provide added security for government workers, there has been long-standing discontent with the system and tension and conflict between government workers and elected officials ever since.

For many years, public health organizations operated under a command-and-control approach to management. If a problem was assigned to the public health organization, it sought to acquire the resources needed to deal with that problem. Resources were deployed directly from the organization; this approach worked well when the major problems called for environmental engineering solutions or communicable disease control expertise. As problems became more complex, encroaching on the territory of other health and human service agencies, command-and-control approaches brought only limited success. To resolve delicate turf issues, cooperation with other agencies and collaborative approaches began to supplement more centrally controlled strategies.

External collaborations added to the challenges facing public agency managers as they also grappled with promoting worker efficiency and effectiveness. Management training has never been well supported in the public sector, certainly not to the extent that it has been in the private sector. As a result, public health organizations often are poorly managed; this generates tensions and conflicts between professional staff and administrators brought into an agency to maximize efficiency

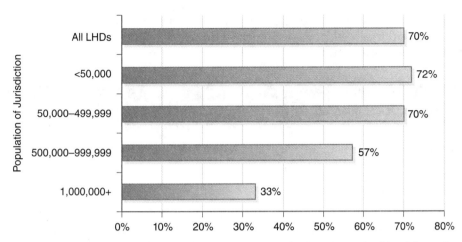

Figure 7-3   Percentage of local health departments with a local board of health in the jurisdiction, by size of population served, United States, 2013

Data from National Association of County and City Health Officials. *2013 National Profile of Local Health Departments.* Washington, DC: NACCHO; 2014.

and effectiveness, as well as between the organization and its community collaborators. For example, there has been a declining proportion of local health department (LHD) heads with medical degrees. For larger health departments (especially those serving populations of 100,000 or more), this trend is partly explained by the employment of nonphysician executives to manage the increasingly complex array of community and clinical services. Clinical professionals in health departments have not always adjusted well to these changes, and the result sometimes takes the form of management and morale problems.

Public health agencies at the state and local levels often have governing or advisory boards to guide their efforts. Seventy percent of LHDs reported the presence of a local board of health in the 2013 National Association of County and City Health Officials' profile, with a notably higher prevalence in smaller local health jurisdictions (see Figure 7-3). Over recent decades, boards have assumed roles less involved with direct agency operations than when initially established. Agency leadership today provides the lion's share of the direction of professional staff, while boards have focused on roles such as approving regulations, advising/approving agency budgets, and hiring the agency director. The role of many local boards of health has shifted from directing to advising the agency, prompting debate as to their role in the modern practice of public health. Nonetheless, public health agencies often have a plethora of advisory boards and committees developed for specific programs or activities. Although the proliferation of these advisory bodies can be seen as unwieldy and sometimes conflicting with the roles of more formally established bodies, such as the board of health itself, these groups also serve to expand participation and communication with professional constituencies. Even when superfluous from a management perspective, these can often be effective constituency-building strategies. Boards of health and various forms of advisory committees provide a link between the organization and the community it serves. Agency and community interests are better served by fostering the utilization of these relationships than by limiting or eliminating them.

OUTSIDE-THE-BOOK THINKING 7-1

How have the roles of local boards of health changed over the past century? What would be the most useful roles for such boards today?

Within public health agencies, leadership positions carry several different responsibilities. The leader manages the agency, interacts with the major stakeholders and constituency groups, and carries out some largely ceremonial functions. The specific authorities of the agency are vested in its director through statutes or ordinances. Within state and LHDs, there has been a steady move away from physician directors of agencies; only one in eight LHDs report having a chief executive officer who holds a medical degree. An evolving literature on leadership is developing within the public health community. The Centers for Disease Control and Prevention (CDC) have established a national public health leadership institute, and nearly two dozen regional and state-based leadership development initiatives were in place in 2014.

Leadership development programs are often organized around concepts such as envisioning the future, inspiring others to act, and generally acting through others. Leadership in public health, however, involves more than individual leaders or individuals in leadership positions. Public health is intimately involved in leadership, serving as an agent of social change by identifying health problems and risks and stimulating actions toward their elimination. Because the work of public health emphasizes both collective and individual leadership, the battery of leadership principles and practices is pertinent throughout public health organizations and systems. In many respects, the tools necessary for 21st-century community public health practice are tools of and for public health leadership.

Nongovernmental organizations have played major roles in public health activities since 1900. As the national network of federal, state, and local public agencies expanded and government assumed more responsibility for health issues, it often assimilated public health initiatives that were developed and supported by nongovernmental organizations. The modern public health system truly represents the work of both government and nongovernmental organizations. Several examples bolster this claim. The Rockefeller Sanitary Committee's Hookworm Eradication early in the 20th century stimulated the development of LHDs; other foundations sponsored health department development and medical education reform. The National Tuberculosis Association worked for tuberculosis (TB) prevention and treatment. The National Consumers League championed maternal and infant health initiatives in the 1920s. In the mid-20th century, the American Red Cross supported nutrition programs and the March of Dimes led the national effort to develop and deploy a successful polio vaccine. In the latter decades of the 20th century, Mothers

Against Drunk Driving grew into a national campaign for stronger laws against drunk driving. Professional organizations and labor unions also worked to promote public health. The American Medical Association advocated better vital statistics and safer foods and drugs. The American Dental Association endorsed water fluoridation, despite the economic consequences to its members. Labor organizations supported safer workplaces in industry. Today, nongovernmental organizations sponsor diverse public health service and research programs, including family planning, human immunodeficiency virus (HIV) prevention, violence prevention, vaccine development, and heart disease and cancer prevention.

Coalitions and Consortia

An increasingly important amalgamation of organizational resources is reflected in collaborative links among various agencies and organizations. Often, these arrangements are described as coalitions or consortia, although other terms are frequently used, and distinctions are often blurred.[5] Coalitions can be formed for short-term efforts or established to address ongoing problems on a long-term basis. They are most likely to be successful when they include representation from all groups affected by a problem and active in efforts to deal with that problem. In general, coalitions and consortia are formal partnerships involving two or more groups working together to achieve specific goals according to a common plan. The rationale for a consortia approach is that the goals are believed to be beyond the capacity of any one participating organization. Goals can take various forms, from communication among members, to public and professional education, to advocating and lobbying for particular policy changes. It is essential that coalition members be in agreement that the problem is best addressed through a coalition approach and that they be comfortable with the scope of activities planned. Building on mutual interests allows a coalition to place expectations and demands on its member organizations.

There are many advantages to working through coalitions and consortia. Collaborative efforts can function more efficiently than single organizations because work plans are shared among collaborating organizations rather than carried out by a single group. This serves to conserve limited resources and provides a pathway for reaching a larger part of the community. When organizations band together around specific goals, their efforts carry greater credibility than when only one or a few organizations are involved. Collaborative efforts are also excellent mechanisms for ensuring a broad range of inputs and perspectives into the policy development process and for facilitating communication and information across agencies and organizations. This offers the added benefit of helping staff from one organization to view problems and possible solutions from a broader perspective than their usual vantage point. By building trust and personal relationships around one issue, collaborative approaches facilitate future collaborations around other issues.

There are no set rules for developing coalitions and consortia, but some general principles and approaches are useful after the decision is made to use a collaborative approach (see Table 7-1). That decision may come from a lead agency determining that a coalition would facilitate achievement of some goal or, in some instances, being required to establish one by a funding organization. On other occasions, an organization may be requested by community leaders or other agencies to organize a

Table 7-1   Key Steps for Coalitions and Other Collaborative Organizations

Step 1: Analyze the program's objectives and determine whether to form a coalition.
Step 2: Recruit the right people.
Step 3: Develop a set of preliminary objectives and activities.
Step 4: Convene the coalition.
Step 5: Anticipate the necessary resources.
Step 6: Define the elements of a successful coalition structure.
Step 7: Maintain coalition vitality.
Step 8: Make improvements through evaluation.

   Data from Contra Costa County Health Services Department Prevention Program. *Developing Effective Coalitions: An Eight Step Guide.* Martinez, CA: Contra Costa County Health Department; 1994.

collaborative effort. Unmet community needs, scandals, and service breakdowns all serve to promote the development of coalitions, as do both informal and formal ties that exist among members.

   Most coalitions have an agency or organization that leads the effort. Lead agencies must have both the credibility and the resources necessary for a coalition to succeed. If it is determined that a coalition is the best mechanism to address a particular goal, the resources needed from the lead agency and other coalition members should be assessed to determine whether the coalition represents the best use of those resources to accomplish that goal. This requires examination of objectives and implementation strategies that might facilitate achievement of the coalition's goals. A range of implementation strategies is available to coalitions, including making advocacy efforts to influence policy and legislation, changing organizational behavior, promoting networks, educating providers, educating the community, and increasing individual knowledge and skills. One or more implementation strategies should be adopted by the coalition on the basis of how well these fit with the community's strengths and weaknesses.

OUTSIDE-THE-BOOK THINKING 7-2

Which factors determine the optimum size for a coalition?

   After the decision is made to develop a coalition, recruitment of the appropriate members is necessary to advance the process. Questions to be addressed include whether membership will consist of individuals or organizations and, if the latter, who should represent a particular organization on the coalition. In some cases, it is desirable to have agency leaders; in others, lower-level staff more familiar with the issues and programs may make better members. The size of the coalition also requires careful consideration. After these issues are decided, preliminary objectives and work plans are developed, and the coalition is convened. At this point, the role of the lead agency in chairing or staffing the coalition should be determined, and resources needed to carry out the coalition's work plan should be identified and made available. Early decisions of the coalition should establish its expected life span, criteria for membership and decision making, and expectations for participation at and between meetings. Constant vigilance is necessary to identify problems internal to the coalition's operation. These can include a loss of interest and participation from some members, tension and conflict over power and leadership of the coalition, a lack of community representativeness, and turnover of coalition members. Frequently, coalition members perceive threats to their organizational autonomy or come to disagree about service priorities or, more specifically, about which members will provide specific services.

Careful assessment of a coalition's strengths and weaknesses, together with a commitment to make a good process even better, is often necessary to maintain the vitality and momentum of even the best coalition. Many of these steps and issues appear to be straightforward and noncontroversial until they are addressed within the context of an actual coalition experience. In virtually all instances, however, coalitions rely on information as well as relationships to achieve their ends.

INFORMATION MANAGEMENT IN PUBLIC HEALTH

In addition to human and organizational resources, information and evidence is a key component of public health infrastructure. The information resources that support public health practice include both the scientific basis of public health and the mountains of data and information needed to assess and address health problems. To some degree, the knowledge base is captured in the competencies for public health professionals across a broad range of analytical, communication, policy development and planning, cultural, basic public health science, and management skills. Although this knowledge base is provided through undergraduate and graduate-level public health education, it can also be acquired through other educational, training, and experiential opportunities.

Information resources to carry out the activities of public health are increasingly abundant and accessible. Several important principles that underlie the effective use of information sets in public health are highlighted in Table 7-2.[6] The need to ensure both flexibility and compatibility within information systems creates a tension that is not always readily resolved. This is apparent in the two general categories of data sets commonly used in public health practice: population- and encounter-based data. It is important to recognize their differences, although there is often great value in using both categories to identify and address health problems.

Encounter- or service-based data are collected for a variety of purposes, including reimbursement, eligibility, and evaluation of care. These data sets are common to programs that provide primary or episodic healthcare services; nutrition services for women, infants, and children; mental health and substance abuse treatment; and many other services. Data and information are collected for individual recipients of these services, which may include important clinical preventive services, such as immunizations or cancer screening. Aggregate data from these service encounters provide useful information on health needs and the health status of a population, including program coverage and penetration rates; however, the population

Table 7-2   Principles of Public Health Information

1. Recognize different types of data: encounter-based data on individuals as they encounter providers and universal data on populations from surveys and environmental monitoring systems.
2. Provide for integrated management to improve meeting individual needs and to portray fully individual participation in multiple, categorical programs.
3. Maintain a service orientation to address the overriding concern of public health information systems.
4. Ensure flexibility so as to adapt to differences in data collection resources at the local level while accommodating data needs to support a broad range of public health programs and objectives.
5. Achieve system compatibility to allow data flow and functioning across systems in a fully compatible fashion.
6. Protect confidentiality to provide better service and to preserve privacy.

Data from Lumpkin JR. Six principles of public health information. *J Public Health Manage Pract.* 1995; 1: 40–42.

is limited to those seeking services and may not be representative of the larger population.

Another category of data describes populations rather than individuals. Examples include national surveys of health status and service utilization, as well as behavioral risk factor surveys of the population that collect information on population samples (composed of individual respondents) that are representative of the entire population. For these data sets, a population is described through the use of sampling techniques. Other data sets capture information on specific health events and outcomes for a defined population, such as cancer incidence registries and vital records systems. For these, data are collected on individuals and aggregated in comparison with a reference population, often derived from census information (e.g., the rate of newly diagnosed lung cancers among women aged 45 to 64 years in a state). Data sets that describe risks or hazards common to a population, such as environmental monitoring data, also contribute to population-based data.

The limitations of encounter-based information systems are apparent when individuals participate in more than one service program. A prenatal care program may have its own information system; the women, infants, and children program serving the same person may have another system; and the lead screening program yet another. The communicable disease program may have separate systems for general communicable diseases, HIV infections, TB, and sexually transmitted diseases. Beyond these health information systems, an individual may also be receiving services from other agencies for mental health, substance abuse, spousal abuse, and Medicaid. Information systems are often problem specific, but individuals generally have multiple problems. Integration of information systems across the entire spectrum of human services programs and needs is essential both to promote efficiency in programs and to characterize the health status and needs of individuals and populations.

Confidentiality and privacy issues pose special challenges for information systems. Federal and state statutes for the collection, sharing, and confidentiality of health statistics may make it impossible for individuals to be identified unless they have consented. Disclosure of personal identifiers should be permitted only to government entities or research projects with written agreements to protect the confidentiality of the information or to a governmental entity for the purpose of conducting an audit, evaluation, or investigation of the agency.

Information and Analytic Techniques

The capacity of the public health system to effectively use information expanded exponentially during the 20th century. Advances occurred in both study design and periodic standardized health surveys. Methods of data collection evolved from simple measures of disease prevalence, such as field surveys, to more complex studies and precise analyses, such as case-control studies, cohort studies, and randomized clinical trials. The first well-developed, longitudinal cohort study was conducted in 1947 among the 28,000 residents of Framingham, Massachusetts, many of whom volunteered to be followed over time to determine incidence of heart disease. The Framingham Heart Study has served as a model for other longitudinal cohort studies, advancing understanding of the multiple risk factors that contribute to disease. The age of modern clinical trials began in 1948 with a study of streptomycin therapy for TB; this study involved randomization, selection criteria, predetermined evaluation criteria, and ethical considerations. In 1950, the first convincing evidence of an association between lung cancer and tobacco use was provided in a case-control study, adding credibility to this important study design. Subsequently, sophisticated statistical tests and analytic computer programs enabled multiple variables collected in large-scale studies to be measured and tools to be developed for mathematical modeling. These advances contributed to the elucidation of risk factors for heart disease and other chronic diseases and the development of effective interventions.

OUTSIDE-THE-BOOK THINKING 7-3

Which factors limit our ability to use the extensive amount of data and information that is currently available? How can these obstacles be overcome?

The first periodic standardized health surveys in the United States began in 1921. In 1935, the first national health survey was conducted among U.S. residents. In 1956, these efforts culminated in the National Health Survey, a population-based survey that evolved from focusing on chronic disease to estimating disease prevalence for major causes of death, measuring the burden of infectious diseases, assessing exposure to environmental toxicants, and measuring the population's vaccination coverage. Other population-based surveys, such as the Behavioral Risk Factor Surveillance System, Youth Risk Behavior Survey, and the National Survey of Family Growth, were developed to assess risk factors for chronic diseases and other conditions. Survey methods used in epidemiologic studies were enhanced by new approaches to sampling and interviewing developed by social scientists and statisticians.

Information and the Assessment Function of Public Health

Information drives the public health core function of assessment in at least three ways.[7] First, public health agencies commonly use surveillance data to monitor community health status and trends and to identify any new health risks or hazards. Second, after health needs and problems are identified, information is needed on the community's resources that are available to address those needs and problems and on the effectiveness of those interventions. Third, information from assessments of health needs and current efforts must be tailored to the needs of decision and policy makers to facilitate more effective interventions. Data sources for the various facets of the assessment function monitor health status and risk factors, identify and evaluate resources, and inform and advise managers, policy makers, and the public. These interrelated purposes demonstrate that information is a critical public health practice resource in applications involving surveillance, planning processes, selection of scientifically based interventions, and health communications.

Information and Surveillance

Public health surveillance activities monitor health status and risk factors in the population. Although surveillance data sets have become both more sophisticated and more accessible in recent years, the most important consideration for their establishment relates to why and how they will be used.

Health data in the United States benefit from national enumerations of the population that are conducted every 10 years. The decennial census was established to ensure fair representation in the U.S. Congress but now also serves as an important source of demographic information on the population. National disease monitoring was first conducted in the United States in 1850 when the federal government began publishing mortality statistics based on death registrations. In the late 19th century, Congress authorized the collection of morbidity reports on cholera, smallpox, plague, and yellow fever for use in quarantine measures and provided funding to expand weekly reporting from states and municipal authorities. The first annual summary of notifiable diseases appeared in 1912, with reports of 10 diseases from 19 states, the District of Columbia, and Hawaii. By 1928, all states were reporting on 29 diseases. In 1950, state and territorial health officers authorized the Council of State and Territorial Epidemiologists to determine which diseases should be reported to the U.S. Public Health Service. The CDC assumed responsibility for collecting and publishing national data on notifiable diseases in 1961. As of 2014, more than 60 infectious diseases were notifiable at the national level (see Table 7-3).

Numerous sources of data are available for epidemiologic surveillance data. These range from well-known data sets, such as birth and death records, to lesser known and used sources, such as school and work absenteeism reports. Several important data sources are operated through the CDC's National Center for Health Statistics, which maintains systems for the following:

- Vital Statistics (births, deaths, fetal deaths, induced abortions, marriages, divorces, follow-back surveys to gather additional information)
- National Health Interview Survey (amount, distribution, and effects of illness and disability, using a multistage probability sample)

Table 7-3   Nationally Notifiable Infectious Diseases, United States, 2014

Anthrax
Arboviral diseases, neuroinvasive and non-neuroinvasive
Babesiosis
Botulism
Brucellosis
Chancroid
Chlamydia trachomatis infection
Cholera
Coccidioidomycosis
Congenital syphilis
Cryptosporidiosis
Cyclosporiasis
Dengue virus infections
Diphtheria
Ehrlichiosis and anaplasmosis
Giardiasis
Gonorrhea
Haemophilus influenzae, invasive disease
Hansen's disease
Hantavirus pulmonary syndrome
Hemolytic uremic syndrome, post-diarrheal
Hepatitis A, acute
Hepatitis B, acute
Hepatitis B, chronic
Hepatitis B, perinatal infection
Hepatitis C, acute
Hepatitis C, past or present
HIV infection (AIDS has been reclassified as HIV Stage III)
Influenza-associated pediatric mortality
Invasive pneumococcal disease
Legionellosis
Leptospirosis
Listeriosis
Lyme disease
Malaria
Measles
Meningococcal disease
Mumps
Novel influenza A virus infections
Pertussis
Plague
Poliomyelitis, paralytic
Poliovirus infection, nonparalytic
Psittacosis
Q fever
Rabies, animal
Rabies, human
Rubella
Rubella, congenital syndrome

(continues)

Table 7-3   Nationally Notifiable Infectious Diseases, United States, 2014 (*Continued*)

Salmonellosis
Severe acute respiratory syndrome–associated coronavirus disease
Shiga toxin-producing *Escherichia coli*
Shigellosis
Smallpox
Spotted fever rickettsiosis
Streptococcal toxic-shock syndrome
Syphilis
Tetanus
Toxic shock syndrome (other than streptococcal)
Trichinellosis
Tuberculosis
Tularemia
Typhoid fever
Vancomycin-intermediate *Staphylococcus aureus* and Vancomycin-resistant *Staphylococcus aureus*
Varicella
Varicella deaths
Vibriosis
Viral hemorrhagic fever
Yellow fever

Data from Centers for Disease Control and Prevention, 2014.

- National Medical Care, Utilization, and Expenditure Survey (use of and expenditures for medical services, conducted in 1980 but not repeated since)
- National Ambulatory Medical Care Survey (location, setting, and frequency of ambulatory care encounters)
- National Health and Nutrition Examination Survey (direct physical, physiologic, and biochemical data from a national sample)
- National Hospital Discharge Survey (characteristics of patients, lengths of stay, diagnoses, procedures, and patterns of patient use by type of hospital)

Surveillance is multifaceted in that information is collected at a variety of levels. Surveillance information used in environmental public health applications illustrates this point. For any environmental agent that is considered to be a hazard, surveillance efforts can measure its effects at various steps in its chain of causation. For example, the agent's presence in the environment can be assessed, and its route of exposure can be measured through surveillance efforts that can be considered hazard surveillance. Beyond hazard surveillance, exposure surveillance can track actual exposures between the host and agent, the frequency in which the agent reaches its target tissue, and the early production of adverse effects. In addition, outcome surveillance can measure the actual adverse effects after these become clinically apparent. Together, these three levels of surveillance activities provide a more complete picture of the problem and allow for a more rational strategy for its control and for evaluating whether control strategies are working.

Most data sets are neither complete nor completely accurate. Each has problems and issues related to completeness, accuracy, and timeliness. For example, key denominator information provided through census enumerations undercounts important subpopulations that are often at greater risk of adverse health effects. Even the data set often considered to be the most complete—birth and death records—includes some important data elements that are underreported or inaccurately recorded, including maternal behaviors, length of gestation, and congenital anomalies of newborn infants. Death records also suffer from variability in determining cause of death and, specifically, in identifying true underlying causes, such as tobacco or alcohol.

Vital records represent yet another example of an important federal health policy being operationalized through the states; there is no national mandate for uniform reporting of births and deaths. Through a voluntary and cooperative effort with the states, a national model of these records is implemented by the states and localities, stimulated in part by federal grants for a national cooperative health statistics system.

Access to information and data for surveillance purposes has improved steadily with advanced technology for electronic management and transfer. Today, reports including a mix of text, tables, and figures are available from an increasing number of federal and state sources through a variety of electronic modes, especially via the World Wide Web. Surveillance systems are a major component of the public health preparedness activities that are described in a separate chapter.

Information and Planning

Although there are various forms of planning, each relies heavily on data and information resources. In public health, planning information is widely employed for purposes of community health planning, agency strategic and operational planning, and program planning and management.

The community health planning role is new for many local governmental public health agencies. From the mid-1960s through the mid-1980s, community health planning was carried out through a national program of state and local planning agencies. The Comprehensive Health Planning Act of 1966 and the National Health Planning and Resource Development Act of 1974 established the framework for these structures and activities. At the state level, state health departments generally coordinated the development of state health plans, in part through the generation of local health plans. These local plans were developed by agencies known as health systems agencies, whose role was to organize and coordinate community participation in the development and implementation of the local plans. In large part, this form of planning focused on resources within the health system, assessing the availability of facilities, health manpower, and specific services. Where resources were lacking, plans were established to increase supply. Where resources were underused, plans sought to increase demand. As consumer majorities sat on planning boards at both the state and local levels, the focus was on resource planning rather than on needs-based planning.

Largely because of their focus on resources, inability to effectuate change, and widespread provider resentment of consumer-dominated processes, political support for this effort waned, and the federal program was repealed. Very soon thereafter most of the local health planning agencies also disappeared, leaving a significant void. LHDs, with a few exceptions, had not been very involved in community health planning and found it difficult to pick up the slack. LHDs often lacked staff with the skills and expertise in community health planning: Many information sources resided at levels of government outside their direct control, and they simply did not see it as part of their job description at a time when demands for serving the uninsured and addressing the AIDS epidemic were at their doorsteps. These factors contributed to the need for the development of tools such as APEXPH (Assessment Protocol for Excellence in Public Health) and MAPP (Mobilizing for Action through Planning and Partnerships), the Planned Approach to Community Health, Model Standards, and the series of national *Healthy People* initiatives described in other chapters.

OUTSIDE-THE-BOOK THINKING 7-4

Is health planning at the community level necessary? If so, who should be responsible? How can duplication and replication of community health planning be averted?

The framework of planning objectives in the *Healthy People* process promoted greater consistency among state health plans. Most states use measures drawn directly from the *Healthy People* process; however, this also led states to replicate the lack of emphasis on mental health, substance abuse, environmental health, and occupational health issues that have marked the earlier iterations of *Healthy People*. In some states, these objectives are addressed in separate planning processes or not at all. States found that baseline data were generally available for state planning efforts modeled on *Healthy People 2020*, but they also found that such data were far less available at the county, city, or neighborhood levels. Planning efforts relied heavily on vital records and, to a lesser extent, on behavioral risk factor and notifiable disease data. Only infrequently were sources such as youth behavioral surveys, hospital discharge data, or morbidity data used in state planning processes during the early 2000s. Stimulated by renewed interest in community-level health planning in the latter part of the decade, however, this situation has gradually improved.

APEXPH/MAPP and other community needs assessment processes call for a variety of mortality, morbidity, and risk factor information, as well as data and information on available resources to address priority health problems. Information describing the health status and needs of the local population is often available from federal and state sources, but more frequently, these sources must be supplemented with more locally developed information. The lessons from earlier attempts at consumer-directed local health planning demonstrate that community health planning is as much a political process as it is an objective process based on statistical data. Diversity in values and perspectives within a community cannot be homogenized through the use of what so-called experts consider objective data. These past failures make it all the more difficult for LHDs seeking to reenter this minefield.

Information resources also support the strategic and operational planning activities of an organization. Strategic planning, as examined in the discussion of 21st-century community public health practice, seeks to identify external and internal trends that might influence the agency's ability to carry out its mission and role. Operational planning looks to maximize the use of available resources to achieve particular objectives that have been established for a specific period of time, generally 1 to 2 years.

At the heart of public health interventions for improving the quality of life and reducing preventable mortality and morbidity are scientifically sound strategies and approaches. Although the scientific basis for public health interventions has always been highly valued, the formal application of rigorous assessments to the evidence for effectiveness is a relatively new undertaking for public health. Considerable progress has been made on this front since 1990. The program management chapter discusses the principles, strategies, and tools that will drive public health interventions in the early 21st century.

FISCAL MANAGEMENT IN PUBLIC HEALTH

The financial resources available for public health activities can be viewed as both inputs and outcomes of the system. They are clearly inputs in that they represent an economic measure of the human, organizational, and informational resources described in this chapter, as well as the physical facilities, equipment, and other inputs that do not fit nicely into any of the other categories. The financial resources provided for public health activities, however, also represent the perceived worthiness or value of these activities in comparison with other public policy goals. In this light, financial resources are a product of public health activities and an expression of their value in the eyes of society. In either interpretation, however, it is useful to quantify their levels and assess changes over time.

Fiscal Dimensions of the Public Health System

It is challenging to link financial expenditures directly to the core functions and essential public health services (EPHS) framework. As we have seen in previous chapters, the essential public health services framework includes both population-based and personal health activities. The public sector sponsors many but not all of the activities included in the essential public health services framework. Some personal health services provided through public sector resources fall into the essential public health services framework, such as those assuring the provision of care when otherwise unavailable, while others do not. In the public sector, agencies other than official health agencies provide essential public health services. For example, mental health, substance abuse, environmental protection, and emergency management agencies contribute as well. As a result, the essential public health services framework is not easily delineated and measured through the use of financial and accounting systems. Although precise determinations may not be possible, current national health expenditure tracking systems allow for reasonable approximations of public health activity expenditures in the United States.

The economic dimensions of the U.S. health system merit repeating here, including total national health expenditures ($3 trillion in 2015) and the amount identified for government public health activities ($75 billion in 2012).[8] The government public health activity category captures much of the nation's spending for essential public health services, although there are additional essential public health service activities imbedded in several other government-sponsored programs and in entities outside government altogether. Examples of the latter include public information and education campaigns of voluntary health organizations such as heart, lung, cancer, and diabetes associations. Examples of the former include maternal and child health programs, environmental health activities, school health, and mental health, alcohol, and substance abuse programs operated by federal and state agencies. These activities are included in categories other than the public health activity category of the national health accounts.

Adjustments to the total government public health activity spending figures are necessary to approximate essential public health services expenditures. The rationale for computing an adjusted total government public health activity spending level is that several important public health programs and services that fall within the essential public health services framework are not captured in the government public health activity category. These include maternal and child health services, mental health, substance abuse prevention, and environmental protection activities, all of which contribute to the spectrum of essential public health services in many communities.

An important subset of both public health activity and essential public health services expenditures support population-based public health activities, which are activities directed toward the community or an entire population rather than toward specific individuals. Population-based public health activities are a core component of the public health system. Although there is no agreed-upon method for calculating population-based public health expenditures, several sources estimate it to be approximately one-fourth of essential public health services spending, or about 1% of total national health expenditures.[9–12] The largest share (approximately 70%) of essential public health services spending supports personal healthcare activities to link individuals to healthcare services and to provide such services if otherwise unavailable.

An assessment of essential public health services spending in Florida for 2005–2006 demonstrated similar findings. Expenditures for enabling access and assuring care (EPHS 7) comprised 69% of state and local public health spending, with the remaining 31% split among the other nine essential public health service categories. Federal sources supported the majority of expenditures only for EPHS 7. Federal and state–local sources equally shared the burden for mobilizing partnerships (EPHS 4), while state–local sources supported the majority of spending for the other eight essential public health service categories. Figure 7-4 summarizes these findings.[13]

More than two-thirds of population-based service expenditures in the states are derived from nonfederal sources, reinforcing the observation that state and local governments bear the brunt of the burden for funding public health activities in the United States. Who currently pays the bills says much about the likelihood for expansion of public health efforts in the future. Shrinking tax bases of state and local governments, and mounting political opposition to tax increases of any kind do not augur well for future increases in state and local public health resources.

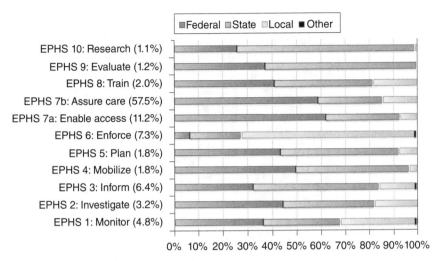

Figure 7-4 Federal, state, local, and other funds supporting essential public health services, Florida, 2005–2006

Data from Brooks RG, Beitsch LM, Street P, Chukmaitov A. Aligning public health financing with essential public health service functions and national health performance standards. *J Public Health Manage Pract.* 2009;15(4):299–306

These expenditure estimates for essential public health services, public health activity, and population-based services fail to capture public health spending by nongovernmental public health agencies. It is estimated that nongovernmental organizations are responsible for approximately one-fourth to one-third of the total performance of essential public health services in the community.[14] This important contribution to the national public health effort is often overlooked and underappreciated.

Based on 2012 data, Figure 7-5 and Table 7-4 summarize estimates of the fiscal resources supporting public health core functions and essential services, using the findings and assumptions described in this section. All factors considered, a reasonable estimate is that approximately $120 billion—or 4.3% of national health expenditures—supported activities related to public health core functions and essential services in 2012. About $25 to $30 billion funded population-based services, and the remaining $90 to $95 billion supported personal care. This amounts to less than $100 per person per year (or about $0.25 per person per day) for population-based services and about $380 per person per year (or just over $1.00 per person per day) for the entire package of essential public health services. Public health's infrastructure serves the U.S. population for less than the cost of one can of cola per day.

Financial Management in Public Health

Financial management skills are important in all organizations, especially for midlevel and senior managers. Key financial management skills for public health professionals and managers include understanding and constructing budgets,

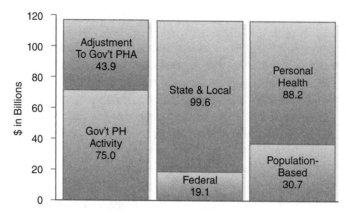

Figure 7-5   Estimated total essential public health services-related expenditures by funding category, source, and type of service, United States, 2012

Governmental public health activity and adjustment to governmental public health (see text for programs included). Data from Centers for Medicare and Medicaid Services, Office of the Actuary, National Health Statistics Group.

interpreting financial data and communications, and assessing and correcting an organization's financial status.[15]

Budgets are financial tools for systematically converting the objectives of an organization into plans for acquiring revenues and controlling expenditures. Most organizations utilize several different types of budgets. An operating or cash budget identifies anticipated revenues and expenditures and, for some organizations,

Table 7-4   Estimated Expenditures for Essential Public Health Services, by Source of Funds, United States, 2012

	Federal	*State and Local*	*Total*
Governmental public health activity	$10.8 B	$64.1 B	$75.0 B
Additional governmental public health spending (maternal and child health, substance abuse, mental health, school health, other state and local)	$8.3 B	$35.5 B	$43.9 B
Total public health spending	$19.1 B	$99.6 B	$118.9 B
Population-based public health activity component of total EPHS expenditures			$30.7 B
Personal health component of total EPHS expenditures			$88.2 B

Note: Dollars in billions (B)

Governmental public health activity and adjustment to governmental public health (see text for programs included). Data from Centers for Medicare and Medicaid Services, Office of the Actuary, National Health Statistics Group.

borrowing and lending needs. Separate budgets for revenues and expenditures contribute to the overall operating budget. Accounts receivable are an especially important component of an organization's revenue as they represent expected or anticipated revenue that is not yet available as cash. Health and human service providers often carry substantial levels of account receivables while waiting for government agencies to reimburse for services already rendered. This can place a significant cash flow burden on an organization, requiring that it borrow money to meet payrolls, pay bills, and invest in growth opportunities. A capital budget for an organization plans income and expenditures related to long-term assets such as buildings, vehicles, and sophisticated equipment.

Several examples of financial management tools are offered here as tables. Table 7-5 provides an example of a budget request for a new project. Table 7-6 presents an example of an annual budget for an organization, and Table 7-7 is

Table 7-5   Budget Request Example

Name of Project Date Proposed Budget (based on a 12-month budget)	
A. Direct Salaries and Wages *Personnel* Position title and name • Annual salary • Percent time on project • Months on project • Funding request for this position • Justification for each position	Total $ XXXX
B. Direct Staffing Fringe Benefits *Direct Staffing Fringe Benefits* Agency fringe benefit rate X total direct salaries.	Total $ XXXX
C. Consultants *Consultant Costs* This category is appropriate when hiring an individual or organization to give professional advice or services (training, expert consultant, etc.) for a fee but not as an employee of the grantee organization. • Name of consultant • Organizational affiliation • Nature of services to be rendered • Number of days of consultation (basis for fee) • Expected rate of compensation (travel, per diem, other related expenses; list a subtotal for each consultant in this category) • Method of accountability If this information is unknown for any consultant at the time the application is submitted, the information may be submitted at a later date as a revision to the budget. In the body of the budget request, a summary justification should be provided of the proposed consultants and amounts for each.	Total $ XXXX

(continues)

Table 7-5   Budget Request Example *(Continued)*

D. Equipment *Equipment Requested* • Identify each different equipment type • Number • Unit cost • Subtotals • Justification	Total $ XXXX
E. Supplies *Consumable Supplies Requested* • Identify each different type of consumable supplies • Number • Unit cost • Subtotals • Justification	Total $ XXXX
F. Travel Dollars requested in the travel category should be staff travel only. Travel for consultants should be shown in the consultant category. In-state travel and out-of-state travel should be calculated separately. • Persons and cost per trip for in-state travel • Persons and cost per trip for out-of-state travel with assumptions for type of travel, accommodations, daily allowance (per diem) costs, registration fees, etc. • Justification	Total $ XXXX
G. Other This category contains items not included in the previous budget categories, such as telephone, postage, and printing. Individually list each item requested and provide appropriate justification related to the project objectives. Some of these may be self-explanatory (telephone, postage, rent) unless the unit rate or total amount requested is excessive. If not, include additional justification. For printing costs, identify the type and number of copies of documents to be printed (e.g., procedure manuals, materials for marketing campaign).	Total $ XXXX
H. Contractual Costs A summary should be provided for each proposed contract and the subtotal for each. • Name of contractor • Method of selection • Period of performance • Scope of work • Method of accountability • Itemized budget and justification	Total $ XXXX
I. Total Direct Costs Sum all of the direct cost categories.	Total $ XXXX
J. Total Indirect Costs Indicate the method of calculating indirect costs (e.g., indirect costs = x% of direct costs).	Total $ XXXX
K. Grand Total Requested Sum the total direct and indirect cost categories.	Total $ XXXX

Table 7-6 Annual Budget Example

	1st Quarter	2nd Quarter	3rd Quarter	4th Quarter	TOTAL
Revenue					
Grants	245,000	205,000	233,000	225,000	908,000
Contracts	159,000	180,000	165,000	175,000	679,000
Other	74,000	69,000	80,000	77,000	300,000
Total revenue	478,000	454,000	478,000	477,000	1,887,000
Expenditures					
Payroll wages	283,050	282,825	282,825	283,300	1,132,000
Payroll taxes	35,192	16,217	35,217	34,142	120,768
Fringe	64,158	64,158	64,158	64,158	256,632
Total payroll	382,400	363,200	382,200	381,600	1,509,400
Consultants and Contracts					
Audit	7,875	7,875	7,875	7,875	31,500
Attorney fees	2,397	2,397	2,397	2,397	9,588
Other	1,050	1,050	1,050	1,050	4,200
Total consultants and contracts	11,322	11,322	11,322	11,322	45,288
Travel					
Local	2,256	2,256	2,256	2,256	9,024
Out-of-town	2,372	2,373	2,372	2,372	9,489
Total travel	4,628	4,629	4,628	4,628	18,513
Space					
Rent	22,500	22,500	22,500	22,500	90,000
Heat	8,719	2,718	2,719	8,719	22,875
Utilities	4,781	4,783	4,782	4,779	19,125
Total space	36,000	30,001	30,001	35,998	132,000
Equipment					
Copy rental	3,503	3,503	3,503	3,503	14,012
Postage	3,497	3,497	3,497	3,497	13,988
Repair/replace	2,436	2,437	2,435	2,432	9,740
Total equipment	9,436	9,437	9,435	9,432	37,740
Consumables					
Office supplies	2,307	2,020	2,711	2,307	9,345
Training supplies	2,411	2,700	2,016	2,408	9,535
Total consumables	4,718	4,720	4,727	4,715	18,880
Other					
Postage	2,340	2,230	2,301	2,300	9,246

(continues)

Table 7-6   Annual Budget Example   (*Continued*)

	1st Quarter	2nd Quarter	3rd Quarter	4th Quarter	TOTAL
Telephone	3,205	3,107	3,072	3,125	12,509
Insurance	8,047	8,102	8,275	8,101	32,525
Dues/subscriptions	2,102	2,307	2,237	2,115	8,761
Staff development	1,985	1,573	1,705	1,640	6,903
Security	2,300	2,304	2,301	2,303	9,208
Miscellaneous	1,871	2,148	2,059	2,019	8,097
Total other	21,850	21,780	21,950	21,669	87,249
Unapplied					
Contingency	9,435	9,435	9,435	9,435	37,740
Total unapplied	9,435	9,435	9,435	9,435	37,740
TOTAL	479,789	454,524	473,698	478,799	1,886,810
(SURPLUS DEFICIT)	−1,789	−524	4,302	−1,799	190

Table 7-7   Quarterly Budget Report Example

	Budget	Actual	Variance
Revenue			
Grants	245,000	243,000	−2,000
Contracts	159,000	161,000	2,000
Other	74,000	73,000	−1,000
Total revenue	478,000	477,000	−1,000
Expenditures			
Payroll wages	283,050	284,725	−1,675
Payroll taxes	35,192	36,633	−1,441
Fringe	64,158	63,051	1,107
Total payroll	382,400	384,409	−2,009
Consultants and Contracts			
Audit	7,875	7,875	0
Attorney fees	2,397	2,397	0
Other	1,050	1,075	−25
Total consultants and contracts	11,322	11,347	−25

Table 7-7   Quarterly Budget Report Example (*Continued*)

	Budget	*Actual*	*Variance*
Travel			
Local	2,256	1,974	282
Out-of-town	2,372	1,841	531
Total travel	4,628	3,815	813
Space			
Rent	22,500	22,500	0
Heat	8,719	8,821	−102
Utilities	4,781	4,870	-89
Total space	36,000	36,191	−191
Equipment			
Copy rental	3,503	3,521	−18
Postage	3,497	3,394	103
Repair/replace	2,436	2,064	372
Total equipment	9,436	8,979	457
Consumables			
Office supplies	2,307	2,170	137
Training supplies	2,411	2,314	97
Total consumables	4,718	4,484	234
Other			
Postage	2,340	2,299	41
Telephone	3,205	3,303	−98
Insurance	8,047	7,798	249
Dues/subscriptions	2,102	2,012	90
Staff development	1,985	1,500	485
Security	2,300	2,270	30
Miscellaneous	1,871	1,953	−82
Total other	21,850	21,135	715
Unapplied			
Contingency	9,435	8,527	908
Total unapplied	9,435	8,527	908
TOTAL	479,789	478,887	902
(SURPLUS DEFICIT)	−1,789	−1,887	−98

an example of a quarterly budget report for this same organization. Public health professionals should be able to construct a simple budget and identify problems and issues in their agency's overall operating budget and periodic budget reports.

PERFORMANCE MANAGEMENT IN PUBLIC HEALTH

Effective and successful public health organizations track the work they produce and the results they achieve—the basic definition of performance measurement. These organizations then build on performance measurement activities to achieve internal quality improvement goals and to demonstrate accountability to external stakeholders. Performance management integrates an organization's use of standards, measurement, and performance improvement to change institutional capacities, processes, and priorities and to more effectively address the needs of the communities they serve. A growing compendium of practical tools is emerging to assist organizations in institutionalizing performance management strategies and activities. The Public Health Accreditation Board's recently launched voluntary national health department accreditation program (discussed in a previous chapter) takes a giant step toward greater deployment of quality improvement strategies that can strengthen organizational performance and enhance public accountability.

Public health leaders and managers face issues related to performance at many different levels, including the performance of individuals, programs, agencies, inter-organizational collaborations, and the overall public health system itself. Although these levels represent different dimensions of public health performance, each can be assessed using common approaches that focus on the work produced and the results achieved. Performance measurement is an important management tool with an impressive record of improving performance throughout the public, voluntary, and private sectors. These accomplishments derive from fundamental principles of improvement science: To improve something we must be able to control it; to control it we must be able to understand it; and to understand it we must be able to measure it.[16]

Drawing on a growing body of literature and practical tools, the Turning Point Performance Management National Excellence Collaborative delineated four key elements of managing public health performance.[17,18] The collaborative viewed performance management as the active use of performance data in making management decisions, integrating four fundamental components:

1. Applying appropriate standards: the identification and establishment of organizational or system performance standards, targets and goals, and relevant indicators
2. Actually measuring key aspects of performance: the application and use of performance indicators through appropriate data collection and information management practices
3. Reporting and interpreting measurements: documentation and reporting of progress toward meeting standards and targets and sharing of such information through feedback
4. Making changes based on information derived from measuring performance (quality improvement): establishment of a program or process to manage

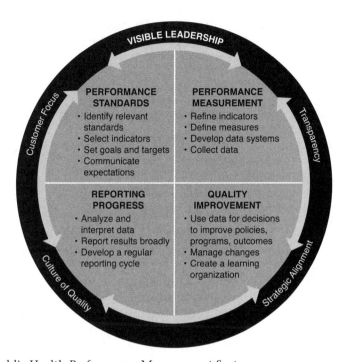

Figure 7-6 Public Health Performance Management System

Reproduced from Public Health Foundation, Turning Point: Performance Management Project and Publications. Available at www.phf.org. Accessed September 12, 2014.

change and achieve quality improvement based on performance standards, measurements, and reports

The performance management model illustrated in Figure 7-6 integrates these fundamental components into a coherent model for understanding and managing complex public health programs, organizations, and systems. Key organizational characteristics supporting successful performance management initiatives include visible leadership, alignment with strategic intent, customer focus, a quality of culture within the organization, and transparency and are also integrated into this model.[19]

Performance measurement lies at the heart of this framework. Performance measurement is the selection and use of quantitative measures to reflect critical aspects of activities, including their effect on the public and other public health customers. Stated simply, it is the regular collection and reporting of data to track work that is performed and results that are achieved.

An effective performance measurement process incorporates stakeholder input; promotes top leadership support (enhancing an organizational culture of quality improvement); creates a clear mission statement; develops long-term goals and objectives; formulates short-term goals and interim measures; devises simple, manageable approaches, and provides support and technical assistance to those involved in the process. In this light, performance measurement serves several important purposes, providing information concerning the capacity to perform, results of current efforts, and effectiveness of current performance. Potential organizational benefits from measuring performance include the following:

- Clear goals and objectives
- Identification of strengths and weaknesses
- Opportunities for collaborative approaches internally and externally
- Clearer lines of accountability
- Improved quality
- Better tracking of progress over time
- More effective communication
- Better resource allocation and deployment
- Strengthened organizational effectiveness

Performance measurement focuses on what is occurring, but it does not extensively address why or how. Evaluative research (often called program evaluation) provides more in-depth assessment of the conceptualization, design, implementation, and utility of interventions. Performance measurement can be viewed as one component of a comprehensive evaluation, but its primary purpose is to inform managers so that changes can be instituted within the life cycle of a set of activities. In sum, performance measurement is a management and oversight tool to facilitate positive change and improvement in performance.

The terminology used in performance measurement can be inconsistent and confusing. In general, a performance measure is the specific quantitative representation of a capacity, process, or outcome that is deemed relevant to the assessment of performance. In public health, performance measurement most frequently occurs within the context of a particular program (e.g., childhood immunizations or retail food safety). However, the performance of an agency (e.g., a state or local health department), partnership, or community public health system are also appropriate targets of performance measurement. In public health practice, the term *performance measurement* characterizes the selection and use of quantitative measures of public health system capacities, processes, and outcomes to inform public health leaders and managers and the public about critical aspects of public health performance.

Performance measures that are used to determine whether or to what extent a performance standard is achieved are often called performance indicators. For example, a performance standard might call for a comprehensive community health assessment to be completed every 3 years. Performance indicators for this standard could take one of several forms. The administrator of the local public health agency could be asked whether this standard was met, or more objectively a review team might look for a completed assessment at the time of a site visit as empirical evidence. The agency administrator's response (yes or no) and the actual document are both performance indicators in this example and serve as evidence to determine whether the standard has been achieved. The quality and usefulness of performance indicators rely on several key attributes, including validity, reliability, specificity, credibility, understandability, availability, and potential for misuse. The interaction between performance standards and performance measures is captured in the first two quadrants of the performance management framework described earlier.

Performance measures provide useful information concerning the capacity to perform, process performance (including outputs), and ultimate results (effect/outcomes). Useful individually, performance measures provide richer information when multiple dimensions are measured and related to one another. For example, relating capacities to outcomes (such as the cost effectiveness or cost per case of disease prevented) is a common approach to assessing the effectiveness of an activity or intervention. Similarly, measures relating capacities to processes (as in the cost per unit of service delivered) provide useful insights into efficiency. Ideally, measuring and relating measures for all of these dimensions provide the most useful information for improving performance.

OUTSIDE-THE-BOOK THINKING 7-5

What are the ultimate performance measures for a public health organization? Would they differ from the ultimate performance measures for a state–local public health system?

Performance measurement and performance improvement initiatives proliferated in the public sector in the final decades of the 20th century, fueled, in part, by the potential for improving the quality of public programs and services. Federal agencies have been subject to the Government Performance and Results Act since the mid-1990s; state and local governments have adopted a variety of accountability systems.[20,21] Likewise, performance measurement has gained widespread acceptance in the health sector among both public and private sector organizations. Similarly, accreditation programs based on principles of performance measurement are in place for a wide variety of healthcare organizations and settings, including community networks providing health services.

Paralleling these developments, specific interest in performance measurement within the public health system matured steadily during the 20th century, especially after the Institute of Medicine's sentinel 1988 report, *The Future of Public Health*.[22] This interest was advanced by aspirations of improving quality, enhancing accountability, and strengthening the science base of public health practice, embracing challenges articulated in *The Future of Public Health*.[23-25]

HEALTHY PEOPLE 2020 PUBLIC HEALTH INFRASTRUCTURE OBJECTIVES

Only 1 of the more than 500 national health objectives included in the *Healthy People 1990* and *Healthy People 2000* processes directly addressed the national public health infrastructure. That objective (from *Healthy People 2000*) called for 90% of the population to be served by an LHD that was effectively carrying out public health's core functions. The pursuit of this objective during the 1990s focused attention on the infrastructure capacity that must be in place for this target to be achieved. As a result, a more comprehensive panel of objectives related to the public health infrastructure was established for the *Healthy People 2010* and *2020* national health objectives (see Table 7-8). These infrastructure objectives address the workforce,

Table 7-8   *Healthy People 2020* Public Health Infrastructure Objectives

Workforce

1. Increase the proportion of federal, tribal, state, and local public health agencies that incorporate the core competencies for public health professionals into job descriptions and performance evaluations.
2. (Developmental) Increase the proportion of tribal, state, and local public health personnel who receive continuing education consistent with the core competencies for public health professionals.
3. Increase the proportion of Council on Education for Public Health (CEPH)-accredited schools of public health, CEPH-accredited academic programs, and schools of nursing (with a public health or community health component) that integrate the core competencies for public health professionals into curricula.
4. Increase the proportion of 4-year colleges and universities that offer public health or related majors and/or minors.
5. (Developmental) Increase the proportion of 4-year colleges and universities that offer public health or related majors and/or minors that are consistent with the core competencies of undergraduate public health education.
6. Increase the proportion of 2-year colleges that offer public health or related associate degrees and/or certificate programs.

Data and Information Systems

1. Increase the proportion of population-based *Healthy People 2020* objectives for which national data are available for all major population groups.
2. Increase the proportion of *Healthy People 2020* objectives that are tracked regularly at the national level.
3. (Developmental) Increase the proportion of *Healthy People 2020* objectives for which national data are released within 1 year of the end of data collection.
4. Increase the number of states that record vital events using the latest U.S. standard certificates and reports.

Public Health Organizations

1. Increase the proportion of tribal and state public health agencies that provide or assure comprehensive laboratory services to support essential public health services.
2. Increase the proportion of public health laboratory systems (including state, tribal, and local) that perform at a high level of quality in support of the 10 essential public health services.
3. Increase the proportion of tribal, state, and local public health agencies that provide or assure comprehensive epidemiology services to support essential public health services.
4. Increase the proportion of state and local public health jurisdictions that conduct a public health system assessment using national performance standards.
5. (Developmental) Increase the proportion of tribal, state, and local public health agencies that have implemented a health improvement plan and increase the proportion of local health jurisdictions that have implemented a health improvement plan linked with their state plan.
6. (Developmental) Increase the proportion of tribal, state, and local public health agencies that have implemented an agency-wide quality improvement process.
7. (Developmental) Increase the proportion of tribal, state, and local public health agencies that are accredited.

Data from U.S. Dept. of Health and Human Services. *Healthy People 2020 Public Health Infrastructure Objectives.* Available at http://www.healthypeople.gov/2020/topicsobjectives2020/objectiveslist .aspx?topicId=35. Accessed September 11, 2014.

organizational, and informational dimensions of the public health infrastructure described in this chapter.[26] Several of these objectives are identified as "developmental," which indicates the lack of national baseline data at the beginning of the decade and the need for the development of data collection and tracking systems. The inability to develop information systems to track progress for the majority of the public health infrastructure objectives for 2010 suggests that the national agenda for measuring and strengthening the public health infrastructure has a long way to go.[27]

OUTSIDE-THE-BOOK THINKING 7-6

Review the *Healthy People 2020* national health objectives for the public health infrastructure. Identify the one that should be the highest priority. Justify your selection.

CONCLUSION

Public health infrastructure includes the inputs and ingredients of the public health system that are blended together to carry out public health's core functions and essential public health services. Although these can be lumped and split in a variety of ways, several key elements are easily recognized. The first of these is the workforce of public health, an army of individuals committed to improving population health, although relatively few have had other than on-the-job training for their roles. The diversity of this workforce in terms of educational and experiential backgrounds represents both a major strength and a potential weakness to focus and direct their collective efforts. Facilitating the contributions of the workforce are the organizations in which they work. These organizations exist at all levels of government, as well as in all sectors of the community. The relationships between and among the agencies, organizations, institutions, and individuals committed to this work are more often informal and collaborative than formalized and centrally directed. Leadership within and across organizations to assess and address health issues and needs in the community is essential to initiate the community problem identification and problem-solving activities that can foster the changes necessary for improved health outcomes. The workforce, the organizations, and their leadership rely heavily on information for identifying problems, determining interventions, and tracking progress toward agreed-upon objectives. Information also drives the human resources management, financial management, and performance management activities of public health organizations and systems. Together, these essential ingredients of the public system formulate the system's capacity to act in serving the public health. The public health infrastructure has evolved to provide the elements necessary for successful public health interventions: organized and systematic observations through morbidity and mortality surveillance, well-designed epidemiologic studies and other data to facilitate the decision-making process, and individuals and organizations to advocate for resources and to ensure that effective policies and programs were implemented and conducted properly. In the 21st century, public health is a complex collaboration among federal, state, and local governments, nongovernmental organizations, and community members. This infrastructure, and the essential public health services that it provides, represents a small portion of the national economy and only approximately 3% to 5% of all health-related expenditures, but its contribution to improved health status and its potential for realizing further gains and closing current gaps suggest that it is worth its weight in gold.

REFERENCES

1. Roper WL, Baker EL, Dyal WW, et al. Strengthening the public health system. *Public Health Rep.* 1992; *107*: 609–615.

2. Kennedy VC, Moore FI. A systems approach to public health workforce development. *J Public Health Manage Pract.* 2001; *7*: 17–22.

3. Moore FI. *Functional Job Analysis: Guidelines for Task Development and Job Design.* Geneva, Switzerland: World Health Organization; 1999.

4. National Board of Public Health Examiners. *CPH: Certified in Public Health.* Available at https://www.nbphe.org/getcertified.cfm. Accessed September 22, 2014.

5. Cohen L, Baer N, Satterwhite P. *Developing Effective Coalitions: An Eight Step Guide.* Martinez, CA: Contra Costa County Health Services Department; 1994.

6. Lumpkin JR. Six principles of public health information. *J Public Health Manage Pract.* 1995; *1*: 40–42.

7. Keppel KG, Freedman MA. What is assessment? *J Public Health Manage Pract.* 1995; *1*: 1–7.

8. Centers for Disease Control and Prevention, National Center for Health Statistics. *Health, United States, 2013.* Hyattsville, MD: National Center for Health Statistics; 2014.

9. Sensenig AL. Refining estimates of public health spending as measured in national health expenditure accounts: the United States experience. *J Public Health Manage Pract.* 2007; *13*: 103–114.

10. Eilbert KW, Barry M, Bialek R, et al. *Measuring Expenditures for Essential Public Health Services.* Washington, DC: Public Health Foundation; 1996.

11. Eilbert KW, Barry M, Bialek R, et al. Public health expenditures: developing estimates for improved policy making. *J Public Health Manage Pract.* 1997; *3*: 1–9.

12. Barry M, Centra L, Pratt E, et al. *Where Do the Dollars Go? Measuring Local Public Health Expenditures.* Washington, DC: Public Health Foundation; 1998.

13. Brooks RG, Beitsch LM, Street P, et al. Aligning public health financing with essential public health service expenditures and national public health performance standards. *J Public Health Manage Pract.* 2009; *15*(4): 299–306.

14. Mays GP, Miller CA, Halverson PK, et al. Availability and perceived effectiveness of public health activities in the nation's most populous communities. *Am J Public Health.* 2004; *94*: 1019–1026.

15. Costich JF, Honore PA, Scutchfield FD. Public health financial management needs: report of a national survey. *J Public Health Manage Pract.* 2009; *15*(4): 307–310.

16. Harrington HJ. *The Improvement Process: How America's Leading Companies Improve Quality.* New York: McGraw-Hill; 1987.

17. Turning Point Program National Office. *Performance Management in Public Health: A Literature Review.* Seattle, WA: Turning Point; 2002.

18. Turning Point Program National Office. *From Silos to Systems: Using Performance Management to Improve the Public's Health.* Seattle, WA: Turning Point; 2003.

19. Public Health Foundation. *Turning Point: Performance Management Project and Publications.* Available at http://www.phf.org/resourcestools/Pages/Turning_Point_Project_Publications.aspx. Accessed September 12, 2014.

20. Wholey J, Newcomer K. Clarifying goals, reporting results. *New Direct Eval.* 1997; *75*: 91–98.

21. Perrin EB, Durch JS, Skillman SM, eds. *Health Performance Measurement in the Public Sector: Principles and Policies for Implementing an Information Network*. Washington, DC: National Academy Press; 1999.

22. Institute of Medicine. *The Future of Public Health*. Washington, DC: National Academy Press; 1988.

23. Perrin EB, Koshel JJ, eds. *Assessment of Performance Measures for Public Health, Substance Abuse, and Mental Health*. Washington, DC: National Academy Press; 1997.

24. Office of Disease Prevention and Health Promotion. *Enabling Performance Measurement Activities in the States and Communities*. Seattle: University of Washington, School of Public Health and Community Medicine; 1998.

25. Durch JS, Bailey LA, Stoto MA, eds. *Improving Health in the Community: A Role for Performance Monitoring*. Washington, DC: National Academy Press; 1997.

26. U.S. Department of Health and Human Services. *Healthy People 2020*. Washington, DC: U.S. Department of Health and Human Services; 2010.

27. U.S. Department of Health and Human Services. *Healthy People 2010: Mid-Course Review, Chapter 23, Public Health Infrastructure*. Washington, DC: U.S. Department of Health and Human Services; 2006.

Chapter 8

Managing Public Health Interventions

LEARNING OBJECTIVES

Given a prevalent public health problem (disease or condition), develop a strategy for designing, implementing, and evaluating an evidence-based intervention. Key aspects of this competency expectation include being able to:

- List general categories of public health programs and services.
- Describe the difference between community prevention and clinical preventive services.
- Describe the major steps in the planning, implementation, and evaluation of a public health program.
- Describe how and when planning and evaluation occur during the life of a program.
- Define and develop outcome, impact, and process objectives.
- Describe the relationships among activities, process measures, impact measures, and outcome measures in the evaluation of a program.
- Explain the difference between doing things right and doing the right things within the context of a public health intervention.

Public health practice affects everyone in the community in one way or another. Still, the image that the public most commonly associates with public health is the provision of medical care—mostly treatment—to low-income populations. Although this image is understandable, for public health professionals, it is disconcerting.

There are several reasons why this image is prevalent. Many people equate public health with what public health agencies do, and public sector agencies play an important safety-net role in serving individuals who otherwise lack access to care. This vital safety-net role often overshadows the population-based activities of these agencies. In fact, the major share of public health resources supports personal care as opposed to population-based interventions.

Public perceptions as to the primary products of public health practice differ from those of most public health practitioners who believe that population-based interventions are the heart and soul of public health practice, however, public

---

233

health professionals also know that public health is broader than what public health agencies do and that both the public and private sectors provide preventive as well as treatment interventions.

Preventive interventions that target individuals are considered clinical prevention; those that target populations are considered community prevention. Although population-based prevention is usually ascribed to public sector efforts, this should not imply that disease prevention and health promotion are offered only through the public sector or that future shifts in the level and proportion of these strategies offered by public and private providers are unlikely; however, the public appears to understand and highly value personal care, both curative and preventive. Its understanding of population-based interventions is much less complete, although public opinion polls provide evidence that these interventions are also highly valued.

Just as people wish to be known as much for their aspirations as for their deeds, public health seeks to be identified with the wide variety of strategies that promote, protect, and maintain health. These strategies, in the form of various interventions, are often organized as programs. Programs represent identifiable products of the public health system's functioning. This chapter examines various forms of public health interventions, as well as key steps in their planning, development, and evaluation. Key questions addressed in this chapter include the following:

- What are the important interventions and programs of public health?
- Which characteristics distinguish clinical preventive interventions from population-based interventions?
- How are public health interventions planned and evaluated?

INTERVENTIONS, PROGRAMS, AND SERVICES

The outcomes of the public health system result from carrying out the system's important processes. The important processes of public health, embodied in the essential public health services framework, affect outcomes both directly and indirectly. They directly affect outcomes by identifying important health problems and mobilizing efforts to address those problems. Interventions occur in a variety of forms, including statutes, regulations, policies, and programs intended to improve health status. Many interventions are organized into programs consisting of component processes that together seek to achieve specific outcomes. In this light, public health processes contribute to both the generation and operation of programs. As such, programs are understandable and useful constructs that link public health practice with specific outcomes.

Programs are collections of activities that have common objectives; lumping and splitting otherwise discrete programs can result in different formulations. For example, measles immunizations and measles surveillance can be considered as either separate programs or as components of a single program, depending on the formulation of their program objectives. A separate measles immunization program might have an objective to achieve a 90% immunization rate among 2- to 3-year-old children in a particular community. A separate measles surveillance program's objective might be to investigate newly reported cases of measles within 48 hours. Both of these could be considered as part of a more comprehensive measles prevention and control program whose objective might be stated as seeking a reduction in the incidence of measles by some percentage from the current rate.

Programs also provide an understandable framework for describing the scope and content of public health practice and for cataloging public health expenditures. Organizations generally develop budgets and track expenditures on a program-by-program basis. As a result, information on the economic dimensions of public health programs is available at a variety of levels. Nevertheless, public health practice is more than an aggregation of programs, and public health organizations are more than 40 different companies under one roof, as one health officer described his agency in the early 1990s before reengineering the agency from a program focus to one emphasizing public health's core functions.

Programs and their component processes are sometimes referred to as services if some benefit is bestowed on the individual or groups targeted for those interventions. Other processes of programs may be performed to support the provision of services. Some public health services, such as childhood immunizations, can be classified as clinical services if directly aimed at protecting or improving individual well-being. Others, such as the fluoridation of public water supplies, can be considered population-based services if directed toward a group of individuals or the entire population.

This connotation of services represents one aspect of what programs do, although programs are often known for the services that are provided through them. For example, immunization programs are commonly thought of as vaccinations given to individuals, although the actual shots given represent only one activity of that program. Public education, provider education, outreach, compliance determination, recordkeeping, and follow up are also activities of immunization programs. Together, these make up a program whose best known services are vaccinations. The terms *programs* and *services* are often used interchangeably when public health activities are reported. The use of the term *services* in the essential public health services framework further muddies the water because these are not services in the same way as the clinical preventive and population-based services described previously.

Data from the National Association of County and City Health Officials' (NACCHO) profiles of local health departments (LHDs) provide one measure of the prevalence of public health activities and services as well as the level of involvement by LHDs.[1] Table 8-1 summarizes information from NACCHO's 2013 survey as to the prevalence of specific public health activities and services in jurisdictions served by LHDs. The percentage of jurisdictions in which a particular activity or service is available does not imply that the LHD is the entity providing that service. A variety of configurations are possible: the LHD directly providing the service; the LHD contracting with another organization to provide the service; the LHD both directly providing and contracting for the service; another local governmental agency providing the service; a state agency providing the service; multiple governmental agencies providing the service; nongovernmental organizations providing the service; or the LHD and nongovernmental organizations providing the service.

The services most frequently provided directly by LHDs are highlighted in Figure 8-1. These include a variety of immunization, infectious disease prevention and control, and environmental health activities. Nutrition services and school and day care inspections are also among the most frequently provided services by LHDs.

Table 8-1 Public Health Activities and Services Provided by Local Health Departments (LHDs), United States, 2013

Category	Provided by 0–39% of LHDs	Provided by 40–59% of LHDs	Provided by 60–79% of LHDs	Provided by 80–100% of LHDs
Immunizations				• Adult immunizations • Childhood immunizations
Screening for diseases and conditions	• Cardiovascular disease	• Cancer • Diabetes • HIV/AIDS	• High blood pressure • Blood lead • Sexually transmitted diseases	• Tuberculosis
Communicable disease treatment	• HIV/AIDS	• Sexually transmitted diseases	• Tuberculosis	
Maternal and child health	• Early Periodic Screening, Diagnosis, and Treatment services • Obstetrics • Prenatal care • Well child care	• Family planning	• Women, Infants, and Children Program • Maternal and child health home visits	
Other health services	• Behavioral and mental health • Home health • Oral health • Substance abuse			
Population-based primary prevention services	• Injury • Mental illness • Substance abuse • Violence	• Chronic disease • Physical activity • Unintended pregnancy	• Nutrition and obesity • Tobacco use	
Surveillance and epidemiology	• Behavioral risk factors • Injury	• Chronic disease • Syndromic surveillance	• Environmental health • Maternal and child health	• Communicable and infectious diseases

Table 8-1 Public Health Activities and Services Provided by Local Health Departments (LHDs), United States, 2013 (*Continued*)

Category	Provided by 0–39% of LHDs	Provided by 40–59% of LHDs	Provided by 60–79% of LHDs	Provided by 80–100% of LHDs
Environmental health	• Air pollution • Collection of unused pharmaceuticals • Hazardous waste disposal • Hazmat response • Indoor air quality • Land use planning • Pollution prevention • Noise pollution • Radiation control • Surface water protection	• Groundwater protection • Vector control	• Food safety education	
Regulation, inspection, and/or licensing	• Cosmetology businesses • Health-related facilities • Food processing • Housing inspections • Milk processing • Mobile homes • Public drinking water • Solid waste haulers • Solid waste disposal • Tobacco retailers	• Campgrounds and RVs • Hotels and motels • Lead inspection • Private drinking water • Public swimming pools • Septic tank installation • Schools and day care centers • Smoke-free ordinances	• Food service establishments	
Other public health activities	• Animal control • Asthma prevention and/or management • Correctional health • Emergency medical services • Laboratory services • Medical examiner's office • Occupational safety and health • School-based clinics • School health • Veterinary public health	• Outreach and enrollment for medical insurance • Vital records		

Data from the National Association of County and City Health Officials. *2013 National Profile of Local Health Departments*. Washington, DC: NACCHO; 2014.

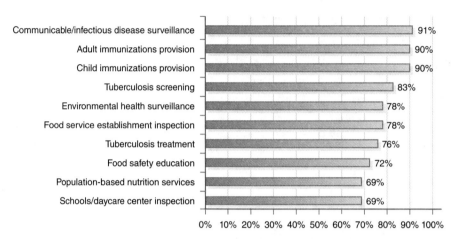

Figure 8-1   The 10 activities and services provided by the largest percentage of LHDs.

Data from National Association of County and City Health Officials. *2013 National Profile of Local Health Departments*. Washington, DC: NACCHO; 2014.

Figure 8-2 identifies the most frequent public health activities that are provided through a contract involving the LHD and another entity. Although increasing somewhat in recent years, the level of contracting for public health activities is far below that of the LHD directly offering these services. Laboratory services are the only public health activity for which contracting is used in more than 10% of jurisdictions.

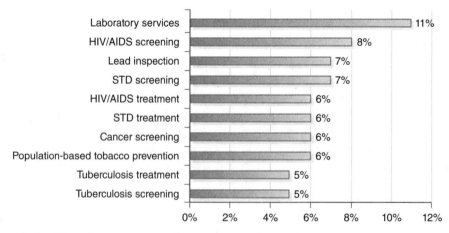

Figure 8-2   The 10 activities and services performed under contract by the largest percentage of LHDs.

Data from National Association of County and City Health Officials. *2013 National Profile of Local Health Departments*. Washington, DC: NACCHO; 2014.

Public health activities and services can also be provided by other local governmental agencies. Animal control, land use planning, hazmat response, and emergency medical services lead this list with more than half of jurisdictions relying on a local governmental agency other than the health department for these services.

OUTSIDE-THE-BOOK THINKING 8-1

What are some important factors in a community that determine which public, voluntary, or private sector organizations provide specific public health programs and services?

Nongovernmental agencies also play major roles in providing a variety of public health activities and services in the community. These agencies are especially critical for comprehensive primary care, obstetrical care, home health services, oral health care, mental health, and substance abuse services.

There are many different combinations and permutations of service delivery from one community to another. These patterns also change over time, with LHDs today more likely to provide surveillance for behavioral risk factors, injuries, and communicable diseases than 20 years ago.[1,2] Notably, LHDs are now less likely to offer laboratory services; home health care; animal control; Early Periodic Screening, Diagnosis, and Treatment services; prenatal care; and public drinking water protection services. Several recent trends explain the lower levels of involvement of LHDs in many of these activities. One is that fewer LHDs are now involved in providing clinical services as other healthcare providers have become more engaged with serving low-income populations through expansions of Medicaid eligibility and State Children's Health Insurance Programs. Another trend is the increased involvement of nongovernmental organizations in addressing community health problems as a result of the growth and maturation of community-wide planning initiatives.

Categorizing the Programs and Services of Public Health

Aggregating programs into categories that focus on broad outcomes provides additional insights into the products of public health practice. External audiences who think of public health in terms of programs and services, rather than internal processes, readily understand this approach. The mega-outcome categories included in the Public Health in America statement (discussed in previous chapters) represent what public health does and offer a clear and comprehensive aggregation of the aspirations of the public health system to do the following:[3]

- Prevent epidemics
- Protect the environment, workplaces, housing, food, and water
- Prevent injuries
- Promote healthy behaviors
- Respond to disasters
- Ensure the quality, accessibility, and accountability of health services

Each of these categories includes a mixture of preventive interventions targeted both to populations and to individuals. Preventing epidemics includes efforts such as disease surveillance, disease investigation, contact tracing, case management, prophylactic treatment, laboratory services, and immunizations. Environmental protection includes air and water quality monitoring and permitting, food, housing and workplace safety standards enforcement, toxic waste permitting and hazardous conditions monitoring, environmental risk assessment services, toxicology evaluation services, laboratory services, and enforcement activities. Injury prevention includes injury surveillance, trauma network services, public education and awareness campaigns, child car seat loaner programs, and so forth. Promoting healthy behaviors includes behavioral risk factor monitoring, fitness programs, comprehensive school health education, worksite health promotion, community-wide risk reduction programs, media involvement, health education, parenting education, and information clearinghouses and other referral sources. Disaster response includes disaster planning, emergency medical system maintenance, trauma networks, disaster management drills, and emergency information system establishment. Ensuring the quality, accessibility, and accountability of health services can include health professions licensing and certification, medical facilities licensing and certification, laboratory services quality assurance, hospital outcomes monitoring, personal services outcomes monitoring, personal services availability assessment, patient satisfaction assessment, cost-effectiveness studies, and automated and linked database management.

Using the health system framework presented in an earlier chapter, these programs and services can also be described in terms of their intervention strategy, level of prevention, practice domain, and target population. Intervention strategies include health promotion, specific protection, early identification and treatment, disability limitation, and rehabilitation. By level of prevention, interventions can be classified as primary, secondary, or tertiary. By practice domain, interventions can be furnished by either public health or medical care practitioners. Interventions are also grouped by their target population, either individuals or populations.

As demonstrated in Table 8-1, the activities available to carry out public health's core functions are extensive. Some are clinically oriented preventive services for individuals; others are population-based programs and services. The clinical preventive services emphasize early case findings and other aspects of primary care, whereas population-based programs and services largely involve a variety of health promotion and specific protection services. There is considerable overlap between the two, especially for specific protection and early case-finding services.

Evidence-Based Clinical Preventive Services

Clinical preventive services include screening tests, counseling interventions, immunizations, and prophylactic regimens for individuals of all age groups and risk categories. Although many of these interventions have been widely accepted and deployed by practitioners, there have been increasing concerns as to whether they truly improved clinical outcomes. Since the 1980s, both the Canadian Task Force on Preventive Health Care and the U.S. Preventive Services Task Force (USPSTF) have reviewed information on the effectiveness of specific clinical preventive services.[4] At the heart of this examination are five key questions:[5]

1. How important is the target condition?
2. How important is the risk factor?
3. How accurately can the risk factor or target population be identified?
4. Is the preventive service effective?
5. Do the benefits of implementation outweigh the costs?

The importance of the target condition is assessed using measures of frequency and severity. Incidence and prevalence are two key measures of frequency, whereas mortality, morbidity, and survival rates are useful measures of severity. The importance of a risk factor is determined by its frequency (incidence and prevalence) and measures of the magnitude of the relationship between the risk factor and the target condition, such as absolute and attributable risk. Absolute risk measures the incidence of the target condition in the population with the risk factor. Attributable risk measures the amount of the risk that is attributable to one particular risk factor.

Risk factor or target population accuracy depends on measures of sensitivity (the proportion of persons with a condition who correctly test positive), specificity (the proportion of persons without a condition who correctly test negative), and positive predictive value (proportion of positive test results that are correct). For screening tests, the criteria consider the accuracy and effectiveness of early detection. For counseling interventions, the criteria relate to the efficacy of risk reduction and the effectiveness of counseling. Efficacy of vaccines is the primary criterion for evaluating these biologic interventions. For chemoprophylaxis, the criteria relate to efficacy, as well as to the effectiveness of counseling. Recommendations for clinical preventive services were first published in 1989 and revised periodically for the various age and risk status groups. The current edition of these recommendations is an ongoing process involving reexamination of previous recommendations and consideration of new ones. In order to expedite their translation into practice, recommendations are now released soon after the task force concludes its examination of a specific clinical preventive service.

The USPSTF grades its recommendations (A, B, C, D, or I) based on the strength of evidence and magnitude of net benefit (benefits minus harms). An "A" grade means that the USPSTF strongly recommends that clinicians provide the service to eligible patients. The USPSTF found good evidence that the service improves important health outcomes and concluded that benefits substantially outweigh harms. A grade of "B" means that the task force recommends that clinicians provide the service to eligible patients based on at least fair evidence that the service improves important health outcomes and that benefits outweigh harms. A grade of "C" means that the USPSTF makes no recommendation for or against routine provision of the service based on at least fair evidence that the service can improve health outcomes but after concluding that the balance of benefits and harms is too close to justify a general recommendation. A "D" grade means that the task force recommends against routinely providing the service to asymptomatic patients based on at least fair evidence that the service is ineffective or that harms outweigh benefits. Finally, an "I" grade means that the USPSTF concludes that the evidence is insufficient to recommend for or against routinely providing the service. In these cases, evidence that the service is effective is lacking, of poor quality, or conflicting, and the balance of benefits and harms cannot be determined.

Assessments of the effectiveness of preventive services are made in part by examining the quality of the scientific evidence available for specific interventions. Evidence from properly designed randomized controlled trials is most heavily weighted in this process followed, in order, by evidence from controlled trials without randomization, well-designed cohort or case-control studies (preferably multicenter studies), multiple time series or uncontrolled studies, and expert clinical opinion.

This grading scheme became even more important with the enactment of comprehensive health reform legislation in 2010 affecting individuals in private health insurance plans as well as those served by Medicare and Medicaid. One provision of the health reform package stipulates that group health plans and health insurance issuers offering group or individual health insurance coverage shall provide coverage for but cannot impose any cost-sharing requirements for evidence-based items or services that carry a rating of A or B in the current USPSTF recommendations. Similarly, other health reform provisions waive any coinsurance requirements for most preventive services for Medicare recipients, resulting in Medicare paying 100% of these costs. These include personalized prevention plan services, initial preventive physical examinations, and any recommended preventive services that are graded A or B by the USPSTF. Medicaid state options for diagnostic, screening, preventive, and rehabilitation services now include all clinical preventive services graded A or B by the USPSTF, as well as all immunizations recommended by the Advisory Committee on Immunization Practices of the Centers for Disease Control and Prevention (CDC). States covering these services in their state Medicaid plans would have the percentage of federal support for their state Medicaid programs increased by 1%.

A summary of the recommendations made by the task force as of 2014 is provided in Table 8-2. These recommendations were not intended to serve as standards of care; rather, they stand as statements as to the quality of the evidence available to justify the use of practices as effective preventive interventions. The USPSTF recommends that clinicians discuss these preventive services with eligible patients and offer them as a priority. All of these services have received an A (strongly recommended) or a B (recommended) grade from the task force.

The effectiveness of immunizations has been well established through reductions of more than 99% for diseases that include poliomyelitis, rubella, diphtheria, and pertussis. Several screening tests have also contributed to reductions in disease mortality and morbidity. For example, hypertension screening has contributed to a 67% reduction in stroke mortality since 1968, and newborn screening for both congenital hypothyroidism and phenylketonuria and cervical cancer screening through Pap tests have greatly reduced the burden of these diseases. Chemoprophylaxis, especially for diseases such as tuberculosis, has also contributed to reductions in mortality and morbidity in recent decades. Despite the successes with these forms of clinical preventive services, the greatest potential lies in changing personal behaviors. In the clinical setting, counseling, often supported with screening tests, appears to be the clinical preventive service with the greatest potential.[4]

Complementing the scientific assessment of efficacy (answering the question "does it work?"), the task force has increasingly focused on assessment of economic benefits and costs (answering the question "is it worth it?"). These economic

Table 8-2 Clinical Preventive Services Recommended by the U.S. Preventive Services Relevant for Implementation of the Affordable Care Act as of January 2014

Topic	The USPSTF recommends...	Grade
Abdominal aortic aneurysm screening: men	... one-time screening for abdominal aortic aneurysm by ultrasonography in men ages 65 to 75 years who have ever smoked.	B
Alcohol misuse: screening and counseling	... that clinicians screen adults age 18 years or older for alcohol misuse and provide persons engaged in risky or hazardous drinking with brief behavioral counseling interventions to reduce alcohol misuse.	B
Anemia screening: pregnant women	... routine screening for iron deficiency anemia in asymptomatic pregnant women.	B
Aspirin to prevent cardiovascular disease: men	... the use of aspirin for men ages 45 to 79 years when the potential benefit due to a reduction in myocardial infarctions outweighs the potential harm due to an increase in gastrointestinal hemorrhage.	A
Aspirin to prevent cardiovascular disease: women	... the use of aspirin for women ages 55 to 79 years when the potential benefit of a reduction in ischemic strokes outweighs the potential harm of an increase in gastrointestinal hemorrhage.	A
Bacteriuria screening: pregnant women	... screening for asymptomatic bacteriuria with urine culture in pregnant women at 12 to 16 weeks' gestation or at the first prenatal visit, if later.	A
Blood pressure screening in adults	... screening for high blood pressure in adults age 18 years and older.	A
BRCA risk assessment and genetic counseling/ testing	... that primary care providers screen women who have family members with breast, ovarian, tubal, or peritoneal cancer with one of several screening tools designed to identify a family history that may be associated with an increased risk for potentially harmful mutations in breast cancer susceptibility genes (*BRCA1* or *BRCA2*). Women with positive screening results should receive genetic counseling and, if indicated after counseling, BRCA testing.	B
Breast cancer preventive medications	... that clinicians engage in shared, informed decision making with women who are at increased risk for breast cancer about medications to reduce their risk. For women who are at increased risk for breast cancer and at low risk for adverse medication effects, clinicians should offer to prescribe risk-reducing medications, such as tamoxifen or raloxifene.	B
Breast cancer screening	... screening mammography for women, with or without clinical breast examination, every 1 to 2 years for women age 40 years and older.	B
Breastfeeding counseling	... interventions during pregnancy and after birth to promote and support breastfeeding.	B

(*continues*)

Table 8-2   Clinical Preventive Services Recommended by the U.S. Preventive Services Relevant for Implementation of the Affordable Care Act as of January 2014 (*Continued*)

Topic	The USPSTF recommends…	Grade
Cervical cancer screening	… screening for cervical cancer in women ages 21 to 65 years with cytology (Pap smear) every 3 years or, for women ages 30 to 65 years who want to lengthen the screening interval, screening with a combination of cytology and human papillomavirus (HPV) testing every 5 years.	A
Chlamydial infection screening: nonpregnant women	… screening for chlamydial infection in all sexually active nonpregnant young women age 24 years and younger and for older nonpregnant women who are at increased risk.	A
Chlamydial infection screening: pregnant women	… screening for chlamydial infection in all pregnant women age 24 years and younger and for older pregnant women who are at increased risk.	B
Cholesterol abnormalities screening: men 35 and older	… screening men age 35 years and older for lipid disorders.	A
Cholesterol abnormalities screening: men younger than 35	… screening men ages 20 to 35 years for lipid disorders if they are at increased risk for coronary heart disease.	B
Cholesterol abnormalities screening: women 45 and older	… screening women age 45 years and older for lipid disorders if they are at increased risk for coronary heart disease.	A
Cholesterol abnormalities screening: women younger than 45	… screening women ages 20 to 45 years for lipid disorders if they are at increased risk for coronary heart disease.	B
Colorectal cancer screening	… screening for colorectal cancer using fecal occult blood testing, sigmoidoscopy, or colonoscopy in adults beginning at age 50 years and continuing until age 75 years. The risks and benefits of these screening methods vary.	A
Dental caries prevention: preschool children	… that primary care clinicians prescribe oral fluoride supplementation at currently recommended doses to preschool children older than age 6 months whose primary water source is deficient in fluoride.	B
Depression screening: adolescents	… screening adolescents (ages 12 to 18 years) for major depressive disorder when systems are in place to ensure accurate diagnosis, psychotherapy (cognitive behavioral or interpersonal), and follow up.	B
Depression screening: adults	… screening adults for depression when staff-assisted depression care supports are in place to assure accurate diagnosis, effective treatment, and follow up.	B
Diabetes screening	… screening for type 2 diabetes in asymptomatic adults with sustained blood pressure (either treated or untreated) greater than 135/80 mm Hg.	B

Table 8-2   Clinical Preventive Services Recommended by the U.S. Preventive Services Relevant for Implementation of the Affordable Care Act as of January 2014 (*Continued*)

Topic	The USPSTF recommends...	Grade
Falls prevention in older adults: exercise or physical therapy	... exercise or physical therapy to prevent falls in community-dwelling adults age 65 years and older who are at increased risk for falls.	B
Falls prevention in older adults: vitamin D	... vitamin D supplementation to prevent falls in community-dwelling adults age 65 years and older who are at increased risk for falls.	B
Folic acid supplementation	... that all women planning or capable of pregnancy take a daily supplement containing 0.4 to 0.8 mg (400 to 800 µg) of folic acid.	A
Gestational diabetes mellitus screening	... screening for gestational diabetes mellitus in asymptomatic pregnant women after 24 weeks of gestation.	B
Gonorrhea prophylactic medication: newborns	... prophylactic ocular topical medication for all newborns for the prevention of gonococcal ophthalmia neonatorum.	A
Gonorrhea screening: women	... that clinicians screen all sexually active women, including those who are pregnant, for gonorrhea infection if they are at increased risk for infection (i.e., if they are young or have other individual or population risk factors).	B
Healthy diet counseling	... intensive behavioral dietary counseling for adult patients with hyperlipidemia and other known risk factors for cardiovascular and diet-related chronic disease. Intensive counseling can be delivered by primary care clinicians or by referral to other specialists, such as nutritionists or dietitians.	B
Hearing loss screening: newborns	... screening for hearing loss in all newborn infants.	B
Hemoglobinopathies screening: newborns	... screening for sickle cell disease in newborns.	A
Hepatitis B screening: pregnant women	... screening for hepatitis B virus infection in pregnant women at their first prenatal visit.	A
Hepatitis C virus infection screening: adults	... screening for hepatitis C virus (HCV) infection in persons at high risk for infection. The USPSTF also recommends offering one-time screening for HCV infection to adults born between 1945 and 1965.	B
HIV screening: nonpregnant adolescents and adults	... that clinicians screen for HIV infection in adolescents and adults ages 15 to 65 years. Younger adolescents and older adults who are at increased risk should also be screened.	A
HIV screening: pregnant women	... that clinicians screen all pregnant women for HIV, including those who present in labor who are untested and whose HIV status is unknown.	A
Hypothyroidism screening: newborns	... screening for congenital hypothyroidism in newborns.	A

(continues)

Table 8-2 Clinical Preventive Services Recommended by the U.S. Preventive Services Relevant for Implementation of the Affordable Care Act as of January 2014 *(Continued)*

Topic	The USPSTF recommends...	Grade
Intimate partner violence screening: women of childbearing age	... that clinicians screen women of childbearing age for intimate partner violence, such as domestic violence, and provide or refer women who screen positive to intervention services. This recommendation applies to women who do not have signs or symptoms of abuse.	B
Iron supplementation in children	... routine iron supplementation for asymptomatic children ages 6 to 12 months who are at increased risk for iron deficiency anemia.	B
Lung cancer screening	... annual screening for lung cancer with low-dose computed tomography in adults ages 55 to 80 years who have a 30 pack-year smoking history and currently smoke or have quit within the past 15 years. Screening should be discontinued once a person has not smoked for 15 years or develops a health problem that substantially limits life expectancy or the ability or willingness to have curative lung surgery.	B
Obesity screening and counseling: adults	... screening all adults for obesity. Clinicians should offer or refer patients with a body mass index of 30 kg/m^2 or higher to intensive, multicomponent behavioral interventions.	B
Obesity screening and counseling: children	... that clinicians screen children age 6 years and older for obesity and offer or refer them to comprehensive, intensive behavioral interventions to promote improvement in weight status.	B
Osteoporosis screening: women	... screening for osteoporosis in women age 65 years and older and in younger women whose fracture risk is equal to or greater than that of a 65-year-old white woman who has no additional risk factors.	B
Phenylketonuria screening: newborns	... screening for phenylketonuria in newborns.	A
Rh incompatibility screening: first pregnancy visit	... Rh (D) blood typing and antibody testing for all pregnant women during their first visit for pregnancy-related care.	A
Rh incompatibility screening: 24- to 28- weeks' gestation	... repeated Rh (D) antibody testing for all unsensitized Rh (D)-negative women at 24- to 28-weeks' gestation, unless the biological father is known to be Rh (D)-negative.	B
Sexually transmitted infections counseling	... high-intensity behavioral counseling to prevent sexually transmitted infections (STIs) in all sexually active adolescents and for adults at increased risk for STIs.	B
Skin cancer behavioral counseling	... counseling children, adolescents, and young adults ages 10 to 24 years who have fair skin about minimizing their exposure to ultraviolet radiation to reduce risk for skin cancer.	B
Tobacco use counseling and interventions: non-pregnant adults	... that clinicians ask all adults about tobacco use and provide tobacco cessation interventions for those who use tobacco products.	A

Table 8-2 Clinical Preventive Services Recommended by the U.S. Preventive Services Relevant for Implementation of the Affordable Care Act as of January 2014 (*Continued*)

Topic	The USPSTF recommends...	Grade
Tobacco use counseling: pregnant women	... that clinicians ask all pregnant women about tobacco use and provide augmented, pregnancy-tailored counseling to those who smoke.	A
Tobacco use interventions: children and adolescents	... that clinicians provide interventions, including education or brief counseling, to prevent initiation of tobacco use in school-aged children and adolescents.	B
Syphilis screening: non-pregnant persons	... that clinicians screen persons at increased risk for syphilis infection.	A
Syphilis screening: pregnant women	... that clinicians screen all pregnant women for syphilis infection.	A
Visual acuity screening in children	... vision screening for all children at least once between the ages of 3 and 5 years to detect the presence of amblyopia or its risk factors.	B

Data from *USPSTF A and B Recommendations*. U.S. Preventive Services Task Force. http://www.uspreventiveservicestaskforce.org/uspstf/uspsabrecs.htm.

evaluations provide an additional dimension to the review of clinical preventive services that takes on greater importance in a world of finite resources, conflicting claims, and competing demands on decision makers.

Notwithstanding the demonstrated effectiveness of many clinical preventive interventions, they remain underused. Reasons for the failure to provide clinical preventive interventions often relate to reimbursement practices, provider education and practice patterns, and the pluralistic and fragmented health system in the United States. In addition to these factors, the proliferation of recommendations as to appropriate use of these interventions has created confusion and uncertainty among many health providers as to exactly what should be done and when. Further complicating the picture are underlying suspicions and uncertainty among health providers as to whether interventions such as counseling are effective in the first place. The process developed by the USPSTF sought to address these last two concerns directly.

The review of evidence leading to the age- and risk group-specific recommendations of the task force was accompanied by several important findings. The task force concluded that interventions addressing patients' personal health practices are vitally important in view of the major health risks and problems currently facing the U.S. population. Providers must take on a greater role in assisting their patients to reduce risks in their daily lives. In short, personal health behaviors are a legitimate and important clinical concern, and both clinicians and patients should share decision making regarding possible interventions. In determining that many screening tests are effective, the task force also found that many are not. These unproved and ineffective services must be avoided and their costs averted as clinicians become more selective in ordering tests and providing preventive services. Most important, the task force concluded that many opportunities for delivering preventive services were being missed, especially for persons with limited access to care.

Another important conclusion of the USPSTF was that, for some health problems and risks, community-wide preventive interventions are more effective than clinical services. This does not diminish the role of clinical providers, however, because their standing in the community can do much to advance community interventions and link them more effectively with the provision of clinical services.

Evidence-Based Community Preventive Services

Scientifically sound strategies and approaches are essential for public health interventions to be successful in improving quality of life and reducing preventable mortality and morbidity. Public health practitioners have always highly valued the science base for public health practice, but only recently has the evidence for the effectiveness of community-based interventions been subjected to rigorous scrutiny. This effort is modeled on the work of the USPSTF, which reviewed data and information related to the provision of clinical preventive services to assess what works and what does not. The clinical practice guidelines that emerged from that process have been widely accepted and have served to raise the standard of practice for clinical preventive services for specific age groups.

For preventive interventions, the job only begins with demonstrating efficacy: that an intervention works well under ideal circumstances. Although an intervention may be efficacious, it may not work somewhere else because of the particular conditions and circumstances that exist there. Such an intervention would not be considered effective: that is, it would not have the results intended. Many different social, ethical, legal, and distributional factors may limit effectiveness in a particular setting.[6] Figure 8-3 illustrates the life cycle of a preventive intervention, from its development through basic research to its eventual widespread intervention. In between, applied research activities and community demonstrations are necessary to provide a complete picture of its effectiveness in terms of its influence on outcomes, economic considerations, and safety.

Although these analyses have been applied to clinical preventive services for more than a decade, efforts to apply them to community prevention activities are of more recent vintage. In 1995, the first steps were taken toward the development of practice guidelines for public health using similar principles.[6]

An assessment of the feasibility of such an undertaking was completed through the Council on Linkages Between Academia and Public Health Practice. The conclusions and recommendations of this assessment are presented in Table 8-3; they indicate strong support for developing population-based practice guidelines. The primary purpose of guidelines for community preventive services is to provide public health practitioners, their community partners, and policy makers with information needed for informed decision making on the most effective public health strategies, policies, and programs for their communities. Where interventions are found to be effective, this process then examines their cost effectiveness, benefits and harms, generalizability, and barriers to implementation. This

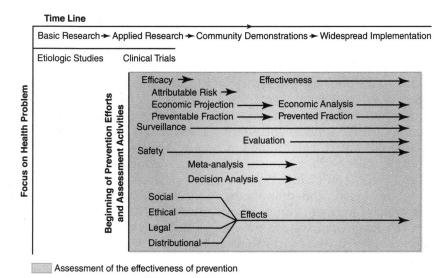

Figure 8-3 Natural history of the development of an effective prevention strtegy and temporal relationship to the types of assessment activities.

Reproduced from Teutsch S. A framework for assessing the effectiveness of disese and injury prevention. *MMWR*. 1992;41(RR-3).

Table 8-3 Practice Guidelines for Public Health: Recommendations for Assessment of Scientific Evidence, Feasibility, and Benefits

1. Public health practice guidelines are feasible, based on scientific evidence and other empirical information.
2. The potential benefits of public health practice guidelines are immediate and far reaching.
3. Each set of guidelines should have a carefully circumscribed scope.
4. Guidelines should be flexible rather than proscriptive.
5. Guidelines should be dynamic.
6. All major stakeholders should be involved as the guidelines are developed.
7. Critical questions are an efficient tool to structure the evidence-collection process.
8. A'database search for scientific studies is a useful first step.
9. Additional sources of documentary evidence should be tapped and systematically evaluated.
10. Empiric evidence from state and local public health programs should be sought, evaluated, and incorporated into the guidelines.
11. Development of guidelines will stimulate needed research.
12. Guidelines should be pilot tested before dissemination, then continuously evaluated.

Data from Council on Linkages Between Academia and Public Health Practice. Practical Guidelines for Public Health: Assessment of Scientific Evidence, Feasibility and Benefits. Washington, DC: Council on Linkages, U.S. Public Health Services; October 1995.

information provides the basis for evidence-based recommendations on the use of specific community preventive interventions.

Population-based community prevention focuses on assessing and addressing common, as well as emergent, health problems and needs. It is both an investment strategy and a tool for protecting and enhancing community health status. Several forces have accelerated interest in a more evidence-based approach to community prevention that complements recent advances in evidence-based medicine and clinical preventive services in order to assess what works and what does not. The increasing chronic disease burden is one of those forces necessitating greater interest in preventive (reducing incidence and prevalence) strategies that focus on education and behavioral change rather than on new treatment modalities. Lessons learned in terms of environmental interventions and public policy changes in laws, regulations, and enforcement can be extended to new threats and other conditions. Changes in the healthcare system are also needed in order to promote and target effective clinical preventive services to reach more of those who would benefit from such services.

The progress made after 1950 in identifying risk factors associated with chronic diseases and injuries is sometimes called the second epidemiologic revolution. With the importance of heart disease, stroke, cancer, diabetes, chronic lung diseases, and injuries as major contributors to morbidity and mortality, health promotion programs have grown in number and scope over the past 2 decades. Examples include injury risk reduction through seat belts, education to prevent tobacco use, campaigns against drinking and driving, nutrition education (fat intake), fitness campaigns, smokeless tobacco use, stress management, and programs promoting safe sex and abstinence. Risk or harm reduction strategies often seek to reduce, rather than totally eliminate, risk factors in a population by focusing on multiple strategies and by not considering the risk behavior from a moral or value-laden perspective.

Commercial marketing concepts and techniques are increasingly used in community prevention efforts. Often termed *social marketing*, target audiences are identified for purposes of influencing voluntary behaviors or policy makers. Social marketing techniques promote the acceptance, rejection, maintenance, or modification of specific health or care-seeking behaviors by offering or reinforcing incentives and/or consequences that serve the self-interest of individuals in the target group.[7] This consumer-driven focus is rapidly gaining acceptance among public health professionals and organizations.

Although viewed as important for health purposes, and increasingly emphasized by public and voluntary organizations, these services have not been widely embraced by providers and organizations in the private sector. To some extent, this has occurred because insurance plans have not covered these services and because they are not viewed as valued by the public. As a result, providers have not sought to advertise or otherwise promote them. Instead, disease-specific services emphasizing sophisticated, high-technology services, including screening tests, have been used to attract patients and market share.

The convergence of these considerations led to the development of the Task Force on Community Preventive Services and the establishment of *The Guide to Community Preventive Services*[8] (referred to here as *The Community Guide*). *The Community Guide identifies strategies that work to promote healthy lifestyles, prevent* disease, and increase the number of people who receive appropriate preventive counseling and screening. *The Community Guide* provides decision makers with recommendations regarding population-based interventions to promote health and to prevent injury, disease, disability, and premature death. These recommendations target communities and healthcare providers and focus on changing risk behaviors; reducing the prevalence of diseases, injuries, and impairments; and addressing environmental and ecosystem challenges.

Systematic reviews are conducted for specific interventions within each health topic addressed in *The Community Guide*. The assessment evaluates evidence of effectiveness and translates that into a recommendation or a finding of insufficient evidence. Importantly, a determination that evidence is insufficient does not mean that there is evidence of ineffectiveness. Table 8-4 summarizes the task force's conclusions as of 2014 regarding community preventive services that work.

Community preventive services embody the two basic strategies for primary prevention: health promotion and specific prevention and foster appropriate use of various tools for secondary prevention. These strategies are largely targeted to populations—the entire population or specific groups. These services constitute public health practice regardless of whether they are provided by public or private sector

Table 8-4   Topics Addressed by Task Force on Community Preventive Services Recommendations as of March 2014

Adolescent health
Alcohol—excessive consumption
Asthma
Birth defects
Cancer
Cardiovascular disease
Diabetes
Emergency preparedness
Health communication
Health equity
HIV/AIDS, sexually transmitted infections, pregnancy
Mental health
Motor vehicle injury
Nutrition
Obesity
Oral health
Physical activity
Social environment
Tobacco
Vaccination
Violence
Worksite

Data from The Guide to Community Preventive Services, *Task Force on Community Preventive Services*. Accessible at www.thecommunityguide.org. Retrieved March 14, 2014.

organizations and providers. It is not essential that all community preventive services be provided by the public sector, although some specific services can be organized and provided only through that route (e.g., fluoridation of water supplies).

It is likely that, as more communities become engaged in community-wide health improvement initiatives across the United States, there will be greater recognition of the need for community prevention services geared toward chronic diseases and a variety of behavioral health problems. During the 20th century, public health priorities shifted away from communicable disease control, environmental hazards, and maternal and child health services toward chronic disease prevention, injuries, violence, mental health, and substance abuse as community health priorities.[9]

OUTSIDE-THE-BOOK THINKING 8-2

Which are the best sources for identifying evidence-based public health interventions?

Evidence-based public health practice presents formidable challenges for several important reasons. Frequently relying on cross-sectional and quasi-experimental designs that lack a true comparison or control group, the quality of evidence for public health interventions is often limited in comparison with the evidence for medical interventions. In addition, there is a longer time period between intervention and outcome for many public health activities. Still, there are a variety of tools available to public health practitioners to assist in determining when public health action is warranted, including meta-analysis, risk assessment, economic evaluation, public health surveillance, and expert panels and consensus conferences.[10,11] Basic steps useful for enhancing evidence-based public health practice are illustrated in Figure 8-4 and Table 8-5. These include the following:[10]

- Developing an initial, concise, operation statement of the issue
- Determining what is known through the scientific literature
- Quantifying the issue
- Developing program or policy options
- Developing an action plan for the program or policy
- Evaluating the program or policy

It is clear that the needs of science and public policy differ in terms of their standards of evidence. Scientists would prefer that many true hypotheses go unproven rather than to "prove" one false hypothesis. Public health professionals, however, often cannot wait until definitive evidence is available. Evidence-based practice does not demand that judgment be suspended until all of the evidence is in or that only "gold standard" evidence is acceptable.

For decades, the tobacco industry dismissed evidence of the causal link between tobacco use and lung cancer as inconclusive because it was based largely on observational studies. This objection resonated with research scientists but did not deter public health activists from planning and implementing anti-tobacco interventions.

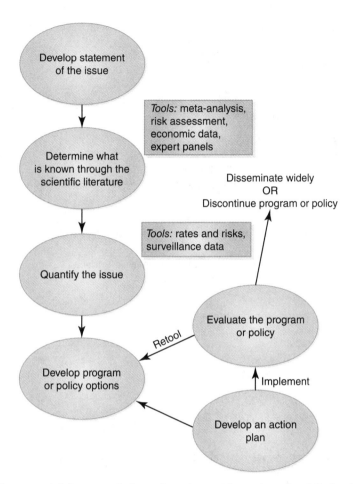

Figure 8-4 A sequential framework for enhancing evidence-based public health

Reproduced from Brownson RC, Gurney JG, Land GH. Evidence-based decision making in public health. *J Pub Health Manage Pract.* 1999;5(5):86–97.

PROGRAM MANAGEMENT IN PUBLIC HEALTH

Program management in public health includes the myriad activities involved with the design, development, implementation, and evaluation of interventions addressing public health problems. Effective program management is an organized response requiring a carefully designed problem statement, the availability of an appropriate intervention, and the capacity to deliver that intervention in a specific setting. Each of these is an essential component of an organized response. The challenge is to bring these elements together and direct them toward the solution of problems. Public health program management seeks to organize and direct public health workers, scientifically sound interventions, and appropriate strategies toward specific health problems.[12] The ultimate aim is to eliminate or reduce these problems to the maximum extent possible (effectiveness) and to achieve these results

Table 8-5   Quantitative and Qualitative Factors in Public Health Decision Making

Factor-Specific Questions

Size of the problem
- Is it important?
- What is the public health burden?

Problem preventability
- What is the efficacy?
- Can it work at least in ideal circumstances?
- What do we know about the biological plausibility? Is it logical (theory based)?

Intervention effectiveness
- What is the effectiveness?
- Does it work in real-world settings? Would it work in the settings being considered (is it generalizable)?
- How much less effective would it be compared with ideal settings?
- Is there better evidence for alternative interventions?

Benefits and harms
- What are all of the consequences of the intervention?
- What are the trade-offs?

Intervention cost
- Is it affordable?

Comparison of benefits and costs
- What is the value?
- How does it compare to other alternatives?

Incremental gain
- What are the additional costs and benefits (value) compared with what is already being done (if anything)?

Feasibility
- Are adequate time and money available?

Acceptability
- Is it consistent with community priorities, culture, values, and the political situation?

Appropriateness
- Is it likely to work in this specific setting?
- Are there ways to better understand the context for intervention in various populations?

Equitability
- Does it distribute resources fairly?

Sustainability
- Are resources and incentives likely to support conditions to maintain the intervention?

Data from Anderson LM, Brownson RC, Fullilove MT, et al. Evidence-based public health policy and practice: promises and limits. *Am J Prev Med.* 2005; 28: 226–230.

with the minimum resources necessary (efficiency). Effectiveness and efficiency are the primary criteria by which programs are judged or evaluated.

Management revolves around resource allocation and utilization. The resources of public health include the human, organizational, informational, fiscal, and other supportive resources. To use these resources both effectively and efficiently, there must be a process that carefully examines the problem for the pathways most likely to yield successful results. There are two cardinal sins of program management: failing to achieve program objectives when adequate resources are available and using more resources than are necessary to achieve a program's objectives. The first situation is more commonly viewed as poor management than the second, although from a management point of view each results in resources being wasted. When program management is improperly or only partially applied, resources and technology are underused, and problems are not fully addressed or resources and technology are inefficiently used, resulting in excess resource consumption and opportunity costs.

Program management calls for the development of a program hypothesis. This is best understood when programs are considered at the level of their basic elements, namely, the specific activities or tasks that are undertaken. The program hypothesis in its simplest form is a logic model; if the designated activities are successfully undertaken, the program's goals and objectives will be successfully addressed. For health programs, we expect that these activities will change characteristics of individuals or populations such that factors contributing to the level of the health problem will improve. With improvements in these various factors affecting the health problem, we expect that the level of the health problem itself will also be improved. Depending on how many intervening levels of factors there might be, we expect that improvement at one level will result in improvements at higher levels. These terms will be defined and clarified later; the major point here is that rational programs use logic models in order to address directly the chain of causation that creates the health problem being targeted by the program.

OUTSIDE-THE-BOOK THINKING 8-3

How are planning and evaluation related to program implementation?

The management cycle is often described as consisting of three phases: planning (deciding what to do and how to do it), implementation (acting to accomplish what has been planned), and evaluation (comparing the results of what was accomplished with what was intended).[12] Very often, planning, implementation, and evaluation have been viewed as linear processes. First, we plan. Then we implement. Finally, we evaluate what has occurred. In this linear model, we stop planning when we begin implementing, and we do not evaluate until after we have implemented our program. This approach views planning and evaluation as discrete, independent functions carried out at different points in the life span of a program. There are few fallacies more dangerous to sound management than this one! It is critical that

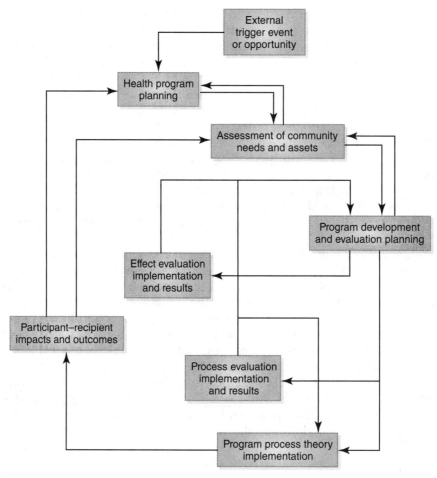

Figure 8-5   The planning and evaluation cycle.

Reproduced from Issel LM. *Public Health Program Planning and Evaluation: A Practical, Systematic Approach for Community Health.* Sudbury, MA: Jones and Bartlett; 2004.

planning and evaluation be viewed as interrelated and interdependent processes working together at varying levels of emphasis throughout the life of a program. Rather than a linear process, program management should be viewed as a cyclical process in which one step logically leads to the next and feedback obtained at all steps is used to revise the directions established in preceding steps. This relationship is illustrated in Figure 8-5, which is reprinted from Michele Issel's excellent text on public health program planning and development.[13]

Program management centers on the development of objectives. Unfortunately, objectives are all too often viewed as the products of planners alone. Program management in public health and other areas is simply too important for objectives to be left to the planners! Objectives are more than abstract targets for achievement. Although they are often characterized as the blueprint of a program, they actually serve more as a road map than as a blueprint. Objectives point the program toward a specific destination and, at the same time, set its speed and establish its mile markers. Objectives guide program administration and establish the framework and strategy for program evaluation. Rather than serving primarily as a tool for program planning, they guide all aspects of program planning, administration, and evaluation.

Linking Planning and Evaluation

A practical definition of planning views it as the application of rational decision making to the commitment of future resources. Planning is as much an art as it is a science. Planners do not have any special abilities to predict or foresee the future, and planning does not result in certainty as to what will happen. Rational planning serves to reduce but not entirely eliminate risk. The management purpose behind planning must be kept in mind: it is to make the most efficient use of resources. As a result, planning should not be judged solely by the accuracy of its predictions or even by whether planning targets, such as objectives, are met. Instead, planning should be judged on the basis of whether it helps an organization to achieve the best possible results in a changing environment. It is rare for programs to be carried out exactly as they were designed. Change occurs constantly among the external and internal factors that affect both the problem and programs designed to address the problem. Ongoing planning serves to recognize changes and modify implementation strategies accordingly. The ability of a program to evaluate itself continuously determines how quickly and effectively it can respond to changing conditions.

The key to the process of evaluation is the ability to ask the right questions. All too often, little thought is given to an evaluation strategy until the program is already in place and decision makers or funders begin to ask for evidence of its benefit. In short, evaluation is an afterthought. As a result, programs scurry around, asking this question: What are we doing that we can measure? Unfortunately, very little can be done at this point. Evaluation strategies should be developed and agreed upon before programs are implemented, and they should be based on asking a quite different question: What do we need to measure to know what we are doing? We return to these issues in greater detail as we discuss planning and evaluation in subsequent sections of this chapter. The point here is that these are not to be considered as bookends for program implementation; rather, they should be carried out concurrently and continuously. When this is done, planning and evaluation contribute substantially to a rational decision-making system in which managers are more likely to ask the right questions and direct resources toward the most promising intervention activities.

Key Questions for Managers

There are five key questions that guide the program management process:[12]

1. Where are we?
2. Where do we want to be?
3. Should we do something?
4. What should we do?
5. How do we know that we are getting there?

Table 8-6 Key Questions for Managers of Public Health Programs

Where are we?
- State the problem.
- Identify the appropriate intervention.
- Specify resources.
- Project the future level of the problem.

Where do we want to be?
- Identify the desired outcome objective.

Should we do something?
- Discontinue current efforts?
- Maintain current efforts?
- Implement a new intervention?

What should we do?
- Analyze the problem for determinants and contributing factors.
- Determine the intervention point most likely to succeed.
- Develop impact and process objectives, activity measures, work plan, and budget.
- Develop an expected outcome objective.

How do we know that we are getting there?
- Track progress toward achieving activity measures and process objectives (doing things right).
- Track progress toward achieving impact and outcome objectives (doing the right things).

Modified from *Program Management: A Guide for Improving Program Decisions*. Atlanta, GA: USPHS-CDC-PHPPO; 1984.

These questions provide managers with much of the essential information needed to make better decisions. They focus attention on the essential components of any decision process: the starting point, the ending point, and the intermediate measurements. The logic and the rational nature of this process can be tracked through decision models, such as those developed by the CDC for public health program managers. In Table 8-6, the five questions serve as a road map of the program manager's major duties and tasks.

Even with a road map, journeys require a destination or goal. For public health programs, goals are generalized statements expressing a program's intended effect on one or more health problems. Goals are often described as timeless statements of overall aspirations; these generally serve to establish boundaries for the program's operational activities, but they also serve as the philosophic justification for a program's existence. It is unusual for program managers to be involved in the establishment of goals. Higher authorities, such as boards, legislative bodies, or even funding sources, usually establish these. Despite being somewhat abstract and externally developed, goals serve a valuable purpose for public health programs. Goals need to be clearly stated, and they need to be understood by all program staff, if only to serve as a common bond and continuous reminder of the program's aspirations.

Where Are We?

The essence of decision making at any level is deciding either to do something or to do nothing. A rational decision to do or not do something calls for a thorough assessment of the current situation based on asking this question: Where are we? Determining the current status of things assists the manager in several ways. It provides information that can be later used to decide whether action should be taken. It also serves to describe the dimensions of a potential problem in terms of which groups might be more affected and establishes a baseline for comparisons over time.

In examining where things stand, it is important to assess in detail the problem, the interventions capable of addressing the problem, and the resources available to deploy those interventions. Although these three elements need to be considered together in determining the current situation, the availability of an effective intervention is absolutely essential from the program management perspective. Without a potentially effective intervention, it makes little sense to plan and implement a program. The availability of an effective intervention refers to the current level of sophistication of the knowledge and techniques for its coordinated application. It is the science and knowledge base for developing and justifying a technical approach for accomplishing a goal. The specific intervention approach could be drawn from any of the categories of health interventions strategies described in the public health and the health system chapter (health promotion, specific protection, early case finding and treatment, disability limitation, and rehabilitation) and from recommendations as to effectiveness from the U.S. Task Force on Clinical Preventive Services and the Task Force on Community Preventive Services. As a result, the intervention could be based on medical sciences, physical sciences, or social sciences. Sometimes referred to as the state of the art, this knowledge or technical information convinces program managers that a particular health problem can be addressed.

OUTSIDE-THE-BOOK THINKING 8-4

Why is defining the health problem so important in program management?

In addition to the capability to intervene, there are two other considerations in assessing where things currently stand. These are the level of a health problem and the capacity or resources to intervene. A health problem is defined here as a situation or condition of people (expressed in health outcome terms, such as *mortality*, *morbidity*, or *disability*) that is considered undesirable and is likely to exist in the future unless additional interventions are implemented. The heart of any intervention strategy lies in the definition of the problem. The development of objectives and intervention strategies flows naturally from a careful and precise statement of the problem. Problem statements come in all formats and lengths, and they vary significantly in their complexity. Still, all good problem statements present a clear, concise, and accurate description of the condition to be controlled or prevented in a target population. The more carefully that a problem is stated, the more likely it is that it can be accurately measured.

Planning processes look to the future. Above all, planning is concerned with future resource allocation; therefore, decisions will need to address the anticipated future level of problems rather than their current levels. It makes little sense to throw additional resources at a problem if that problem's level is declining and the level of the problem in the future may not be deemed unacceptable. This would constitute at least a partial waste of resources, something that is to be avoided with good management practices. Even a decreasing level of a problem may merit additional resource allocation if that level is judged to be unacceptable or if additional resources might accelerate the decrease.

Looking to both the past and the future is necessary to describe a problem adequately because its trends are an important aspect of its description. Tracking problems over time also helps to project their future levels through trend analysis techniques. Often, however, tracking the level of a problem provides only an incomplete picture of changes over time. It is also important to track changes and trends in the problem's major determinants. For example, changes in low birth weight (a major determinant of infant mortality) should be examined alongside infant mortality rates, and changes in tobacco use should be tracked alongside lung cancer rates. Projecting future levels of a problem on the basis of trends in the problem and its determinants is fraught with uncertainty and is imprecise at best. Nonetheless, it is both useful and rational in informing decisions that will allocate resources to achieve specific results.

In addition to trends and projections of levels, the process of problem specification calls for assessment of the size, scope, and distribution of a problem, beginning with a clear definition of the problem in terms of its nature and etiology, its magnitude and extent in terms of its incidence and prevalence, its affected populations in terms of specific populations at risk (by age, gender, race, occupation, or other risk factors), and its time and place of occurrence. In some respects, this reads like the major components of a news story in terms of who, what, when, where, and how much.

Just as problems need to be carefully specified in determining where we are, resources also need to be assessed for their trends over time in terms of financial resources, as well as human resources (number, types, and skills), organizational resources, information resources, facilities, equipment, and other materials. Tracking both the problem and the resources over time allows for reasonable predictions to be made as to the effects (if any) of resources on the problem and what might be expected at various future resource levels. This information facilitates the development of realistic outcomes.

Where Do We Want to Be?

Determining where you are allows for a comparison with where you want to be. In answering this question, we make an effort to identify the level at which a problem will be considered acceptable at some point in the future. This is the level at which a current problem will no longer be considered a problem, and it is very much dependent on how carefully and comprehensively the problem has been described. If a problem is well defined in terms of what, how much, who, when, and where, priorities can be established so that resources can be most efficiently used to achieve program results. Specific measurable objectives can also be established on the basis of these components of the problem description. The term *desired outcome objective* refers to the level to which a health problem should be reduced and/or maintained within a specified time period. It is meant to be long term (generally 2 or more years), realistic (achievable through the intervention strategies proposed), and measurable. Outcome objectives are designed to measure directly the level of the health problem; they include a statement of how much and when the program should affect the health problem. An outcome objective is a quantitative measurement of the health problem at some future date and is something that the manager believes the program can and should accomplish. To establish meaningful outcome objectives, the three key ingredients are the availability of effective interventions, the resources and capacity to implement these interventions, and projections for the future level of the health problem. By assessing the past and current relationships among capability, capacity, and outcomes, we can project realistic and measurable outcome objectives for various levels of program activity.

Should We Do Something?

The purpose of asking the first two questions (where are we? and where do we want to be?) is to force a decision as to whether something additional needs to be done. When where you are (and are likely to be) differs from where you would like to be, change is indicated. Change can take one of two forms: doing more or doing less. As a result, there are three options in terms of resource allocation and deployment: reduce (or even eliminate) current efforts, maintain current efforts, or implement a new intervention.

Discontinuing current efforts may be called for if the health problem has already reached or is projected to reach desirable levels such that further resource allocation is unnecessary. From a manager's point of view, this represents an opportunity to save or redirect resources rather than to waste them.

A second option is to continue to provide the same level of resources if that level will achieve the desired outcome level by the target achievement date. The decision for a maintenance level should never become automatic; an active, analytic decision-making process should precede it. If the expected level of the problem falls within the acceptable range and resources are available, maintenance of the current level of effort is appropriate.

Interventions are called for when the projected level of the problem exceeds the desired outcome objective and when the capability and capacity to intervene are available. With the availability of technology and resources, the trick is to determine the best implementation strategy that will use these to achieve the desired outcome. How a program gets from where it is to where it wants to be requires that decisions be made as to which specific strategies and activities are to be used. There are generally at least several strategies for affecting the level or extent of a health problem. The decisions to be made are based on which options are likely to be most successful and how much of the program's resources should be devoted to each strategy. A program's intervention strategy determines how a program's resources are to be deployed to achieve the desired outcome objective. The logic behind this is simple: If the strategies and activities are carried out as planned, the problem will be reduced to the expected level on schedule. Many uncertainties and unforeseen circumstances can prevent an intervention strategy from succeeding as planned. These can be viewed as analogous to the difference between efficacy (will it work?) and effectiveness (will it work here?). In any event, an intervention strategy is as much a hypothesis as it is a plan. It remains to be proven, and the likelihood of unforeseen problems and obstacles increases when the problem is inadequately defined and analyzed.

What Should We Do?

When the problem has been clearly and concisely stated, when the capability to intervene exists, and when the capacity to deploy the interventions is on hand, an intervention strategy can succeed. Success will further depend on how thoroughly the problem has been analyzed so that its major determinants and their contributing factors are identified. This analysis provides information as to which approaches are most likely to be effective and allows for matching of program resources with activities that will address key contributing factors.

Consistent with the health problem analysis model described in the health from an ecological perspective chapter, measures of health problems should be stated in terms of health outcomes, such as mortality, morbidity, disability, incidence, and prevalence. Determinants are risk factors that, on the basis of scientific evidence or theory, are thought to influence directly the level of a specific health problem. Contributing factors are those factors that directly or indirectly influence the level of determinants. Analysis should continue until all pertinent direct determinants and their associated contributing factors have been identified. The direct determinants are then examined to determine which offer the greatest chance of success in achieving the desired outcome. For some determinants, there are either no or only partly effective interventions. Those that offer the best chances for success are selected as points of intervention.

In addition to the expected outcome objective, other levels of objectives guide the intervention process. The outcome objective relates to the level of the health problem. Similarly, some objectives relate to determinants, and still others relate to the contributing factors (see Tables 8-7 and 8-8).

Impact objectives address the level to which a direct determinant is to be reduced within a specified time period. They are generally intermediate (1 to 5 years) in terms

Table 8-7   Levels of Program Management and Planning

Goal	Defined Operational and Philosophical Parameters
• Outcome objective	• Projected future level of the health problem
• Impact objective	• Projected future level of a direct determinant
• Process objective	• Projected future level of a contributing factor
• Activities	• Actual tasks performed by program personnel

Modified from *Program Management: A Guide for Improving Program Decisions*. Atlanta, GA: USPHS-CDC-PHPPO; 1984.

Table 8-8   Characteristics of Program Objectives

Term	Time Period	Description	Measurement
Outcome objective	Usually long-term	Related to health problem	Degree of accomplishment; addresses doing the right things
Impact objective	Intermediate	Related to direct determinants and risk factors	Degree of accomplishment; addresses doing the right things
Process objective	Short-term	Related to contributing factors	Degree of accomplishment; addresses doing things right
Activities	Usually short-term	Describes the use of program resources	Accomplishment (yes/no); addresses doing things right

Modified from *Program Management: A Guide for Improving Program Decisions*. Atlanta, GA: USPHS-CDC-PHPPO; 1984.

of time, and they are both realistic and measurable. An impact objective measures a determinant and states how much and when the program will affect the determinant. It is the quantitative measurement of the determinant at some future date.

Just as impact objectives measure determinants, process objectives measure contributing factors. For a program to function as planned, achieving process objectives will lead to achieving impact objectives, which, in turn, will result in achieving the outcome objective. Process objectives are shorter term than outcome or impact objectives. They are of short term (usually 1 year), realistic, and measurable.

The establishment of process objectives initiates two additional steps, one focusing on developing a work plan for the activities necessary to address the process objectives and one revisiting the outcome objective. The former activity is seldom overlooked because it is essential in order to complete the program planning process. The latter activity, however, is often forgotten, resulting in programs operating with outcome objectives that cannot be achieved. The rationale for revisiting the outcome objective is that the intervention strategy selected, together with its process objectives and activity measures, is likely to be only partially successful in reducing the outcome objective to the desired level. Programs are seldom able to achieve the entire improvement called for in the desired outcome objective. As a result, an expected outcome objective is established by reassessing the probability of achieving the desired outcome objective within the estimated time frame for the program. The expected outcome objective represents an estimate of an important future event that can and should be accomplished through the program's actual efforts and within the resources available.

Completing the program-planning process requires the establishment of a work plan with specific activities and tasks that carry out the program's process objectives. Program resources are attached to these activities, and tasks and activity measures are used to track progress. Activity measures are generally very short term (often expressed in weeks or months) but are also realistic and measurable. The program budget is expended in carrying out these activities and tasks. These work statements are short term (less than 1 year), realistic, and measurable, and they describe what is to be done, by whom, when, and where. A budget is very much an operational plan for financial expenditures to support the actions agreed upon in the program plan.

As noted previously, the program plan is based on a logic model, a set of theoretical links or assumptions involving the problem and its determinants, contributing factors, activities, and resources. Program resources are deployed through specific activities that serve to modify contributing factors, resulting in achievement of process objectives. Achievement of the process objectives affects the determinants, resulting in the achievement of impact objectives. Achievement of the impact objectives reduces the level of the health problem, resulting in the achievement of the expected outcome objective.

How Do We Know That We Are Getting There?

To answer the last question—how do we know that we are getting there?—we examine the effectiveness of program design and implementation. Key to any evaluation strategy is the establishment of measurable checkpoints, or milestones, in both time and direction. These assist the manager in determining whether the program is moving in the right direction and whether it will arrive at its destination on time. Both the strategy and the importance of continuously assessing the effectiveness of a program are summed up in the well-known observation that it is more important to be doing the right things than it is to be doing things right. Evaluation focuses on both.

OUTSIDE-THE-BOOK THINKING 8-5

What are outcome, impact, and process objectives, and how do they contribute to program evaluation?

Evaluation was previously characterized as asking the right questions. With a well-analyzed problem statement and the selection of an appropriate intervention strategy, asking the right questions should be straightforward. The key questions are as simple as this: Was the outcome objective achieved? Were the impact objectives achieved? Were process objectives achieved? Were program activities performed as planned? Evaluation within this framework calls for measuring the actual results and comparing them with the intended results. Information on intended results is derived from the program plan, whereas data and information on the actual results must be provided by the program's information system. Goals, objectives, activities, and other standards establish the level of the intended results for comparison.

The intervention strategy represents a causal hypothesis that must be continuously reassessed because circumstances and conditions may change in ways that affect the initial assumptions and links. Evaluation is essential before decisions are made as to whether efforts should be expanded, reduced, or even maintained. In 1999, the CDC developed guidelines for public health professionals to use in program evaluations.[14] These guidelines focus less on the technical aspects of program evaluation than on six essential elements and four broad standards for program evaluations. The six steps include the following:

1. Identify stakeholders, including program implementers, those served or affected, and those who will use the results of the program evaluation.
2. Describe the program, including a clear description of need, expectations for the program, the logic model behind the program, resources to be used, activities to be implemented, and its stage of development and how it fits into the larger organizational and community context.
3. Focus the evaluation design, including a clearly stated purpose for the evaluation (its uses and users), as well as its specific evaluation questions and methods.
4. Gather credible evidence, including indicators that translate the general concepts of the program into specific measures; consider important sources of evidence, collect only what is needed, and use accepted data-gathering and management techniques.
5. Justify conclusions, including analysis, synthesis, interpretation, and recommendations consistent with values of stakeholders.
6. Ensure the use of and share lessons learned, including preparation for addressing both positive and negative findings and adequate mechanisms for feedback, follow up, and dissemination with stakeholders.

These broad evaluation standards help determine whether an evaluation is well designed and working to its full potential. They are very much interrelated to the essential steps in the evaluation, as illustrated in Table 8-9. The standards address four key questions:

1. Is the evaluation useful (utility)?
2. Is the evaluation practical (feasibility)?
3. Is the evaluation ethical (propriety)?
4. Is the evaluation correct (accuracy)?

Table 8-9 Centers for Disease Control and Prevention Evaluation Steps and Relevant Standards

	Utility	Feasibility	Propriety	Accuracy
1. Identify stakeholders	✓		✓	
2. Describe program			✓	✓
3. Focus evaluation design		✓	✓	✓
4. Gather credible evidence	✓			✓
5. Justify conclusions	✓			✓
6. Ensure use, share lessons learned	✓		✓	✓

Modified from Centers for Disease Control and Prevention. Framework for program evaluation in public health. *MMWR*. 1999; 48(RR-11): 1–41.

There are several dimensions for evaluating preventive interventions. These include a program's reach (proportion of the target population that participated in the intervention), efficacy (success rate if implemented as intended), adoption (proportion of all potential settings that will adopt this intervention), implementation (extent to which the intervention is implemented as intended in the real world), and maintenance (extent to which a program is sustained over time).[15] Failure to assess impact in all five dimensions can contribute to inefficient use of resources, suboptimal influence on health outcomes, and limited research opportunities.

Effectiveness represents the ability to produce an intended result and achieve expected outcomes. When a program fails to achieve its expected outcomes, the cause of that failure must be identified. Programs may not be effective for several reasons that relate to the various levels of the program's objectives and activities: its outcome objectives, its impact objectives, its process objectives, and its activity measures.

In reverse order, activity measures may not be achieved if resources are lacking or if personnel fail to carry out their tasks. This results in activity measures not being met. If the activity measures are closely linked to their associated process measures, these also will not be met. Failure to address a program's activity measures and process objectives successfully means that a program is not doing things right. Successfully carrying out activity measures and achieving process objectives, on the other hand, means that a program is doing things right. Even when a program is doing things right, however, it may not be doing the right things. Doing the right things means that program outcome and impact objectives are achieved. Four combinations of program effectiveness can occur:

1. Programs can be doing the right things and doing things right. These are well-designed and well-managed programs that merit emulation.
2. Programs can be doing the right things, even though things are not being done right. The link between the program's process objectives and activity measures and the program's outcome and impact objectives has been poorly identified. These programs are neither well designed nor well managed. It is not possible to link program activities and resources to the outcomes achieved.
3. Programs can be neither doing the right things nor doing things right. These programs are poorly designed and executed on all accounts.
4. Programs can be doing things right but not doing the right things. Here, activity measures and process objectives are achieved but impact and outcome objectives are not. Although the program staff may be satisfied with its performance, the program as a whole cannot be satisfactory. This situation occurs when a problem is inadequately analyzed. It can be argued that these programs, although poorly designed, are at least partly well managed.

As suggested in these various scenarios, programs can suffer from invalid assumptions or incomplete strategies linking process objectives to impact objectives or linking impact objectives to an expected outcome objective. Pinpointing the location of a program's weaknesses in design or implementation calls for continuously assessing the validity, reliability, and completeness of the intervention strategy.

"Doing things right" refers to the performance of activities and the achievement of process objectives. It is measured through process evaluation. Process objectives can be unmet for two reasons: (1) lack of resources, which calls for reassessing the impact and process objectives in order to align them with the available resources (lower expectations or locate additional resources), or (2) lack of performance, which calls for reassessing the program personnel in terms of motivation, skills, and knowledge (hire, fire, train, or motivate). If process objectives are being met, the program is doing things right.

"Doing the right things" refers to the achievement of impact and outcome objectives and measures the program's effectiveness. If the impact objectives are not being achieved but the process objectives are, the manager must reexamine the assumed relationship between contributing factors and the determinants, revise the intervention strategy, and develop a new work plan. If the expected outcome objective is not being achieved but the impact objective is, the manager must reexamine the assumed link between the determinants and the health problem, revise the intervention strategy, and develop a new work plan. If a program is doing things right (activities and process objectives) but is not achieving its projected impact or outcome, the only conclusion is that the program is not doing the right things. If the expected outcome objective is being achieved, the manager must reassess the need for the program and begin the management cycle again.

The three-level objective and evaluation procedure (process, impact, and outcome) facilitates locating the source of problems when a program does not achieve its expected outcome[12] (see Figure 8-6). Many programs start off with a focus on achieving outcomes but rapidly shift to a focus on accomplishing their activities and process measures. This is an example of outcome displacement in that outcomes are displaced as the driving force of programs by lower-level activities. Because every program needs to succeed, a program defines its success by doing things right, even if those things do not lead to the outcomes that the program was designed to produce. If a program cannot succeed in terms of outcome, it will shift its objectives to those it can achieve. Activities and processes then become the program's purpose

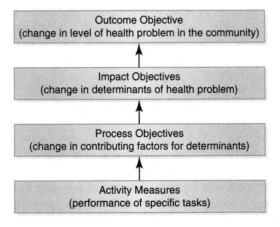

Figure 8-6 Multilevel program evaluation.

Modified from *Program Management: A Guide for Improving Program Decisions*. Atlanta, GA: USPHS-CDC-PHPPO; 1984.

and are accepted as surrogates for achieving the program's objectives. An analogous situation is apparent in the larger health system, where health outcomes have been displaced as objectives by processes such as access to medical care or the perceived quality of specific medical services.

OUTSIDE-THE-BOOK THINKING 8-6

What is the difference between doing things right and doing the right things in public health practice?

This simple program management system works well in public health for many reasons. It is rational, flexible, and adaptable to most programs and allows for easily understood comparisons between programs. In addition, it fosters communications within an organization and serves to prevent outcome displacement. Most important, it provides a road map and mile markers for managers so that they can maintain a steady course along the road to achieving the program's stated outcome objectives.

CONCLUSION

The question "What have you done for me recently?" conveys the expectation for services that permeates society. Interventions and the programs that orchestrate their implementation have become the hallmark of public health. Most people define public health in terms of the interventions that they most frequently encounter. Because personal health services represent such a large share of public health expenditures and because many of public health's population-based services are neither as visible nor as direct as clinical services, a common perception is that public health mainly provides clinical services for those without access to other providers.

There are several ways to categorize or classify the interventions and programs that result from collective efforts to identify and address health needs and risks in the community. One approach separates population-based community preventive from clinical preventive interventions. This approach is based largely on the different emphases of public health and medical practitioners. The interfaces between the two modes of practice are extensive and increasing.

Organizing and orchestrating these interventions are accomplished through program-management methods that begin with and revolve around careful definition of health problems. Analysis of carefully defined health problems allows for the establishment of three levels of objectives for the problem, as well as its determinants and contributing factors. Outcome, impact, and process objectives, together with the specific tasks necessary to carry out the process objectives, constitute a framework for tracking progress and modifying program strategies and activities. This program management system helps programs to keep their "eyes on the prize" rather than allowing them to shift their emphases from their intended outcomes to their day-to-day tasks.

REFERENCES

1. National Association of County and City Health Officials. *2005 National Profile of Local Health Departments*. Washington, DC: National Association of County and City Health Officials; 2006.
2. National Association of County and City Health Officials. *1992–1993 National Profile of Local Health Departments*. Washington, DC: National Association of County and City Health Officials; 1995.
3. Public Health Functions Steering Committee. *Public Health in America*. Washington, DC: U.S. Public Health Service; 1994.
4. U.S. Preventive Services Task Force. *Guide to Clinical Preventive Services*. 2nd ed. Washington, DC: U.S. Department of Health and Human Services; 1995.
5. Teutsch S. A framework for assessing the effectiveness of disease and injury prevention. *MMWR*. 1992; *41*(RR–3).
6. Council on Linkages Between Academia and Public Health Practice. *Practice Guidelines for Public Health: Assessment of Scientific Evidence, Feasibility and Benefits*. Washington, DC: Council on Linkages Between Academia and Public Health Practice; 1995.
7. Grier S, Bryant CA. Social marketing in public health. *Annu Rev Public Health*. 2005; *26*: 319–339.
8. Task Force on Community Preventive Services. *The Guide to Community Preventive Services*. Available at http://www.thecommunityguide.org. Accessed October 10, 2007.
9. Illinois Department of Public Health. *Challenge and Opportunity: Public Health in an Era of Change*. Springfield: Illinois Department of Public Health; 1996.
10. Brownson RC, Gurney JG, Land GH. Evidence-based decision making in public health. *J Public Health Manage Pract*. 1999; *5*: 86–97.
11. Brownson RC, Baker EA, Leet TL, et al. *Evidence-Based Public Health*. New York: Oxford University Press; 2002.
12. Dyal WW. *Program Management: A Guide for Improving Program Decisions*. Atlanta, GA: USPHS-SDC-PHPPO; 1990.
13. Issel LM. *Public Health Program Planning and Evaluation: A Practical Systematic Approach for Community Health*. Sudbury, MA: Jones and Bartlett; 2004.
14. Centers for Disease Control and Prevention. Framework for program evaluation in public health. *MMWR*. 1999; 48: RR–11.
15. Glasgow RE, Vogt TM, Boles SM. Evaluating the public health impact of health promotion interventions: the RE-AIM framework. *Am J Public Health*. 1999; *89*: 1322–1327.

Public Health Emergency Preparedness and Response

LEARNING OBJECTIVES

Given an emergency situation with public health implications (such as H1N1 influenza, massive flooding, or bioterrorism threats), identify the critical components necessary for an effective response. Key aspects of this competency expectation include being able to:

- Differentiate among the various types of public health emergencies and disasters, including their definitions and related terminology.

- Describe why emergencies and disasters are problems in which the public health system must be an integral participant across a range of activities.

- Describe the roles, responsibilities and competencies expected of public health workers in emergency preparedness and response.

- Define terrorism and bioterrorism and identify category A, B, and C biologic agents and their unique characteristics and relevance to bioterrorism events and threats.

- Describe recent governmental public health initiatives for public health emergency preparedness and response.

PUBLIC HEALTH ROLES IN EMERGENCY PREPAREDNESS AND RESPONSE

Public health crossed the threshold of the new century as an admittedly important but poorly understood contributor to American society. Despite its contributions to population health status and quality of life throughout the 20th century, the visibility and economic valuation of public health activities remained low. This situation changed rapidly after the terrorist attacks on the World Trade Center and Pentagon on September 11, 2001, and the bioterrorism events spreading anthrax through the United States postal system the following month. The nation responded quickly in the aftermath of these events, elevating terrorism, bioterrorism preparedness, and emergency response to the top of the national agenda. Within months, several billion dollars were made available to federal, state, and local public health agencies for public health preparedness and response activities, with additional funding allocated annually thereafter. This explosion of attention, resources, and expectations typifies the history of public health in America—a dramatic health-related event spotlights a largely neglected public health infrastructure resulting in a rapid infusion of resources to resuscitate the system.

This chapter describes the decisions made and actions taken to enhance public health emergency preparedness and response, as well as some of the successes, failures, and lessons learned along the way. The intent is to chronicle why and how public health emergency preparedness and response is emerging as one of the hallmarks of public health practice in 21st century America. Toward that end, this chapter focuses on several key questions:

- What is public health preparedness?
- What are the key components of preparedness?
- Is the public health system adequately prepared?
- What is needed to become fully prepared?

The core functions and essential public health services framework for modern public health responses are organized around six major functions:

- Preventing epidemics and the spread of disease
- Protecting against environmental hazards
- Preventing injuries
- Promoting and encouraging healthy behaviors
- Responding to disasters and assisting communities in recovery
- Ensuring the quality and accessibility of health services[1]

Although only one of these functions explicitly refers to public health's role in responding to emergencies, all six drive the public health approach to emergency preparedness and response. Public health emergency preparedness and response efforts seek to prevent epidemics and the spread of disease, protect against environmental hazards, prevent injuries, promote healthy behaviors, and ensure the quality and accessibility of health services. Each of these is expected by the public and each is evident in effective preparedness and response related to public health emergencies. Together they make preparedness and response a special and particularly critical component of modern public health practice.

For public health emergencies, preparedness and response are inextricably linked.[2] Preparedness is based on lessons learned from both actual and simulated response situations. Effective response is all but impossible without extensive planning and thoughtful preparation. Public health roles in health-related emergencies illustrate both facets.

Public Health Surveillance

Many public health emergencies are readily apparent, but others may not manifest themselves immediately. Effective preparedness and response rely on monitoring disease patterns, investigating individual case reports, and using epidemiologic and laboratory analyses to target public health intervention strategies. For example, foodborne illness outbreaks may involve individuals who remain in the same loca-tion after being exposed, making it easier to identify a common exposure pattern when these individuals seek medical care. Alternatively, an exposure at a convention or family reunion is more difficult to detect because individuals may present for medical care far from the location of exposure. Whether within the same community or in distant locations, it is often difficult for individual medical practitioners to recognize that an outbreak or widespread epidemic is occurring. Prompt recognition and reporting of cases to health authorities is a critical link in the public health chain of protection. New approaches to public health surveillance include biosurveillance and syndromic surveillance, the early detection of abnormal disease patterns and nontraditional early disease indicators, such as pharmaceutical sales, school and work absenteeism, and animal disease events. Multiple large data sets can be mined and analyzed for nontraditional markers of disease, which can lead to more rapid detection and response efforts.

OUTSIDE-THE-BOOK THINKING 9-1

What constitutes vulnerability in populations living in disaster-prone areas? Provide a concrete example from a disaster that has drawn media attention in recent years.

Epidemiologic Investigation and Analysis

Once a disease event is reported, public health agencies can uncover unusual patterns that help identify outbreaks and continuing risks. Public health professionals may use sophisticated analytic tools, such as pattern recognition software and geographic information systems, to determine patterns in disease cases. These surveillance activities help to ensure that disease outbreaks are identified quickly and that appropriate response actions, such as the issuance of health alerts for area providers and communication with response partners, are initiated. Many current disease surveillance systems act in a passive manner (i.e., they rely on providers to initiate disease reports); however, public health agencies are increasingly using active surveillance activities, such as when public health workers proactively seek information from providers and other sources to monitor disease trends. In the event of an actual or threatened public health emergency, active surveillance activities are deployed and/or expanded.

Surveillance activities trigger more extensive and focused epidemiologic investigations in order to determine the identity, source, and modes of transmission of disease agents. Epidemiologic investigations seek to determine what is causing the disease, how the disease is spreading, and who is at risk. Answers to these questions inform efforts to mount rapid and effective interventions. Methods of obtaining epidemiologic information, often characterized as disease detective activities, include contacting patients, obtaining detailed information on location and types of possible exposures, and examining both clinical specimens (such as blood and urine) and environmental samplings (such as food, water, air, and soil). Epidemiologic investigations require trained personnel and, in many cases, are quite intensive in terms of the quantity and quality of human resources needed. Laboratory capacity to support these investigations is critical.

Laboratory Investigation and Analysis

In many situations, laboratories provide the definitive identification of causative agents, both biological and chemical, and through various fingerprinting activities link cases to a common source. Capabilities to identify rare or unusual diseases are often not present in every community, necessitating linkages with higher level laboratories. Specimens may be sent for analysis and confirmation to a regional or state public health laboratory or possibly even to a CDC reference laboratory (laboratories are rated in terms of the level of safety they provide). Some specialized capabilities found at these higher level laboratories include serotyping to determine the antigenic profile of a microorganism and DNA fingerprinting to not only identify the type of microorganism causing an infectious disease but to also pinpoint the particular strain of bacterium or virus involved. In this way, public health authorities can determine if reported disease cases are part of the same outbreak, and therefore linked to a common source. Public health laboratories must rely on specialized protective laboratory equipment and facilities because of the dangerous agents with which they work. Some agents, such as smallpox, require special biocontainment equipment and procedures.

Intervention Through Effective Countermeasures

The primary reason for collecting, analyzing, and sharing information on disease is to control that disease. Expending resources for surveillance and analysis makes little sense if actions do not follow. Interventions that protect individuals from risks associated with environmental hazards are many, including setting standards for health and safety, inspecting food production and importation facilities, monitoring environmental conditions, abating conditions that foster infectious disease (e.g., insect and animal control), and enforcing private-sector compliance with established standards. Disease and injury risks associated with these biologic and chemical hazards, whether naturally occurring or initiated by man, are reduced through rigorous monitoring and enforcement activities. Public health agencies also play a substantial role in remediation of environmental hazards by decontaminating sites and facilities after they are identified. The extent of remediation necessary can vary greatly, just as the nature and extent of the contamination varies with different disease agents and their ability to remain viable outside a human host or animal/insect vector.

Risk Communication

Epidemiologic and laboratory investigations drive the initiation of actions intended to limit the spread of disease and to prevent additional cases in the community. The range of possible actions can be quite broad, including restraining the activities of individuals through isolation and quarantine and imposing temporary or permanent barriers around sources of contamination (e.g., sealing buildings, closing restaurants, and cutting off water supplies). In severe and unusual circumstances, special emergency powers may be put into effect limiting human and animal travel and/or restricting certain types of business activity. In these situations, the importance of effective public education and information activities to communicate risk to the public cannot be overstated. Commonly encountered examples include notices to boil drinking water when contaminated water supplies are suspected and product recalls and food safety advisories for potentially contaminated food products. The dissemination of information on mail handling practices during the anthrax attacks in late 2001 served both public education and risk communication purposes.

Promoting and encouraging healthy behaviors during public health emergencies represents another public health intervention strategy. It is not uncommon in the event of a natural disaster or terrorist attack for the most devastating effects to take the form of social disruption and infrastructure damage. The psychological effects of fear and terror, together with disruption of infrastructure components such as electricity, water, and safe housing, may create more casualties than any initial terrorist's biologic or chemical assault. Such conditions can also foster toxicity and infectious disease threats, such as occurred with the mass evacuation of the area around the World Trade Center leading to the abandonment of food supplies in surrounding homes and restaurants. Public health officials in New York City took steps to secure these premises to avoid the proliferation of rodents and other pests that otherwise could have resulted in secondary health threats.

Preparedness Planning

Organizing responses to emergencies is an important public health role that ensures the availability and accessibility of medical and mental health services. Preparedness and planning cannot eliminate all biologic, chemical, radiation, and mass casualty threats. But coordinated, community-wide planning for emergency medical and public health responses ensures that emergency medical services and medical treatment services are deployed in a rapid and effective manner. Such planning foresees the need for public health measures to be activated in order to ensure the safety of responders and to prevent secondary effects caused by further disease transmission and injury risk. Planning for these coordinated responses includes monitoring available response resources, establishing action protocols, simulating emergency events to improve readiness, training public and private sector personnel, assessing communication capabilities, supplies, and resources, and maintaining relationships with partner organizations to improve coordination. Hazard vulnerability analyses are an especially important planning tool that rate and rank the risk of specific emergencies for communities.

OUTSIDE-THE-BOOK THINKING 9-2

What are the basic functions that public health organizations perform in response to emergencies and disasters? When and how should the organization identify these functions?

Community-Wide Response

Public sector agencies play an important, but not exclusive, role in community-wide responses to emergencies. In many response situations, private sector medical care providers deliver the bulk of the triage and treatment services needed when a mass casualty emergency occurs. Although less involved with direct care, public sector agencies play key roles in coordinating and overseeing the delivery of services as well as communicating with providers, the media, and the public. Supervision of decontamination and triage often falls to public health authorities. Countermeasures such as antibiotics, antitoxins, and chemical antidotes as well as prophylactic medications and vaccines must be obtained, deployed, and delivered. Public health plays an active role in situations necessitating deployment of Strategic National Stockpile (SNS) pharmaceuticals, supplies, and equipment. In some situations, public health professionals also provide direct medical care. Public health also contributes through mobilization of regional and national assets and resources when local resources are overwhelmed. Some emergency situations, such as the anthrax attacks of 2001, prompted public fear and overreactions resulting in mountains of unknown powdery substances being tested and thousands of individuals unnecessarily initiating prophylactic antibiotic treatments. That situation and others over recent years argue that the worried well can stress response systems even more than those actually affected.

Unique Aspects of Bioterrorism Emergencies

Across the spectrum of possible public health emergency scenarios, bioterrorism threats represent a particularly challenging form of public health emergency. Bioterrorism is the threatened or intentional release of biologic agents (viruses, bacteria, or their toxins) for the purpose of influencing the conduct of government or intimidating or coercing a civilian population to further political or social objectives. These agents can be released by way of the air (as aerosols), food, water, or insects. Biologic agents with significant bioterrorism potential are listed in Table 9-1. Category A includes organisms that pose a risk to national security because of several factors. These organisms can be easily disseminated or transmitted from person to person, and they result in high mortality rates and have the potential for major public health impact. In addition, these organisms are likely to cause public panic and social disruption, thereby requiring special action for public health preparedness. Category B agents are the second highest priority organisms. These are moderately easy to disseminate, result in moderate morbidity rates and low mortality rates, and require specific enhancements of the CDC's diagnostic capacity and enhanced disease surveillance. The third highest priority agents fall into Category C and include emerging pathogens that could be engineered for mass dissemination in the future because of availability, ease of production and dissemination, and potential for high morbidity and mortality rates with major public health impact.

Biologic, chemical, radiation, and mass casualty threats that are intentionally inflicted differ from naturally occurring disease and injury threats in a number of important aspects. Central to these differences, bioterrorism is a criminal act requiring its prevention and response to include criminal justice, military, and intelligence

Table 9-1   Biologic Agents with Bioterrorism Potential

Category A
- Anthrax (*Bacillus anthracis*)
- Botulism (*Clostridium botulinum* toxin)
- Plague (Yersinia pestis)
- Smallpox (variola major)
- Tularemia (*Francisella tularensis*)
- Viral hemorrhagic fevers (filoviruses [e.g., Ebola, Marburg] and arenaviruses [e.g., Lassa, Machupo])

Category B
- Brucellosis (Brucella species)
- Epsilon toxin of Clostridium perfringens
- Food safety threats (e.g., Salmonella species, *Escherichia coli* O157:H7, *Shigella*)
- Glanders (*Burkholderia mallei*)
- Meloidosis (*Burkholderia pseudomallei*)
- Psittacosis (*Chlamydia psittaci*)
- Q fever (*Coxiella burnetii*)
- Ricin toxin from Ricinus communis (castor beans)
- Staphylococcal enterotoxin B
- Typhus fever (*Rickettsia prowazekii*)
- Viral encephalitis (alphaviruses [e.g., Venezuelan equine encephalitis, eastern equine encephalitis, western equine encephalitis])
- Water safety threats (e.g., Vibrio cholerae, Cryptosporidium parvum)

Category C
- Emerging infectious diseases such as Nipah virus and hantavirus

Reproduced from Centers for Disease Control and Prevention; 2010.

agencies that are not likely to be familiar with naturally occurring disease outbreaks. Law enforcement agencies, including the Federal Bureau of Investigation, have lead responsibility for responding to a bioterrorism attack. In addition, bioterrorism attacks may involve disease agents that occur infrequently in nature and with which neither public health officials nor clinicians have had much experience. It is increasingly possible to genetically engineer chimeras to create, for example, microorganisms that blend the pathogenic qualities of multiple disease agents. Because such organisms do not exist in nature, they would be completely unknown to public health and medical experts. Attacks related to biologic or chemical threats initiated by a bioterrorist would not likely follow known epidemiologic patterns, diminishing the value of using past experience with disease transmission and manifestation to identify the source or cause.

It is likely that bioterrorists would seek to be covert, expending great energy and attention to ensure the delayed discovery of the disease to maximize the population's exposure. Intentional outbreaks may develop in multiple locations simultaneously, thereby straining local, state, and federal response efforts. With many emerging and reemerging infectious disease threats (e.g., Ebola Virus, Sudden Acute Respiratory Syndrome, West Nile Virus, hantavirus), it is increasingly difficult to

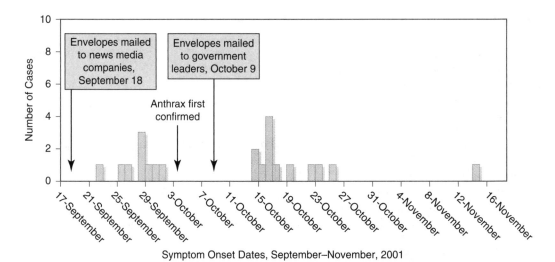

Figure 9-1   Epidemic curve for 22 cases of bioterrorism-related anthrax, United States, 2001.

Reproduced from Jernigan DB, Raghunathan PL, Bell BP, et al. Investigation of bioterrorism-related anthrax, United States, 2001: epidemiologic findings. *Emerg Infect Dis.* 2002; 8(10): 1019–1028.

predict the precise nature of the next public health emergency. It could result from a chance mutation of a microorganism or it could result from the intentional act of terrorists. Multiple threats are possible, necessitating preparedness and response systems that can address a wide variety of unknown and unanticipated hazards. This concept of multiple threats and unknown hazards has led many terrorism experts to advocate for a robust public health infrastructure capable of responding to many different forms of emergencies.

Protecting the public from infectious diseases and other threats is one of the major roles of public health in modern society. This role took on a new meaning after the national security was threatened by the events of September 11, 2001, and the anthrax attacks that were initiated less than a month later. Figure 9-1 and Figure 9-2 summarize the time lines and pathways for the most infamous bioterrorism attack in U.S. history. Initially focused on bioterrorism threats and events, this new role of public health emergency preparedness and response for all types of emergencies and disasters has emerged as central to what public health professionals and organizations are expected to perform in 21st century America.

Workplace Preparedness

Public health emergencies, including those related to terrorism, have many different visages and many different venues. Yet most of the direct victims of terrorism in the United States in recent years have been people at work, including the victims of the bombing of the federal building in Oklahoma City, those who died in the World Trade Center and the Pentagon on September 11, 2001, and the victims who contracted anthrax transmitted through the mail later in that same year.

Acts of terrorism intend to make people feel powerless and believe that they cannot take steps to prevent such incidents or mitigate their consequences. But

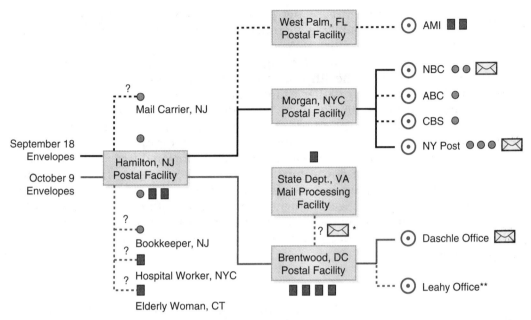

Figure 9-2 Cases of anthrax associated with mailed paths of implicated envelopes and intended target sites, United States, 2001.

Notes: NBC = National Broadcasting Company; AMI = American Media Inc.; CBS = Columbia Broadcasting System.
*Envelope addressed to Senator Leahy found unopened on November 16, 2001, in a barrel of unopened mail sent to Capitol Hill; **dotted line indicates intended path of envelope to Senator Leahy; shaded circle = cutaneous case; shaded rectangle = inhalational case; circle with central dot = intended target; envelope = recovery site of implicated envelope.

Reproduced from Jernigan DB, Raghunathan PL, Bell BP, et al. Investigation of bioterrorism-related anthrax, United States, 2001: epidemiologic findings. *Emerg Infect Dis.* 2002; 8(10): 1019–1028.

experience to date in battling other workplace safety risks suggests that there are steps that can be taken by employers and employees. The workplace is, in effect, a key line of defense for homeland security. This is recognized formally in the formation and scope of responsibilities for the new federal Department of Homeland Security (DHS) as well as in the response of the business community after 2001 in taking tangible steps to enhance security.

NATIONAL PUBLIC HEALTH PREPAREDNESS AND RESPONSE COORDINATION

The terrorist events of 2001 resulted in a series of new national policies and priorities to safeguard American citizens at home. One major development was the creation of the Department of Homeland Security (DHS) with extensive authority and powers related to domestic terrorism and security. In accord with the Homeland Security Act of 2002, several important public health functions were transferred into the new DHS in 2003, including the SNS of emergency pharmaceutical supplies and medical equipment. Responsibilities for SNS were subsequently transferred from DHS to CDC. The new federal agency immediately became part of the American everyday experience through activities providing timely and detailed information about threat levels to the public, government agencies, first responders, transportation hubs, and the private sector.

The establishment of a new federal agency, however, did not substantially alter the configuration of public health responsibilities within the system of operational federalism described in our earlier examination of law, government, and public health. Federal agencies are significant contributors, but public health remains largely a state responsibility, with the bulk of this activity taking place at the local level. For public health emergencies, including national disasters such as Hurricane Katrina in 2005 and bioterrorism events or threats, preparedness and coordinated response across all levels of government are critical. Nonetheless, there are significant issues related to intergovernmental relationships, resource deployment, and financing that make public health emergencies especially difficult challenges for the public health system. The following sections examine key aspects of the structure, operations, and issues in public health emergency preparedness and response at the national, state, and local levels.

Federal Agencies and Assets

Several dozen separate federal departments and agencies have roles in preparing for or responding to public health emergencies, including bioterrorist attacks. Within this constellation of agencies, the Department of Health and Human Services (DHHS) and DHS play the most important public health roles.

Prior to 2003, DHHS was the primary federal agency responsible for the medical and public health response to emergencies (including major disasters and terrorist events). Beginning in 2003, DHHS now shares center stage with the new DHS. DHHS discharges its responsibilities through several operating agencies, including the following:

- Centers for Disease Control and Prevention (CDC): CDC works with state public health agencies to detect, investigate, and prevent the spread of disease in communities. CDC provides support to state public health agencies in a variety of ways, including financial assistance, training programs, technical assistance and expert consultation, sophisticated laboratory services, research activities, and standards development. The Office of Public Health Preparedness and Response coordinates efforts across the various CDC centers, institutes, and offices. CDC now has operational responsibility for deployment of SNS resources during emergencies.
- Health Resources and Services Administration (HRSA): HRSA was the agency originally responsible for a state grant program to facilitate regional hospital preparedness planning and to upgrade the capacity of hospitals and other healthcare facilities to respond to public health emergencies until this program was transferred to the Office of the Assistant Secretary for Preparedness and Response. HRSA is also generally responsible for healthcare workforce development, including grant programs for curriculum development and continuing education for health professionals on bioterrorism preparedness and response.
- Food and Drug Administration (FDA): FDA has responsibilities both for ensuring the safety of the food supply and for ensuring the safety and efficacy of

pharmaceuticals, biologics, and medical devices. FDA fulfills its food safety responsibilities in partnership with the Department of Agriculture, which is responsible for the safety of meat, poultry, and processed egg products.

- National Institutes of Health (NIH): NIH conducts and supports biomedical research, including research targeted at the development of rapid diagnostics and new and more effective vaccines and antimicrobial therapies.
- Office of the Assistant Secretary for Preparedness and Response (ASPR) within DHHS sets overall policy direction and coordinates public health emergency preparedness and response activities across the various DHHS agencies. This office now administers the hospital preparedness program, formerly managed by HRSA.

In 2003, 23 federal agencies, programs, and offices were fashioned into the new federal DHS. The new agency sought to bring a coordinated approach to national security from emergencies and disasters, both natural and man-made. DHS actively promotes an "all-hazards" approach to disasters and homeland security issues. The Federal Emergency Management Agency (FEMA), formerly an independent agency, became one of the major branches of the new DHS responsible for emergency preparedness and response, tasked with responding to, planning for, recovering from, and mitigating against disasters under authority provided by the federal Stafford Act (Table 9-2).

Within DHS, the Emergency Preparedness and Response Directorate coordinates emergency medical response in the event of a public health emergency, including the National Disaster Medical System and the Metropolitan Medical Response Systems (these are described later in this chapter). Other major directorates

Table 9-2 Robert T. Stafford Disaster Relief and Emergency Assistance Act

The Congress hereby finds and declares that (1) because disasters often cause loss of life, human suffering, loss of income, and property loss and damage; and (2) because disasters often disrupt the normal functioning of governments and communities, and adversely affect individuals and families with great severity; special measures, designed to assist the efforts of the affected States in expediting the rendering of aid, assistance, and emergency services, and the reconstruction and rehabilitation of devastated areas, are necessary.

It is the intent of Congress, by this Act, to provide an orderly and continuing means of assistance by the Federal Government to State and local governments in carrying out their responsibilities to alleviate the suffering and damage which result from such disasters by—

1. revising and broadening the scope of existing disaster relief programs;
2. encouraging the development of comprehensive disaster preparedness and assistance plans, programs, capabilities, and organizations by the States and by local government;
3. achieving greater coordination and responsiveness of disaster preparedness and relief programs;
4. encouraging individuals, States, and local governments to protect themselves by obtaining insurance coverage to supplement or replace governmental assistance;
5. encouraging hazard mitigation measures to reduce losses from disasters, including development of land use and construction regulations; and
6. providing Federal assistance programs for both public and private losses sustained in disasters.

Data from FEMA, Public Law 93-288, as amended.

(divisions) of the new DHS include Border and Transportation Security, Science and Technology, Information Analysis and Infrastructure Protection, and Management.

Within DHS, the chief medical officer has primary responsibility for medical issues related to natural and man-made disasters and terrorism. In the aftermath of Hurricane Katrina, the Pandemic and All-Hazards Preparedness Act (PAHPA) of 2006 clarified the roles and responsibilities of DHS and DHHS. Several programs, including the National Disaster Medical System, were moved from DHS to DHHS.

Other federal agencies also carry important responsibilities related to bioterrorism and public health emergency preparedness. The Environmental Protection Agency responds to emergencies involving chemicals and other hazardous substances. The Department of Defense indirectly supports public health preparedness through various research efforts on biologic and chemical weapons, intelligence gathering related to terrorism threats, and civil support functions in the event of an emergency that results in severe social unrest. The Department of Justice has lead responsibility for assessing and investigating terrorist threats, including those related to bioterrorism, and provides funds and assistance to emergency responders (police, fire, ambulance, and rescue personnel) at state and local levels. The Department of Veterans Affairs purchases drugs and other therapeutics for the SNS and operates one of the nation's largest healthcare systems, which could provide critical surge capacity in the event of a mass casualty event. Several other federal agencies, including the Departments of Transportation, Commerce, and Energy, also have potential roles to play in preparing for and responding to a public health emergency.

National Incident Management System

Prior to the establishment of the new DHS, the management of large-scale health events was complicated by the involvement of many different federal agencies. States have established a similar web of agencies to manage disasters and other emergencies, with each developing its own form of an incident management system. In order to ensure greater consistency across states and for interfaces between the federal government and states, a National Incident Management System (NIMS) was prescribed by a presidential directive in 2003 to cover all incidents (natural and unnatural) for which the federal government deploys emergency response assets. The Secretary of Homeland Security is responsible for the development and implementation of NIMS. Its success depends in large part on the establishment of consistent approaches within the states as to roles and responsibilities for both public health agencies and the hospital community (including their supporting healthcare systems) in managing emergencies at the state and regional levels and developing and deploying incident management plans at substate levels.

Bioterrorism and other public health incidents fall within the scope of NIMS. To this end, DHHS has the initial lead responsibility for the federal government and deploys assets as needed within the areas of its statutory responsibility (such as the Public Health Service Act and the Federal Food, Drug, and Cosmetic Act) while keeping the Secretary of Homeland Security apprised regarding the course of the incident and nature of the response operations.

While NIMS is used for all events, the National Response Plan (NRP) is implemented for incidents requiring federal coordination. The NRP is another key provision of the Homeland Security Act of 2002 and Homeland Security Presidential

Directive 5. The purpose of NRP is to align federal coordinating, structures, capabilities, and resources into a unified, all-discipline, and all-hazards approach to domestic incident management. It is based on the premise that incidents are typically managed at the lowest possible geographic, organizational, and jurisdictional level. NRP does not alter or impede the ability of federal agencies to carry out their specific authorities under applicable laws, executive orders, and directives. It establishes the coordinating structures, processes, and protocols required to integrate the specific statutory and policy authorities of various federal departments and agencies in a collective framework for action to include prevention, preparedness, response, and recovery activities. The NRP distinguishes between events that require the secretary of DHS to manage the federal response for incidents of national significance and the majority of incidents occurring each year that are handled by responsible jurisdictions or avenues through other established authorities and existing plans.

Under the NRP, DHS assumes responsibility for coordinating federal response operations, including those involving public health components, under certain conditions. DHS coordinates the federal government's resources utilized in response to or in recovery from terrorist attacks, major disasters, or other emergencies if and when any of the following four conditions applies:

1. A federal department or agency acting under its own authority has requested the assistance.
2. The resources of state and local authorities are overwhelmed and federal assistance has been formally requested by state and local authorities.
3. More than one federal department or agency has become substantially involved in responding to the incident.
4. DHS has been directed to assume responsibility for managing the domestic incident by the president.[3]

For states and local governments to gain full benefit from the emergency response assets of the federal government, states must develop incident management systems that are interoperable with NIMS. Beginning in 2004, adherence to and compatibility with NIMS became a condition of all grants and other awards from federal agencies for any aspect of state or local emergency preparedness and response. NRP compliance was required as well after 2006.

The Pandemic and All-Hazards Preparedness Act (PAHPA) legislation of 2006 and 2013 reauthorized and restructured key components of public health preparedness and response efforts in DHS and DHHS. PAHPA also addressed lessons learned from the flawed federal response to Hurricane Katrina and growing concerns over a possible global flu pandemic. Central to the restructuring of federal roles and responsibilities was the establishment of a national health security strategy for public health emergency preparedness and response, including a full assessment of federal, state, and local public health and medical capabilities. Key elements of the national health security strategy in PAHPA focused on:

- Public health workforce enhancements including revitalization of the Commissioned Corps and loan repayment programs to increase the number of public health professionals working in shortage areas;
- Vaccine tracking and distribution to improve effective distribution of seasonal flu vaccine supplies;

- Enhanced all-hazards medical surge capacity through use of mobile medical assets and federal facilities during emergencies, expanding the Medical Reserve Corps and establishing a single nationwide network of systems for the purpose of advance registration of volunteer health professionals;
- Biomedical research and development for vaccine and drug development to combat pandemic flu emergencies; and
- Grants to state and local government to improve detection and response capabilities for pandemic flu.

Federal Emergency Medical Assets

Several national emergency response assets are available to state and local governments from the new DHS. These include the National Disaster Medical System (NDMS), the Metropolitan Medical Response System (MMRS), and the Strategic National Stockpile (SNS, now under CDC).

The NDMS now operates within the Office of Emergency Preparedness and Response within DHHS. NDMS brings together medical services from DHHS, DHS, Defense, and Veterans Affairs to augment local emergency medical services during a disaster or other large-scale emergency. The NDMS has several operational components, including Disaster Medical Assistance Teams (DMATs), Disaster Mortuary Teams (DMORTs), Federal Coordinating Centers, and Management Support Units.

DMATs are self-sustaining squads of licensed, actively practicing, volunteer professional and paraprofessional medical personnel who provide emergency medical care at the site of a disaster or other emergency. DMATs often triage, stabilize, and prepare patients for evacuation in mass casualty situations. They are sent into these situations to supplement, rather than supplant or replace, local capacity. Once activated, these professionals are federalized, allowing them to practice with their current professional licenses in any jurisdiction. DMORTs include mortuary, dental, and forensic specialists who serve to augment the services of local coroners and medical examiners. Portable temporary mortuaries for mass casualty situations are provided when needed. Management support units provide command, coordination, and communication capabilities for DMATs and DMORTs and other federal assets. Federal Coordinating Centers recruit hospitals to participate in the NDMS and recruit health workers for the DMATs and DMORTs.

The MMRS, involving more than 100 metropolitan communities, integrates existing emergency response systems at the local level, including emergency management, medical and mental health providers, public health agencies, law enforcement, fire departments, emergency medical services, and the National Guard. The MMRS seeks to develop a unified regional response to mass casualty events. MMRS was transferred from DHHS when the new DHS was established in 2003.

The SNS ensures the availability and rapid deployment of life-saving pharmaceuticals, antidotes, other medical supplies, and equipment necessary to counter the effects of nerve agents, biologic pathogens, and chemical agents. The SNS stands ready for immediate deployment to any U.S. location in the event of a terrorist attack using a biologic toxin or chemical agent directed against a civilian population. In the event of a possible bioterrorist attack, a 12-hour push package containing 50 tons of stockpile materials can be immediately dispatched to predetermined

Receipt, Store, and Storage sites identified in state bioterrorism response plans. There are twelve 12-hour push packages centrally located around the United States for immediate deployment. Detailed deployment activities for SNS materials are prescribed in state and local emergency response plans.

Federal Funding for Public Health Preparedness Infrastructure

Although multiple agencies provide federal funding for emergency preparedness, federal support for the public health infrastructure at the state and local levels is provided largely from grants and cooperative agreements with CDC. In 1999, for the first time, CDC awarded more than $40 million for bioterrorism preparedness to states and cities for enhanced laboratory and electronic communication capacity and another $32 million to establish a national pharmaceutical stockpile to ensure availability of vaccines, prophylactic medicines, chemical antidotes, medical supplies, and equipment needed to support a medical response to a biologic or chemical terrorist incident. At the time, these appeared to be large sums. In the wake of September 11, 2001, and the anthrax attacks the following month, increased concerns regarding homeland security led to a $2.1 billion FY 2002 appropriation for CDC's antiterrorism activities, over a 20-fold increase from FY 1999 levels. The FY 2002 supplemental appropriations included nearly $1 billion for grants to states and localities to upgrade state and local capacity. Roughly similar levels of funding were provided throughout the first decade of the new century, although steady reductions marked the years of the second decade. The state and local activities impacted by this funding are described in subsequent sections of this chapter.

STATE AND LOCAL PUBLIC HEALTH PREPAREDNESS AND RESPONSE COORDINATION

State Agencies and Assets

Similar to the federal pattern, states rely on a variety of agencies to deliver public health emergency services. Also similar to the federal model, these functions tend to be concentrated within a limited number of agencies at the state level, with the state health department and state emergency management agency playing the most significant roles. Most state health departments are freestanding agencies (i.e., not part of a larger human services agency), and many have responsibility for emergency medical service systems within the state. However, most states have an environmental health agency that is separate from the state health agency. Although these states may have an environmental health section within the health agency, the environmental health agency is charged with monitoring environmental contaminants and remediation of hazardous conditions. Nearly all states have a separate emergency management agency (patterned after FEMA), and some states have established their own Departments of Homeland Security. In responding to a public health emergency, the state public health agency works collaboratively with the state emergency management agency as well as with the state environmental protection, law enforcement, public safety, and transportation agencies and, in some instances, the National Guard.

States execute their powers and authority to act in public health emergencies through various state public health laws. There are concerns that existing public health laws may be inadequate in some states because they are obsolete and fragmented. A Model Public Health Emergency Powers Act was designed to assist states in examining and enhancing their legal framework for public health emergencies. The model act addresses key issues related to preparedness, surveillance, protection of persons, management of property, and public information and communications.[4]

Considerable differences exist among states in the breadth and depth of services provided within their jurisdictions and the degree to which public health service delivery responsibilities are delegated to local governments. In general, however, state governments are ultimately responsible for ensuring adequate response to a public health emergency and tend to play certain key roles in preparedness and response, regardless of how decentralized a particular public health system might be. Except in the largest metropolitan local public health departments, local public health officials rely on state personnel and capacity for a number of key functions, including advanced laboratory capacity, epidemiologic expertise, and serving as a conduit for federal assistance.

OUTSIDE-THE-BOOK THINKING 9-3

Describe three or more provisions of public health statutes that are important elements of public health emergency response plans.

States participate in an interstate agreement whereby one or more states can provide resources, equipment, services, and other needed support to another state during an emergency incident. This mutual aid agreement, the Emergency Management Assistance Compact (EMAC), covers licensing, credentialing, workers compensation, and reimbursement, allowing personnel to focus on the emergency at hand. EMAC personnel integrate into the existing structures of the requesting state. Of the more than 65,000 personnel deployed to Louisiana, Mississippi, and Alabama for Hurricanes Katrina and Rita in 2005, nearly 4,000 were health and medical personnel.

Incident Command Systems

In order to manage resources effectively and facilitate decision making during emergencies, incident command systems (ICS) are in wide use by police, fire, and emergency management agencies. Initially adopted for the fire service, ICS eliminates many common problems related to communication, terminology, organizational structure, span of control, and other differences across different disciplines and agencies in response to a critical incident. Critical incidents include any natural or man-made event, civil disturbance, or any other occurrence of unusual or severe nature that threatens to cause or actually causes the loss of life or injury to citizens and/or severe damage to property.

In managing critical incidents, clear goals and objectives are established and communicated to responders, response plans are utilized, communications are effective, and resources are utilized in a timely and effective manner. ICS should not be considered an additional set of procedures; rather the system must become part of routine operations, with personnel fully trained in its use and standard operating procedures reflective of the capabilities actually available.

One important key to effective ICS is the ability to size up the incident scene and make the initial call for resources. This allows responders to get control of the incident rather than playing catch-up for the rest of the incident. Appropriate initial size-up prevents unnecessary injury or loss of life, property or environmental damage, and negative perceptions of the responding agencies.

Key components of ICS include:

- Common terminology—Major organizational functions and units are named; in multiple incidents, each incident is named. Common names are used for personnel, equipment, and facilities. Clear terms are used in radio transmissions (e.g., codes, such as "10" codes, are not used).
- Modular organization—ICS develops "top down" from the first unit involved based on the specific incident's management needs. Each ICS is staffed with a designated incident commander (responsible for safety, liaison, and information) with other functions (operations, planning, logistics, finance/administration) staffed as needed.
- Integrated communications—ICS uses a common communications plan and redundant two-way communications.
- A unified command structure—This is necessary when the incident is within a single jurisdiction with multiple agencies involved, or the incident is multijurisdictional, or individuals representing different agencies or jurisdictions share common responsibilities. All agencies involved contribute to the unified command process by determining overall goals and objectives, planning jointly for tactical activities, conducting integrated tactical operations, and maximizing the use of assigned resources.
- Consolidated action plans—Written action plans are necessary when the incident is complex and/or when several agencies and/or jurisdictions are involved. Action plans include specific goals, objectives, and support activities.
- A manageable span of control—The number of subordinates one supervisor can manage effectively should be between three and seven, with five being optimal.
- Designated incident facilities—These include the command post from which all incident operations, direction, control, coordination, and resource management are directed. Command posts can be fixed or mobile but need adequate communications capabilities.
- Comprehensive resource management—This maximizes resource use, consolidates control, reduces communications load, provides accountability, and reduces freelancing.

The emergency management team functions at the emergency operations center (EOC) where it coordinates strategic decisions through the incident command structure. Ideally, the team should be isolated from the confusion, media, and weather during the incident. EOC participants must have adequate authority and decision-making capability. EOC decisions could include issuing curfews, circumventing normal bidding processes, emergency appointments, permanent or temporary

relocation, emergency demolition of unsafe properties, or implementation of pro-
phylaxis to populations. The EOC is supported operationally by incident command
posts in the field, which are responsible for tactical decisions as well as oversight and
command of responders at the scene.

Effective emergency operations plans and standard operating procedures simplify decision making during incidents. Training makes implementation of decisions easier for subordinates. When the level of preparation and practice exercises
is inadequate, emergency operations plans can become overwhelmed by common
incidents and unable to deal with those that are not fully anticipated. In such circumstances, decision making becomes complex and challenging. A comprehensively
planned and frequently exercised organizational system is necessary to overcome
these pitfalls.

As ICS has become increasingly accepted as an effective framework for responding to incidents, its use has extended to other settings. For example, there has been
much progress in development and deployment of hospital emergency ICSs and
tabletop exercises for hospitals. Several states have expanded on the ICS concept to
develop standardized emergency management systems that formally incorporate ICS,
mutual aid agreements, and multijurisdictional and interagency cooperation at the
substate level, resulting in coordinated and unified decisions throughout the state.

Local Agencies and Assets

The front line of response to public health emergencies is at the local level,
where LHDs work collaboratively with other first responders, such as fire and rescue
personnel, emergency medical service providers, law enforcement officers, hazardous materials teams, physicians, and hospitals in preparing for and managing the
consequences of health-related emergencies. Although the relationships between
state and local public health agencies vary greatly from state to state, and even from
local jurisdiction to local jurisdiction within the same state, local government has
significant responsibilities for dealing with emergencies in virtually all states. First
responders play key roles in:

- Recognizing public health emergencies, including those that result from terrorist attacks
- Identifying unique personal safety implications associated with the emergency
  situation
- Identifying security issues that are unique to the event or to the emergency
  medical system response
- Understanding basic principles of patient care based upon the type of emergency event encountered

Focusing on the services most directly related to emergency preparedness and
response, the vast majority of LHDs carry out activities related to epidemiology and
surveillance, communicable disease control, food safety, and restaurant inspections.[5]
Relatively few LHDs operate laboratory services, air quality, animal control, or water
inspections.

In those cases in which the LHD is not responsible for these services, they are
typically delivered by another local government agency (e.g., a fire department or

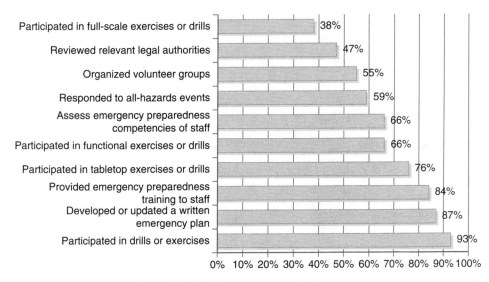

Figure 9-3   Percentage of local health departments with selected emergency preparedness activities in the past year.

Data from National Association of County and City Health Officials, *2013 National Profile of Local Health Departments*. Washington, DC: NACCHO; 2014.

environmental services agency), a private agency (hospital or ambulance service), or the state. Even when services are offered by an LHD, they may be quite limited in terms of scope or hours of availability. For example, although nearly one-half of LHDs report providing laboratory services, these services may be quite limited in nature (e.g., to support tuberculosis and sexually transmitted disease testing). Many LHDs that report having laboratory services are likely to rely on state public health labs for more specialized diagnostic needs.

The state of readiness among LHDs has increased since 2001, when only about one-fourth of LHDs had completed a comprehensive emergency response plan with another one-fourth indicating that planning was underway. Deployment of LHD staff to assist in emergencies is limited by the size and qualifications of the agency's workforce. More than one-half of all LHDs have 20 or fewer staff members.[5] Larger agencies generally have much higher staffing levels and a more comprehensive range of expertise. Figure 9-3 illustrates the range of LHD activities related to emergency preparedness and response in 2013. Nearly 60% of LHDs reported responding to an emergency event in the previous year. Figure 9-4 demonstrates the percentage of LHDs responding to specific events or participating in drills and exercises related to those emergencies. Table 9-3 catalogs the range and types of drills and exercises.

The configuration of LHDs within a state or in a multistate metropolitan area also varies across the country. Several states organize local public health activities at a regional or district level. Other states have virtually hundreds of LHDs that serve towns or townships, some in counties or districts served by a larger LHD. Some communities have no LHD at all. Organizing preparedness and response efforts in these different circumstances presents special problems in terms of multijurisdictional

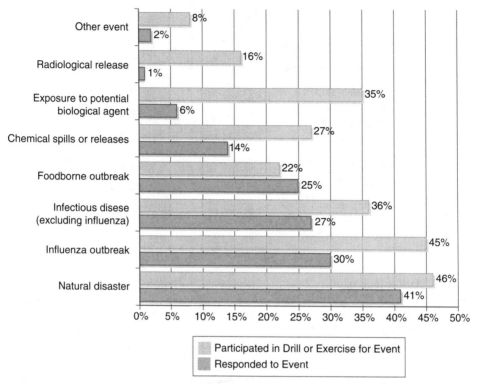

Figure 9-4 Percentage of local health departments responding to a specific all-hazards event or participating in a drill or exercise for that event in the past year.

Modified from National Association of County and City Health Officials, *2013 National Profile of Local Health Departments*. Washington, DC: NACCHO; 2014.

response, surge capacity, backup, and mutual aid agreements. Several capacity assessment and enhancement tools are available from NACCHO and CDC to assist local assessment of readiness.[6-8]

Medical Reserve Corps are locally based volunteer response teams that can be deployed in emergency situations. These multidisciplinary teams often have ongoing relationships with local public health agencies and other community medical care providers that may include volunteer work on health promotion and screening projects or assistance with mosquito control activities in communities where West Nile Virus presents a risk. During emergencies, Medical Reserve Corps teams play predetermined roles such as providing local surge capacity for triage and medical care or assisting with deployment of SNS materials. Several hundred communities already participate in the Medical Reserve Corps program, either through start-up funding from the HRSA or through local resources.

Education and training for frontline workers has been a continuing challenge for local agencies in order for them to assess and address the training needs of key public health professionals, infectious disease specialists, emergency department personnel, and other healthcare (including mental health) providers. Emergency preparedness competencies (Table 9-4) for all public health workers serve as the focal

Table 9-3 Types of Emergency Exercises

Exercise	Activities that can be undertaken by an agency or group of agencies to test their readiness to respond to emergencies or to evaluate the adequacy of their response plan and success of their training program.
Orientation seminar or workshop	An exercise carried out to familiarize new staff with the agency's emergency response activities or current staff to new or changing information or procedures or to bring together response agencies for better understanding and coordination.
Drill	An exercise limited to a specific response activity and conducted to instruct thoroughly through repetition and practice.
Tabletop	An exercise conducted in a conference room setting with situations presented as verbal or written problems or questions intended to generate discussion of actions to be taken based on the emergency plan and standard operating procedures. Basic tabletop exercises use group process to solve problems. Advanced play uses prescripted messages.
Functional	An exercise usually conducted at the site where the event would normally take place such as the command center and designed to evaluate the capabilities of the disaster response system.
Full scale	An exercise designed to test a major portion of the emergency operations plan, evaluate the operational capability of emergency responders in an interactive manner over an extended period of time, and mobilize field personnel and resources.

Adapted from Center for Health Policy, Columbia University School of Nursing. *Defining Emergency Exercises: A Working Guide to the Terminology Used in Practicing Emergency Responses in Communities and Public Health Agencies.* New York, NY: Columbia University School of Nursing, Center for Health Policy; 2004.

point for these assessment, enhancement, and recognition efforts. A more extensive panel of bioterrorism and emergency readiness competencies for various categories of public health workers is also in wide use.[9]

Private Healthcare Providers and Other Partners

In nearly all communities, government agencies play a central role in preparing for and responding to public health emergencies. Often overlooked, however, is the critical contribution made by private sector healthcare providers, pharmaceutical manufacturers, agricultural producers, the food industry, and other private sector interests. An important example is the role played by alert health professionals who are trained to recognize potential emergency situations and report these suspicions to public health officials. Clinicians in Florida played a major role in first identifying and then linking anthrax cases with bioterrorism in 2001. Hospital emergency rooms and physicians' offices are where most individuals who have contracted an infectious disease or are exposed to dangerous chemicals encounter their community's emergency response system. That encounter should trigger an appropriate response if the condition is one that represents a threat to others. Every state has

Table 9-4   Emergency Preparedness Core Competencies for All Public Health Workers

All Public Health Workers must be competent to:
- Describe the public health role in emergency response in a range of emergencies that might arise (e.g., "The department provides surveillance, investigation, and public information in disease outbreaks and collaborates with other agencies in geological, environmental, and weather emergencies").
- Describe the chain of command in emergency response.
- Identify and locate the agency emergency response plan (or the pertinent portion of the plan).
- Describe his/her functional role(s) in emergency response and demonstrate his/her role(s) in regular drills.
- Demonstrate correct use of all communication equipment used for emergency communication (e.g., phone, fax, radio).
- Describe communication role(s) in emergency response—within the agency using established communication systems, with the media, with the general public, and personal (with family, neighbors).
- Identify limits to own knowledge/skill/authority and identify key system resources for referring matters that exceed these limits.
- Recognize unusual events that might indicate an emergency and describe appropriate action (e.g., communicate clearly within chain of command).
- Apply creative problem solving and flexible thinking to unusual challenges within his/her functional responsibilities and evaluate effectiveness of all actions taken.

Public Health Leaders/Administrators must also be competent to:
- Describe the chain of command and management system ("incident command system") or similar protocol for emergency response in the jurisdiction.
- Communicate the public health information, roles, capacities, and legal authority to all emergency response partners—such as other public health agencies, other health agencies, and other governmental agencies—during planning, drills, and actual emergencies. (This includes contributing to effective community-wide response through leadership, team building, negotiation, and conflict resolution.)
- Maintain regular communication with emergency response partners. (This includes maintaining a current directory of partners and identifying appropriate methods for contacting them in emergencies.)
- Ensure that the agency (or the agency unit) has a written, regularly updated plan for major categories of emergencies that respects the culture of the community and provides for continuity of agency operations.
- Ensure that the agency (or agency unit) regularly practices all parts of emergency response.
- Evaluate every emergency response drill (or actual response) to identify needed internal and external improvements.
- Ensure that knowledge and skill gaps identified through emergency response planning, drills, and evaluation are addressed.

Public Health Professionals must also be competent to:
- Demonstrate readiness to apply professional skills to a range of emergency situations during regular drills (e.g., access, use, and interpret surveillance data; access and use lab resources; access and use science-based investigation and risk assessment protocols; identify and use appropriate personal protective equipment).
- Maintain regular communication with partner professionals in other agencies involved in emergency response. (This includes contributing to effective community-wide response through leadership, team building, negotiation, and conflict resolution.)
- Participate in continuing education to maintain up-to-date knowledge in areas relevant to emergency response (e.g., emerging infectious diseases, hazardous materials, and diagnostic tests).

Table 9-4 Emergency Preparedness Core Competencies for All Public Health Workers (*Continued*)

Public Health Technical and Support Staff must also be competent to:
- Demonstrate the use of equipment (including personal protective equipment) and skills associated with his/her functional role in emergency response during regular drills.
- Describe at least one resource for backup support in key areas of responsibility.

Developed by Columbia University School of Nursing, Center for Health Policy under Centers for Disease Control and Prevention/Association of Teachers of Preventive Medicine Cooperative Agreement # TS 0740: Bioterrorism and Emergency Readiness Competencies for all Public Health Workers.

incorporated requirements in state statute that call for physicians, laboratories, and other health providers to notify public health officials when specific notifiable diseases or conditions are encountered. Some states include a general provision that physicians should report "unusual" infectious diseases. Despite these laws and regulations, compliance with disease reporting physicians remains spotty for a variety of reasons. The requirements and the reporting procedures may not be understood by some physicians. Others believe reporting is not worth the time and effort. Reporting from laboratories is more complete, but concerns exist as to whether laboratories serving multiple jurisdictions are fully aware of differences in requirements among the jurisdictions served.

In addition to playing an important role in identifying potential public health emergencies, healthcare providers play a critical role in responding to the medical consequences of those emergencies, especially in mass casualty situations. For the relatively rare disease threats associated with bioterrorism, healthcare providers often have only limited experience dealing with these conditions and look to public health authorities for clinical guidance. Through the development of community-wide emergency response plans, public health agencies, private sector delivery systems, hospitals, physicians, pharmacies, nursing homes, and others are mobilized in the event of an emergency to provide needed treatment to those affected by disease and to provide prophylactic care to those at risk for exposure to disease. State and federal laws that confer tax-exempt status on hospitals typically require those institutions to provide significant community benefit, including the provision of emergency medical services and participation in regional emergency medical service planning. Funds for hospital preparedness, including staff training and preparedness planning, are provided by DHHS and channeled through state health departments.

Other private sector interests also contribute to public health emergency preparedness. Although NIH makes significant investments in the development of new vaccines and antimicrobial agents, pharmaceutical manufacturers represent the primary source of funding for research and development. Efforts to encourage industry interest in the development of vaccines and other countermeasures include incentives such as liability protections, antitrust waivers, patent extensions, and long-term contracts. Similarly, activities to improve the safety and security of the food supply will rely on the agricultural and food production industries to make necessary upgrades to their processes and to seek innovative ways to minimize disease threats.

Public Perceptions and Expectations

The flurry of activity to improve public health emergency preparedness and response capabilities is understandable. The public is highly concerned over the possibility of terrorist attacks of all types. Fears of possible anthrax or smallpox attacks are nearly as high as concerns of conventional explosives, airline hijacking or bombings, and attacks using radioactive, toxic, or hazardous materials as weapons.[10] Among these potential terrorist weapons, concerns persist that smallpox will be used, related in part to the attention placed on smallpox at the national level with the initiation of smallpox preparedness programs that include vaccinations for key medical and first responder personnel. Although the public believes that the country is better prepared for a biologic or chemical attack than it was prior to 2002, the public perceives that the current level of preparedness is not high enough and more needs to be done. Public health leaders have been concerned that the emphasis on bioterrorism would reduce efforts on other public health problems and issues. Figure 9-5 and Figure 9-6 suggest that this concern may be unfounded as evidence

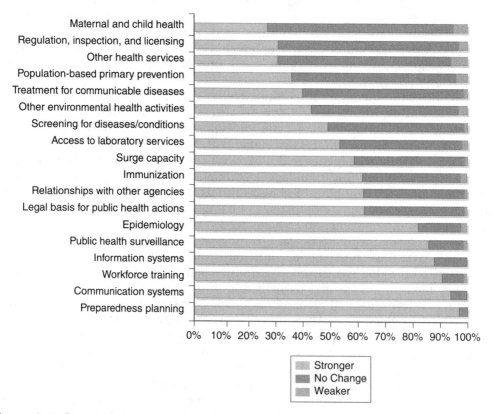

Figure 9-5   Reported change in selected LHD functions beteeen 2002 and 2005 as a result of efforts to imprive emergency preparedness.

Data from National Association of County and City Health Officials. 2005 *National Profile of Local Health Departments*. Washington, DC: NACCHO; 2006.

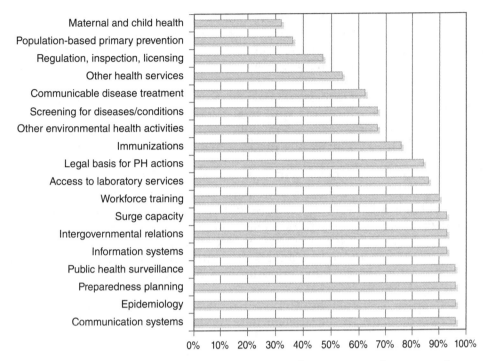

Figure 9-6 Percentage of states reporting stronger infrastructure and programs because of emergency preparedness efforts.

Data from Association of State and Territorial Health Officials (ASTHO). *Profile of State Public Health, Volume One.* Washington, DC: ASTHO; 2009.

suggests that preparedness funding has actually served to strengthen key public health programs as well the public health infrastructure in the United States.

State and Local Preparedness Grants

With the public health infrastructure increasingly viewed as a frontline defense against terrorism and homeland security priority, federal funding for public health purposes increased dramatically beginning in 2002. To put this increase into perspective, total governmental public health activity spending in 2000 was $43 billion, with the federal government accounting for approximately $5 billion.[11]

Beginning in 2002, federal funding increased by more than $2 billion, with about one-half of that amount directed to state and local governments for public health infrastructure improvements. Similar levels were funded through 2010 with reductions implemented thereafter. The infusion of this magnitude of resources afforded the opportunity to address serious and longstanding gaps in public health protection and foster greater consistency and enhanced quality throughout the national network of governmental public health agencies at the federal, state, and local levels.

Public health infrastructure funding was channeled to the states and several large cities (including New York, Chicago, Los Angeles, and Washington, DC) through

CDC. Each state received a minimum award of $5 million plus an additional amount based on a population formula. Activities supported by these funds were to be consistent with federal guidance. In several funding cycles, additional priorities were added, some without additional resources. In 2003, federal guidance incorporated specific smallpox preparedness and response capacities and allowed for costs associated with smallpox preparedness to be covered by grant funds. In 2006, pandemic flu preparedness became a priority with some additional one time funding provided. Amidst the evolution of broader federal policies on national security, CDC guidance since 2011 has focused on increasing specific capabilities at the state and local level.

State and Local Emergency Preparedness Capabilities

In 2011, CDC implemented a systematic process for defining a set of public health preparedness capabilities to assist state and local health departments with their strategic planning. The resulting public health preparedness capabilities established national standards for public health preparedness capability-based planning in order to assist state and local planners in identifying gaps in preparedness, determining the specific jurisdictional priorities, and developing plans for building and sustaining capabilities.

CDC identified 15 public health preparedness capabilities (shown below in their corresponding domains) as the basis for state and local public health preparedness:

Biosurveillance

- Public Health Laboratory Testing
- Public Health Surveillance and Epidemiological Investigation

Community Resilience

- Community Preparedness
- Community Recovery

Countermeasures and Mitigation

- Medical Countermeasure Dispensing
- Medical Materiel Management and Distribution
- Non-Pharmaceutical Interventions
- Responder Safety and Health

Incident Management

- Emergency Operations Coordination

Information Management

- Emergency Public Information and Warning
- Information Sharing

Surge Management

- Fatality Management
- Mass Care
- Medical Surge
- Volunteer Management[12]

The basic strategy was for each jurisdiction to determine the order of the capabilities it would pursue based upon the jurisdictional risk assessment completed as part of the community preparedness capability. Jurisdictions were strongly advised to ensure that they first were able to demonstrate capabilities within the biosurveillance, community resilience, countermeasures and mitigation, incident management, and information sharing domains.

In order to delineate the public health aspects for each capability, CDC adopted the terminology and definitions from the DHS Target Capabilities List, content from the Pandemic and All-Hazards Preparedness Act, and capabilities from the National Health Security Strategy (NHSS) as a baseline. Aligning across national programs, the Pandemic and All-Hazards Preparedness Act emphasizes the need to maintain consistency with other key national programs, specifically the NHSS preparedness goals. PAHPA also directs that the NHSS be consistent with the DHS National Preparedness Guidelines, a major component of which is the Target Capabilities List. The National Preparedness Guidelines represent a standard for preparedness based on establishing national priorities through a capabilities-based planning process. In addition to aligning with the National Preparedness Guidelines, CDC determined that the public health preparedness capabilities should also be aligned with the essential public health services framework. CDC conducted a mapping process, which determined that several of the public health preparedness capabilities aligned with multiple essential public health services. Thus, the state and local preparedness capabilities align with both the DHS target capabilities and the HHS essential public health services, with a focus on public health capabilities critical to preparedness (see Figure 9-7).

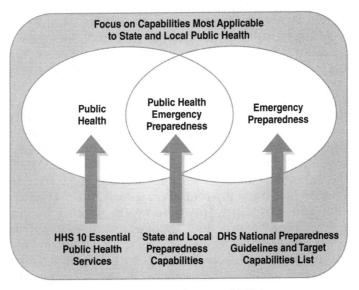

Figure 9-7 Public health emergency preparedness capabilities

Reproduced from Centers for Disease Control and Prevention, Office of Public Health Preparedness and Response. *Public Health Preparedness Capabilities, National Standards for State and Local Planning, March 2011.* Atlanta, GA: CDC; 2011.

The public health preparedness capabilities represent a national public health standard for state and local preparedness that better prepares state and local health departments for responding to public health emergencies and incidents, and supports the accomplishment of the essential public health services. Each of the public health preparedness capabilities identifies priority resource elements that are relevant to both routine public health activities and essential public health services. While demonstrations of capabilities can be achieved through different means (e.g., exercises, planned events, and real incidents), jurisdictions are encouraged to use routine public health activities to demonstrate and evaluate their public health preparedness capabilities.

The content of each public health preparedness capability is based on evidence-informed documents, applicable preparedness literature, and subject matter expertise gathered from across the federal government and the state and local practice community. Each capability includes a definition of the capability and list of the associated functions, performance measures, tasks, and resource considerations.

OUTSIDE-THE-BOOK THINKING 9-4

What is meant by the term "surge capacity," and how is this addressed in public health emergency response plans?

Early Lessons

Effective state and local preparedness programs require hazard and vulnerability analyses, forecasts of the probable health effects, analyses of the availability of needed resources, identification of vulnerable populations, and development of detailed plans for both preparedness and response. Many factors influence the ability of states and localities to complete these tasks. Public health preparedness is particularly challenging because public health and public safety roles differ for federal, state, and local governments. The federal government has primary responsibility for national security, while state and local governments carry the responsibility and financial burden for most other public health responsibilities. At the local level, public health preparedness must be well coordinated with hospital preparedness. Virtually all states now recognize the importance of exercises and drills and there have been a number of national exercises involving the top officials of federal and state government.

Ideally, the infusion of resources to shore up the sagging public health infrastructure would foster positive structural changes in public health systems at the state and local level. The early evidence supports this contention. Yet federal funding is slowly eroding, with the average awards to LHDs in 2013 providing only $1.15 per capita and with smaller LHDs receiving larger per capita awards than LHDs serving more populous communities.[5]

Despite fears that the increased focus on emergency preparedness would weaken other public health duties, this has not occurred. Preparedness is now viewed as an important quality or attribute of an effective public health system rather than as another priority program operating within its own silo. This is the essence of the philosophy that has come to be known as the "dual use," "multiple use," or "all-hazards" strategy. Although still early in the process, some things are clear.

The price for public health preparedness is high, regardless of how it is calculated. In crude dollar terms, its costs reflect a significant increase in the federal investment in governmental public health services provided through governmental public health agencies. This increase will need to be sustained indefinitely, because it primarily supports information, communications, and workforce development systems that are ongoing in nature. It will require commensurate commitment and investment on the part of state and local governments. Otherwise, supplanting will occur in one form or another and the opportunity for federal preparedness funds to leverage other resources will be lost.

The price in terms of federalism and intergovernmental relationships will also be high. States will need to encourage and accept stronger federal leadership on the one hand and generate a better understanding of local needs and priorities on the other. These will need to be fashioned into effective local, regional, state, and multistate efforts in ways that will challenge states to live up to their primary responsibility for the health of their citizens. All this must be done while navigating through a treacherous obstacle course laden with political, economic, and bureaucratic impediments to sustained progress.

The federal government must avoid the pitfall of merely throwing money at the problem, without fostering a national vision of public health preparedness and nurturing the state–local public health systems that must carry out that vision. This will require the federal agencies to be accountable for meaningful capacity and performance standards, consistent credibility as to ends and means, integration both across focus areas and across federal agencies, and leadership rather than either regulatory or advisory approaches to dealing with state–local public health system issues.

Although these are formidable challenges, the opportunities are unprecedented. The boost in federal funding and potential for federal leadership provide a unique opportunity to fashion a more coordinated national public health system. Certainly, the public now expects this, and the price of not being prepared will be even higher.

OUTSIDE-THE-BOOK THINKING 9-5

Choose a public health discipline or occupational group (either your own or one that you are somewhat familiar with) and describe the range of tasks that this discipline may be asked to perform in disaster preparedness and response.

CONCLUSION

Preparing for and responding to emergencies is a well-established role for public health agencies and their workers. This role, highlighted in the Public Health in America statement[1] as one of six critical responsibilities, has often been viewed as one of responding to an occasional natural disaster such as an earthquake, hurricane, or flood. Large-scale events that threaten public health and safety have seldom been intentionally inflicted, until recent examples to the contrary, such as the anthrax mailings in 2001 and the bombings of the federal building in Oklahoma City in the 1990s and the Boston Marathon in 2013. Geopolitical events in the international theater now raise the specter of increased risk for terrorist acts, including bioterrorism, directed against the American population, underscoring the need for sustained preparedness and response capacities at all levels of government.

The cycle of progress in public health preparedness has been remarkably consistent over several centuries in the United States. A terrible epidemic or another form of health-related disaster or threat occurs. Public expectations call for such an event to never occur again. Significant new resources are deployed to raise the level of preparedness and protection. There is no immediate recurrence and the threat seems to dissipate over time. Preparedness, though still important, becomes relatively less important. Eventually, a new threat or event appears, and the cycle repeats itself.

This recurring scenario raises the question as to whether current preparedness efforts represent a new and different strategy that could interrupt this chain of events. Past preparedness efforts focused on a specific threat and diminished as that specific threat diminished. Perhaps a more broadly focused preparedness campaign, one that is valued because it battles many different threats, will fare differently.

REFERENCES

1. Public Health Functions Steering Committee. *Public Health in America*. Washington, DC: U.S. Public Health Service; 1995.
2. Landesmann LY. *Public Health Management of Disasters: The Practice Guide*. Washington, DC: American Public Health Association; 2001.
3. Presidential Homeland Security Directive No. 5, February 28, 2003.
4. The Center for Law and the Public's Health. *The Model State Emergency Health Powers Act*. Baltimore, MD: Georgetown and Johns Hopkins Universities; 2001.
5. National Association of County and City Health Officials. *2013 Profile of Local Health Departments*. Washington, DC: NACCHO; 2014.
6. National Association of County and City Health Officials. *Elements of Effective Local Bioterrorism Preparedness: A Planning Primer for Local Health Departments*. Washington, DC: National Association of County and City Health Officials; 2001.
7. National Association of County and City Health Officials. *Local Centers for Public Health Preparedness: Models for Strengthening Local Public Health Capacity*. Washington, DC: National Association of County and City Health Officials; 2001.
8. Centers for Disease Control and Prevention. *Local Emergency Preparedness and Response Inventory: A Tool for Rapid Assessment of Local Capacity to Respond to Bioterrorism, Outbreaks of Infectious Disease, and Other Public Health Threats and Emergencies*. Atlanta, GA: Centers for Disease Control; 2001.
9. Columbia University School of Nursing, National Association of County and City Health Officials, and Centers for Disease Control and Prevention. 2003. Bioterrorism and Emergency Readiness Competencies for All Public Health Workers. Available at https://training.fema.gov/EMIWeb/downloads/BioTerrorism%20and%20Emergency%20Readiness.pdf. Accessed October 7, 2014.
10. Lake, Snell, Perry, & Associates. *Americans Speak Out on Bioterrorism and U.S. Preparedness to Address Risk*. Princeton, NJ: Robert Wood Johnson Foundation; December 2002.
11. Centers for Medicare and Medicaid Services. National Health Accounts.
12. Centers for Disease Control and Prevention, Office of Public Health Preparedness and Response. *Public Health Preparedness Capabilities: National Standards for State and Local Planning, March 2011*. Atlanta, GA: CDC; 2011.

Public Health Practice: Future Challenges

This text approaches what public health is and how it works from a unified conceptual framework. Key dimensions of the public health system are examined, including its purpose, functions, capacity, processes, and outcomes. Although it is a simple framework, many of the concepts addressed are anything but simple. As a result, much has been left unsaid, and many important issues and problems facing the public health system have been addressed only in passing. This may serve to whet the appetite of those eager to move beyond the basics and ready to tackle emerging and more complex issues in greater depth. The basic concepts included in this text seek to facilitate that process and encourage outside-the-book thinking. Delving into these other issues without the benefit of a broad understanding of the field and how it works, however, can be hazardous in any field of endeavor. For public health workers, continuously fighting off alligators remains the major deterrent to draining the swamp in order to avert the alligator threat in the first place.

The public health achievements of the 20th century demonstrate that the problems facing public health have changed over the past century and argue that we can expect them to continue to change throughout the current century. In retrospect, many past problems appear as though they should have been relatively easy to solve in comparison with those on the public health agenda at the beginning of the 21st century; however, we often forget that last century's problems appeared to be quite formidable to public health advocates 100 years ago. Although formidable, they were eventually deemed unacceptable, initiating the chain of events that resulted in an impressive catalog of accomplishments ranging from infectious disease threats to oral health.

Each public health achievement provides valuable lessons and insights into the obstacles to achieving even further gains that lie ahead. Challenges reside at many levels, especially at the level of preparedness for unforeseen and previously unanticipated threats to the public's health. Melding the expectations for addressing ongoing health problems in the community with those for preparing and responding to new threats leads us to the three key questions addressed in this chapter:

1. What are the lessons learned from the threats and challenges faced by public health in 20th century America?
2. What are the limitations and challenges facing public health in the 21st century?
3. How can these limitations and challenges be overcome?

LESSONS FROM A CENTURY OF PROGRESS IN PUBLIC HEALTH

The remarkable achievements of the 20th century did not completely eradicate the public health problems faced in 1900. Many of these continue to threaten the health of Americans and impede progress toward realizing the life span projections presented in Figure 10-1. New faces for old enemies have appeared in the form of challenges and obstacles to be overcome in the early decades of the 21st century.

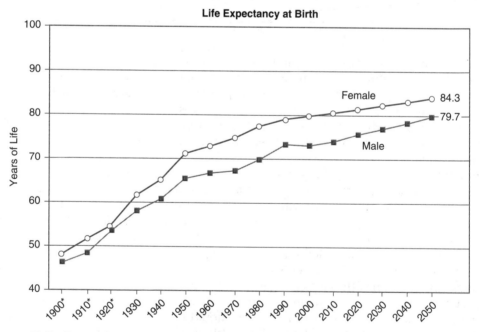

Figure 10-1   Past and projected female and male expectancy at birth, United States, 1900–2050. Reproduced from U.S. Public Health Service. *Healthy People 2010: Understanding and Improving Health.* Washington, DC: PHS; 2000

Infectious diseases, tobacco, maternal and infant mortality, environmental and occupational health, food safety, cardiovascular disease, injuries, and oral health remain high on the list of leading threats to the public's health. Each presents special challenges.

Infectious Diseases

The continuing battle against infectious diseases will be fought on several fronts because of the emergence of new infectious diseases and the reemergence of old enemies, often in drug-resistant forms. For example, infections caused by *Escherichia coli* O157:H7 have emerged as a frequent and frightening risk to the public. Initially identified as the cause of hemorrhagic conditions in the early 1980s, this pathogen was increasingly associated with foodborne illness outbreaks in the 1990s, including a major outbreak in the Pacific Northwest related to *E. coli*-contaminated hamburgers distributed through a national fast food chain.[1] The source of the *E. coli* was cattle. Other outbreaks of this pathogen involved swimmers in lake water contaminated by bathers infected with the organism (Figure 10-2). Because many of the illnesses are minor and both medical and public health practitioners fail to perform the tests necessary to diagnose *E. coli* infections properly, current surveillance efforts greatly underreport the extent of this condition.

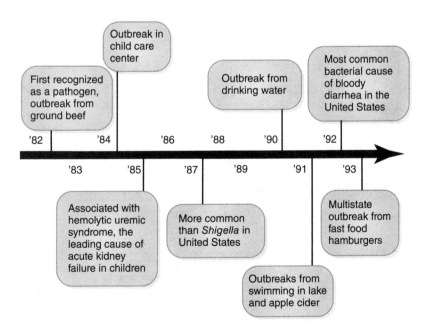

Figure 10-2   Emergence of a public health threat: the *Escherichia coli* O157:H7 time line.

Reproduced from Centers for Disease Control and Prevention. *Addressing Emerging Infectious Disease Threats: A Prevention Strategy for the United States.* Atlanta, GA, CDC; 1994

Multidrug-resistant pathogens represent another emerging infectious disease problem for the public health system. The widespread and, at times, indiscriminate use of antibiotics in agricultural and healthcare settings produces strains of bacteria that are resistant to these drugs. Antimicrobial agents have been increasingly deployed throughout the second half of the 20th century. Slowly, over this period, the consequences of these miracle drugs have been experienced in our communities, as well as our health facilities. The emergence of drug-resistant strains has reduced the effectiveness of treatment for several common infections, including tuberculosis, gonorrhea, pneumococcal infections, and hospital-acquired staphylococcal and enterococcal infections. For tuberculosis, drug resistance and demographic trends, including immigration policies, played substantial roles in this disease's resurgence in the early 1990s. The changing demographics of tuberculosis infections are illustrated in Figure 10-3.

Pathogens, both old and new, have devised ingenious ways of adapting to and thwarting the weapons used to control them. Many factors in society, the environment, and global interconnectedness continue to increase the risk of emergence and spread of infectious diseases. An outbreak of monkeypox virus affecting several states in the United States in 2003 demonstrates how unusual diseases in remote parts of the world can affect Americans virtually overnight (Figure 10-4). In 2014, Middle East Respiratory Syndrome (MERS) made its first appearance in the United States, again illustrating this threat.

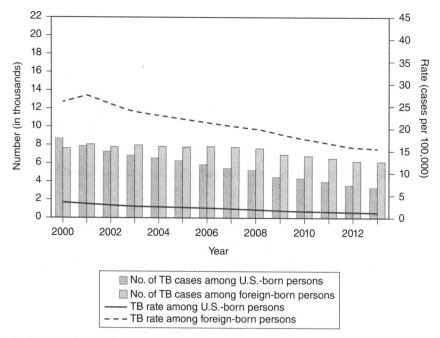

Figure 10-3 Number and rate of tuberculosis cases among U.S.-born and foreign-born persons, by year reported, 2000–2013.

Reproduced from Alami NN, Yuen CM, Miramontes R, Pratt R, Price SF, Navin TR. Trends in tuberculosis, United States, 2013. *MMWR*. 2014; *63*(11): 229–233.

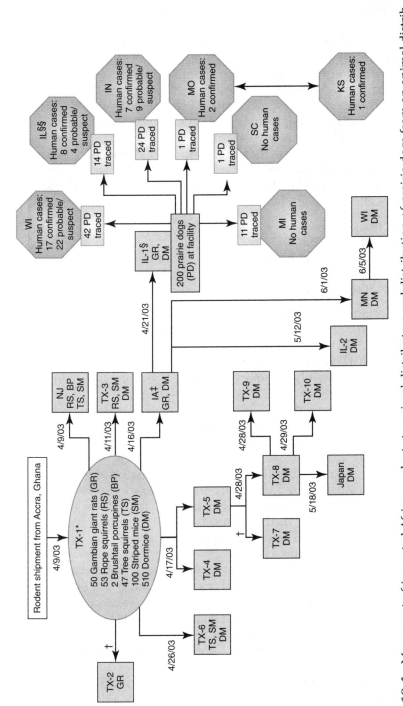

Figure 10-4 Movement of imported African rodents to animal distributors and distribution of prairie dogs from an animal distributor or associated with human cases of monkeypox, 11 states, 2003.

Notes: Illinois (IL), Indiana (IN), Iowa (IA), Kansas (KS), Michigan (MI), Minnesota (MN), Missouri (MO), New Jersey (NJ), South Carolina (SC), Texas (TX), and Wisconsin (WI). Japan is included among sites having received rodents implicated in the outbreak.

*Date of shipment unknown.

* dentified as distributor C in MMWR 2003;52:561–564.
§ dentified as distributor B in MMWR 2003;52:561–564.
‡ dentified as distributor D in MMWR 2003;52:561–564.
§§Includes two persons who were employees at IL-1.

Reproduced from Centers for Disease Control and Prevention. Update: multistate outbreak of monkeypox—Illinois, Indiana, Kansas, Missouri, Ohio, and Wisconsin, 2003. *MMWR.* 2003; 52(27): 642–646.

The potential for global outbreaks and massive pandemics is now on the public health radar screen. An outbreak of severe acute respiratory syndrome hit more than two dozen countries in North America, South America, Europe, and Asia in 2003 before it was contained, but not before taking nearly 800 lives. The possibility of a global pandemic of influenza virus looms as even more frightening because it is impossible to predict when the next influenza pandemic will occur or how severe it will be. Wherever and whenever a pandemic starts, everyone everywhere in the world is at risk. Countries might, through measures such as border closures and travel restrictions, delay arrival of the virus, but cannot stop it.

Health professionals remain concerned that the continued spread of a highly pathogenic avian H5N1 virus across eastern Asia and other countries represents a significant threat to human health. The H5N1 virus has raised concerns about a potential human pandemic because:

- It is especially virulent.
- It is being spread by migratory birds.
- It can be transmitted from birds to mammals and in some limited circumstances to humans.
- Like other influenza viruses, it continues to evolve.

Since 2003, a growing number of human H5N1 cases have been reported in Asia, Africa, and Europe. More than half of the people infected with the H5N1 virus have died. Most of these cases are all believed to have been caused by exposure to infected poultry. There has been no sustained human-to-human transmission of the disease, but the concern is that H5N1 will evolve into a virus capable of human-to-human transmission.

A massive epidemic of Ebola virus disease, a rare and deadly disease previously known as Ebola hemorrhagic fever, led to an unprecedented international response in 2014 after the case count in West Africa (Guinea, Liberia, Nigeria, Sierra Leone) surpassed 20,000 with case fatality rates in the 70% range (see Figure 10-5 and Table 10-1). This explosion of cases occurred after decades of smaller, intermittent outbreaks affecting a dozen countries in Africa. The importation of travel-related cases to the United States and elsewhere outside West Africa in late 2014, leading to cases among several healthcare workers, further demonstrated the global risks associated with uncontrolled local outbreaks and the importance of vigilance and preparedness in dealing with unfamiliar pathogens.

Heightened concerns over the risk of acts of bioterrorism add a new twist to the threats posed by infectious diseases. As noted in our examination of public health emergency preparedness and response, these concerns have raised expectations for public health to serve both national security and personal safety roles.

The influence of infectious diseases in the development of chronic diseases such as diabetes, heart disease, and some cancers further argues that infectious diseases will continue as important health risks in the new century. To battle infectious diseases, the development and deployment of new methods, both in laboratory and epidemiologic sciences, are needed to better understand the interactions among environmental factors as contributors to the emergence and reemergence of infectious disease processes. Also, despite the successes realized in the development and use of vaccines over the past century, substantial gaps persist in the infrastructure

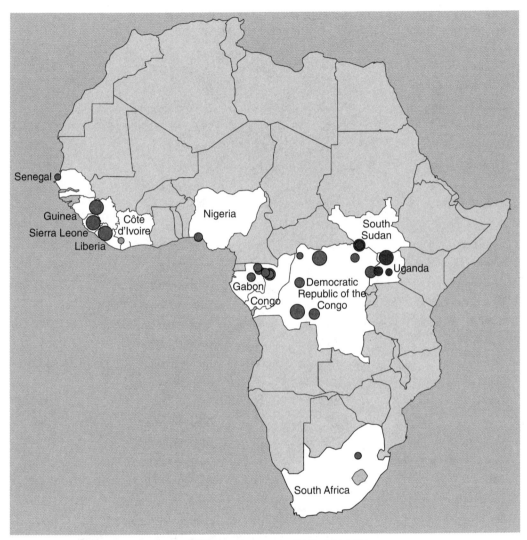

EBOLAVIRUS OUTBREAKS BY SPECIES AND SIZE, 1976-2014

Species	Number of Cases
● Zaire ebolavirus	○ 1-10
● Sudan ebolavirus	○ 11-100
● Tai Forest ebolavirus	○ 101-300
● Bundibugyo ebolavirus	○ Greater than 300 reported cases

0   245   490   980 Miles

Figure 10-5   Cases of Ebola virus disease in Africa, 1976–2014.

Reproduced from Centers for Disease Control and Prevention. Ebola Virus Distribution Map. Available at http://www.cdc.gov/vhf/ebola/outbreaks/history/distribution-map.html. Accessed November 4, 2014.

Table 10-1   Ebola Virus Disease–Known Cases and Outbreaks in Reverse Chronological Order, Various Countries, 1976–2014 (through 11/3/2014)

Country	Cases	Deaths	Species	Year
Dem. Rep. of Congo	66	49	*Zaire ebolavirus*	2014
Multiple countries	13,540	4,941	*Zaire ebolavirus*	2014
Uganda	6*	3*	*Sudan ebolavirus*	2012
Dem. Rep. of Congo	36*	13*	*Bundibugyo ebolavirus*	2012
Uganda	11*	4*	*Sudan ebolavirus*	2012
Uganda	1	1	*Sudan ebolavirus*	2011
Dem. Rep. of Congo	32	15	*Zaire ebolavirus*	2008
Uganda	149	37	*Bundibugyo ebolavirus*	2007
Dem. Rep. of Congo	264	187	*Zaire ebolavirus*	2007
South Sudan	17	7	*Zaire ebolavirus*	2004
Republic of Congo	35	29	*Zaire ebolavirus*	2003
Republic of Congo	143	128	*Zaire ebolavirus*	2002
Republic of Congo	57	43	*Zaire ebolavirus*	2001
Gabon	65	53	*Zaire ebolavirus*	2001
Uganda	425	224	*Zaire ebolavirus*	2000
South Africa	2	1	*Zaire ebolavirus*	1996
Gabon	60	45	*Zaire ebolavirus*	1996
Gabon	37	21	*Zaire ebolavirus*	1996
Dem. Rep. of Congo	315	250	*Zaire ebolavirus*	1995
Côte d'Ivoire (Ivory Coast)	1	0	*Taï Forest ebolavirus*	1994
Gabon	52	31	*Zaire ebolavirus*	1994
South Sudan	34	22	*Sudan ebolavirus*	1979
Dem. Rep. of Congo	1	1	*Zaire ebolavirus*	1977
South Sudan	284	151	*Sudan ebolavirus*	1976
Dem. Rep. of Congo	318	280	*Zaire ebolavirus*	1976

Notes: *Numbers reflect laboratory confirmed cases only. 2014 Democratic Republic of Congo outbreak not related to 2014 outbreak involving multiple countries; Multiple countries in 2014 include Liberia, Sierra Leone, Nigeria, Guinea, United States, Senegal, and Spain as of November 4, 2014.

Data from Centers for Disease Control and Prevention. Available at http://www.cdc.gov/vhf/ebola/outbreaks/history/chronology.html. Accessed November 4, 2014.

of the vaccine delivery system, including the roles played by parents, providers, information technology, and biotech and pharmaceutical companies. Improving the coordination of these elements holds the promise of reducing the toll from infectious diseases in the 21st century.

Tobacco Use

The potential gains to be realized from further reduction of tobacco usage are also apparent. Despite the overall decline in tobacco use among adults over the second half of the 20th century, an alarmingly high prevalence of tobacco use among teens persists, and rates among adults are no longer declining, as they did prior to 1980. These trends suggest that concerns over risks related to exposure to environmental tobacco smoke will continue for many years to come. Disparities in tobacco use by race and ethnicity, together with the growth of demographic groups with high use rates, add yet another dimension to the war against tobacco. New approaches and new products will raise new issues of safety, whereas the increase in tobacco use across the globe will transport old and new challenges around the world.

Maternal and Child Health

Even as maternal and child health outcomes have improved dramatically, there has been little change in the prime determinants of perinatal outcomes—the rate of low birth weight and preterm deliveries. This situation must be addressed to even partially replicate the gains realized in the 20th century. Another important risk factor moving in the wrong direction is the rate of unintended pregnancies. Together, these challenges call for improved understanding of the biologic, social, cultural, economic, psychological, and environmental factors that influence maternal and infant health outcomes and in the effectiveness of intervention strategies designed to address these causative factors.

Motor Vehicle Injuries

The impressive gains realized in reducing motor vehicle injuries have uncovered gaps in our understanding of comprehensive prevention. Challenges include expanding surveillance to monitor nonfatal injuries, detect new problems, and set priorities. Greater research into emerging and priority problems, as well as intervention effectiveness, is also needed, as are more effective collaborations and interagency partnerships. Injuries to pedestrians from vehicles other than automobiles will also challenge public health in the 21st century. The effects of age, alcohol use, seat belt use, and interventions targeting these risks will require greater attention for progress to continue in the battle against motor vehicle injuries.

Cardiovascular Disease

An aging population less threatened by infectious disease and injury will place even more people at risk of ill health related to cardiovascular diseases. Greater attention to research to understand the various social, psychological, environmental, physiologic, and genetic determinants of cardiovascular diseases is needed in the new century. Reducing disparities that exist in terms of burden of disease, prevalence of risk factors, and ability to reach high-risk populations represents another mega challenge. Identifying new and emerging risk factors and their relationships, including genetic and infectious disease factors, will be necessary in both developed and developing parts of the world.

Food Safety

Our understanding of food safety and nutrition made great strides in the 1900s, but both old and new risks will need to be addressed in the new century. Iron and folate deficiencies continue, and many of the advantages related to breastfeeding remain unrealized. The emergence of obesity, often in the midst of food deserts, as an increasingly prevalent condition throughout the population is one of the most startling developments of the late 20th century. Persistent challenges include applying new information about nutrition, dietary patterns, and behavior that promote health and reduce the risk of chronic diseases.

Oral Health

One of the most overlooked achievements of public health in the 20th century was the dramatic decline in dental caries due to fluoridation of drinking water supplies. Ironically, these advances in oral health have contributed to the perception that dental caries are no longer a significant public health problem and that fluoridation is no longer needed. These battles are likely to be fought in political, rather than scientific, arenas, presenting a substantial challenge to public health in the 21st century.

Workplace Safety

Workplaces are now safer than ever before, yet challenges remain on this front, as well. Improved surveillance of work-related injuries and illnesses and better methods of conducting field investigations in high-risk occupations and industries remain formidable challenges. Applying new methods of risk assessment to improve assessment of injury exposures and intervention outcomes, as well as improved research into intervention effectiveness, surveillance methods, and organization of work represent additional challenges for public health practice in the 21st century.

Unfinished Agenda

It is clear that much remains to be done. The national *Healthy People* process articulates this unfinished agenda by identifying important targets and leading indicators of health status for the United States.[2] These health problems persist on the public health agenda, which has now expanded to include new issues related to alcohol and substance abuse, mental health, violence, and risky sexual behaviors. These are now categorized as important public health problems and have taken their rightful place on the public health agenda. Progress toward these leading health indicators documents the challenges that lie ahead. The public health challenges of the 21st century appear daunting, but those of the preceding century must have seemed even more so.

Applying the lessons learned from the recent century of progress in public health to both new and persisting health threats will be necessary to increase the span of healthy life and eliminate the huge disparities in health outcomes that are the overarching goals of the year 2020 national health objectives. The public health challenges of both centuries call for the application of sound science in an environment that supports social justice in health. This remains the most formidable challenge facing public health practice in the 21st century.

OUTSIDE-THE-BOOK THINKING 10-1

What was the most important achievement of public health in the 20th century? Why?
What will likely be the most important achievement of public health in the 21st century? Why?

LIMITATIONS OF 21ST-CENTURY PUBLIC HEALTH

Despite the remarkable achievements of the 20th century, there is much for public health to do in the early decades of the new century. Continued progress is by no means assured because of a new constellation of problems and important limitations of conventional public health efforts. Global environmental threats, the disruption of vital ecosystems, global population overload, persistent and widening social injustice and health inequalities, and lack of access to effective care add to the list of health problems left over from the 20th century.[3] Consider, for example, the implications of the link between social position and health, and a nation growing more and more diverse, with a disproportionate burden of poverty falling on children, minorities, and one-parent families. Further gains in health status may be less related to science than to social policies. For some public health professionals, the limitations of conventional public health are difficult to accept because, in large part, they represent the supporting pillars of the public health enterprise. This reluctance to critically self-assess makes future progress less certain. It is useful to examine these limitations in terms of their relationship to the two major forces shaping public health responses—science and social values.

Among the limitations affecting the science of public health is an undue emphasis on reductionist thinking that seeks molecular-level explanations for social and structural phenomena. Identification of risk factors has been useful for public health efforts, but the emphasis on individual risk factors often obscures patterns that call for multilevel responses. The persistent identification of the association of social deprivation with many of the important health problems of the last century is a case in point. Approaches for reducing coronary heart disease provide another example. Health interventions targeting a reduction in coronary heart disease frequently focus on risk factors at the physiologic level, such as blood pressure control, cholesterol, and obesity and on lifestyle factors at the individual level, including smoking, nutrition, physical activity, and psychosocial factors. However, there are also environmental influences, such as geographic location, housing conditions, occupational risks, and social structure influences, such as social class, age, gender, and race/ethnicity. In this multilevel view of coronary heart disease, interventions that focus on primary and secondary prevention (those addressing the physiologic and individual levels) need to be supplemented by organization-level and community-level interventions (addressing environmental influences) and healthy public policy (addressing the social structure level).

Another limitation of public health's scientific heritage is the penchant for dichotomous thinking and the failure to view health phenomena as continuous. Using coronary heart disease as an example, dichotomous thinking draws attention to individual and physiologic level factors, whereas viewing this condition as continuous encourages a population-wide view and development of interventions that reduce overall incidence and prevalence by affecting frequency distributions in the entire population. A view of health problems as continuous phenomena suggests that efforts be made throughout the population to move the entire frequency distribution for coronary heart disease "to the left," rather than to reduce disease burden only among those groups most heavily impacted. Here it is apparent that science and social values are not pure and mutually exclusive forces.

Discussion and debate over scientific approaches to public health problems are not, however, purely scientific in nature. At the heart of collective actions are collective values as to whether issues affecting individuals are more important than issues affecting communities of individuals and as to the meaning of health itself. Should public health emphasize the health of individuals or the health of communities? In part, these reflect the different perspectives of health described in other chapters. On one hand is a mechanistic view of health as the absence of disease, promoting health interventions that emphasize curative treatment for afflicted individuals. On the other hand is a more holistic view of health that sees health as a complex equilibrium of forces and factors necessary for optimal functioning of that individual. This latter view emphasizes health maintenance and health promotion, often through broad social policies affecting the entire community. Differences in public health systems among societies are largely described by these differences. Some societies, like the United States, focus on individuals using a largely medical treatment approach. Others are more heavily influenced by collectivism and a holistic view of health. At the core of what can be accomplished under either view, however, are basic values and social philosophies that guide the use of the scientific knowledge available at any point in time. These differences in social values also affect perceptions as to what is expected of government and, as a result, the form and leadership of public health efforts. To a large extent, these forces have hastened the development of community public health practice and career opportunities in public health in the United States, a phenomenon described in previous chapters.

THE FUTURE OF PUBLIC HEALTH IN 1988 AND A QUARTER CENTURY LATER

In many respects, the limitations of modern public health are as apparent as its achievements. Persisting, emerging, reemerging, and newly assigned problems will forever challenge public health as a social enterprise. Success will depend on both the structure and the content of the public health response. A continuous, critical, and comprehensive self-examination of the public health enterprise offers the greatest chance for continued success. A series of such self-examinations began with the 1988 report of Institute of Medicine (IOM), *The Future of Public Health*.[4] A comprehensive reexamination, *The Future of the Public's Health in the 21st Century*, was completed in 2002.[5] A companion study of issues related to educating public health professionals was also completed by the IOM in 2002.[ ] These examinations outlined the limitations of public health efforts in the 20th century, but cast these failings as lessons, challenges, and opportunities for public health in the 21st century.

The Future of Public Health, 1988

The IOM's landmark report, completed in 1988, found much of value in the nation's public health efforts, but it also identified a long list of problems. The most serious problem of all was that Americans were taking their public health system for granted. The nation had come to believe that epidemics of communicable diseases were a thing of the past and that food and water would forever be free of infectious and toxic agents. Americans assumed that workplaces, restaurants, and homes were safe and that everyone had access to the information and skills needed to lead healthy lives. They also assumed that all of this could occur even while public health agencies were being increasingly called on to provide health services to nearly 50 million Americans who had no health insurance or were underinsured; however, across the nation, states and localities were failing to provide the resources that would allow both the traditional public health and more recent health service roles to be carried out successfully. When future benefits compete with immediate needs, the results are predictable.

These circumstances fostered the image of a public health system in disarray. Within this system, neither the public nor those involved in the work of public health appreciated the scope and content of public health in modern America. There was little consensus as to the specific responsibilities to be expected from the various levels of government and even less interest in securing such consensus.

Previous chapters document that several formulations in the IOM report have been widely embraced by the public health community. These include statements of the mission, substance, and core functions of public health. The mission has been described simply as ensuring conditions in which people can be healthy. The substance consists largely of organized community efforts to promote health and prevent disease. The IOM report identified an essential role for government in public health in organizing and ensuring that the mission gets addressed. An expanded view of the fundamental functions of governmental public health was articulated in the three core functions of assessment, policy development, and assurance. These represent a more comprehensive view of public health efforts than that conveyed by earlier views that public health primarily furnished services and enforced statutes. The new public health differed in its emphasis on problem identification and resolution as the basis of rational interventions and on working with and through other stakeholders, rather than intervening unilaterally.

Perhaps the most motivating aspect of the IOM report, however, was its characterization of the disarray of public health and the significance of that disarray. The IOM report painted a picture of disjointed efforts in the 1980s to deal with immediate crises, such as the epidemic of human immunodeficiency virus infections and an increasing lack of access to health services and enduring problems with significant social impacts, such as injuries, teen pregnancy, hypertension, depression, and tobacco and drug use. With impending crises on the horizon in the form of toxic substances, mental illness, Alzheimer's disease, and public health capacity, the IOM report found the situation to be grimmer still.

The report found a wide gap between the capacity of the public health system of the 1980s and those of a public health system capable of rising to modern challenges. It charted a course to move ever closer to an optimally functioning system. Several enabling steps were identified:

- Improving the statutory base of public health
- Strengthening the structural and organizational framework
- Improving the capacity for action, including technical, political, management, programmatic, and fiscal competencies of public health professionals
- Strengthening linkages between academia and practice[4]

In the end, the report concluded that working through a multitude of society's institutions, rather than through only traditional public health organizations, is the key to improving the public health system. It is also a daunting task, calling for entering into partnerships with sectors such as education, law enforcement, media, faith, corrections, and business, and fostering change through leadership and influence, rather than through command and control. The barriers to effecting these collaborations are the major obstacles to achieving the aspirations outlined in the *Healthy People* national health objectives. These barriers come in all sizes and shapes and from many different sources. Some are perceived as external barriers; others appear to be more internal.

The IOM report identified important barriers inhibiting effective public health action:

- Lack of consensus on the content of the public health mission
- Inadequate capacity to carry out the essential public health functions of assessment, policy development, and assurance of services
- Disjointed decision making without necessary data and knowledge
- Inequities in the distribution of services and the benefits of public health
- Limits on effective leadership, including poor interaction among the technical and political aspects of decisions, rapid turnover of leaders, and inadequate relationships with the medical profession
- Organizational fragmentation or submersion
- Problems in relationships among the several levels of government
- Inadequate development of necessary knowledge across the full array of public health needs
- Poor public image of public health, inhibiting necessary support
- Special problems that unduly limit the financial resources available to public health[4]

The Future of Public Health, A Quarter Century Later

The IOM advanced these themes through several other reports published in the 1990s and early years of the new century. A brief status report on progress in implementing the 1988 report's major recommendations was completed in the mid-1990s, and a report promoting community health improvement processes appeared later in the decade. A full scale reexamination of the public health enterprise, titled *The Future of the Public's Health in the 21st Century*, was undertaken after the turn of the century and completed in late 2002. That report focused more extensively on multisectoral partnerships with government than had the 1988 report, which mainly emphasized government's role in achieving public health goals.

The 2002 IOM report restated the unique responsibility that government has for promoting and protecting the health of its people. It noted, however, that four factors argue that government alone should not bear full responsibility for the health of the public:

1. Public resources are limited, and public health spending must compete with other valid causes.
2. Democratic societies expressly limit the powers of government and reserve many activities for private institutions.
3. Determinants affecting health derive from multiple sources and sectors, including many social determinants that cannot be addressed by government alone.
4. There is growing evidence that multisectoral collaborations are more powerful and effective than government acting alone.[5]

In light of these factors, the 2002 IOM report examined both the governmental contributions to the public's health and those from other sectors of American society. Recommendations for the governmental enterprise were complemented by recommendations for healthcare providers, business, media, the faith community, and academia. The report proposed six major areas for action:

1. Adopting a population health approach that considers the multiple determinants of health within an ecological framework
2. Strengthening the governmental public health infrastructure, which forms the backbone of the public health system
3. Building a new generation of intersectoral partnerships that also draw on the perspectives and resources of diverse communities and actively engages them in health actions
4. Developing systems of accountability to ensure the quality and availability of public health services
5. Making evidence the foundation of decision making and the measure of success
6. Enhancing and facilitating communication within the public health system (e.g., among all levels of the governmental public health infrastructure, between public health professionals and community members)[5]

Barriers to future progress are apparent in both major IOM reports. Foremost has been the lack of a social-ecological view of health that attempts to understand good and poor health in terms of the multiple factors that interact with each other at the personal, family, community, and population level. Another set of important barriers affecting public health is the prevailing values of the American public—in particular, those restricting the ability of government to identify and address factors that influence health. Social values determine the extent to which government can regulate human behavior, such as through controlling the production and use of tobacco products or requiring bicycle or motorcycle helmet use. These values also determine whether and to what extent family planning or school-based clinic services are provided in a community and determine the content of school health education curricula. Some of these social values find strange bedfellows. For example, many

Americans oppose control of firearms on the basis of principles of self-protection embodied in the U.S. Constitution; gun companies also oppose control, although on the basis of more direct economic considerations.

Economic and resource considerations are common themes, as well. One obvious issue is that most public health activities remain funded from the discretionary budgets of local, state, and federal government. At all levels, discretionary programs have been squeezed by true entitlement programs, such as Medicaid and Medicare, as well as by some governmental responsibilities that have become near entitlements, such as public safety, law enforcement, corrections, and education. The war on terrorism with military campaigns in Iraq and Afghanistan further squeezed the national budget and any chance of significant health or human service initiatives at home. Funding one set of health-related services from governmental discretionary funds while other health services are financed through a competitive marketplace widens the imbalance between treatment and prevention as investment strategies for improved health status. There are powerful economic interests among health sector industries, as well as among industries whose products affect health, such as the tobacco, alcohol, pesticide, and firearms industries. One can only dream that equally powerful lobbies, other than those made up of pharmaceutical companies, might develop for hepatitis or drug-resistant tuberculosis.

All too often, the complex problems and issues of public health, with causes and contributing factors perceived to lie outside its boundaries, lead public health professionals to believe that they should not be held accountable for failure or success; however, many facets of public health practice itself could be further improved. These include relationships with the private sector and medical practice and some internal reengineering of public health processes. Fear and suspicion of the private sector can lead to many missed opportunities. Just as the three most important factors determining real estate values are location, location, and location, it can be argued that the three most important factors for health are jobs, jobs, and jobs. If this is anywhere near true, suspicions of the private sector need to be put to rest. There is little question that employment is a powerful preventive health intervention, in terms of both individual and community health status. Community development activities that bring new businesses and jobs to a community can affect health status more positively than a public health clinic on every corner. Furthermore, businesses have been major forces behind the growth of managed care systems in the United States. Their partnership with public health interests will be essential to secure new resources or to shift the balance between treatment and prevention strategies. Increased partnerships with medical care interests will also be necessary. Unfortunately, there is widespread ignorance of the medical care sector among public health workers.

Among barriers internal to public health agencies is one that often goes unnoticed—the persistent and widespread use of categorical approaches to the deployment of interventions, which often fragments and isolates individual programs, one from another. In addition to the unnecessary proliferation of information, management, and other administrative processes, each program tends to develop its own assortment of interest and constituency groups, including those involving program staff members, who often work to oppose meaningful consolidation and integration of programs.

Another limiting factor is the generalized inability to prioritize and focus public health efforts, despite the wealth of information as to which factors most affect health at the national, state, and even local levels. Time and time again, tobacco, alcohol, diet, and violence have been shown to lie at the root of most preventable mortality and years of potential life lost. Ideally, resource allocation decisions would be made on the basis of the most important attributable risks, rather than being spread around to address, ineffectively, risks both large and small. With scores of priorities, there are really none, and without clear priorities, accountability is seldom expected. Public health has always operated at the interface of science and politics; political issues and compromises are natural. Still, inconsistencies between stated public health priorities and actual program priorities, as demonstrated through funding, are themselves barriers to public understanding and support for public health work. Comprehensive and systematic approaches must replace current silo strategies.

Other factors that influence public understanding and support for public health relate to the transition from conditions caused by microorganisms to those caused by human behaviors. It is more difficult for the public to appreciate the scientific basis for public health interventions when social, rather than physical sciences, guide strategies. This occurs at a time when government is increasingly portrayed as both incompetent and overly intrusive. Largely because governmental processes are considered by the public to be intensely political, the public view of public health processes, including programs and regulations, is that of highly politicized and partly scientific exercises.

There has been considerable debate as to whether the 1988 IOM report accurately captured the problems and needs of the American public health system. In many respects, the report restated the fundamental values and concepts underlying public health in terms of its emphasis on prevention, professional diversity, collaborative nature, community problem solving, loosely attached constituencies, assurance functions, need to draw other sectors into the solution of public health problems, and lack of an identifiable constituency. Taken together, these features appear to represent disarray; however, the cause of this disarray may not lie with public health but rather with our social and governmental institutions, more generally. Posing solutions that restructure the public health system's components may do little more than rearranging the deck chairs on the Titanic would have done.

It may be necessary to more broadly restructure the tasks and functions of public health to deal with modern public health problems. The larger work of public health is to get the threat protection, disease prevention, and health promotion job done right, rather than to get it done through a traditional structuring of roles and responsibilities. Preventing disease and promoting health must be embraced throughout society and its health institutions, rather than existing in a parallel subsystem. There is no evidence to support the contention that public health activities are best organized through public health agencies of government. Other nations have emphasized social policies that have brought them better overall health outcomes for their populations at much lower cost. It is the mission and the effort that are important and not necessarily the organization from which those efforts are generated.

OUTSIDE-THE-BOOK THINKING 10-2

Using an academic grading scale from A to F, how effective is the public health system in the United States? How did you arrive at this rating?

CONCLUSION: THE NEED FOR A MORE EFFECTIVE PUBLIC HEALTH SYSTEM

The perpetual frustration for public health is the gap between what has been achieved and what could have been achieved. The unfulfilled promise of public health should not be viewed as some unfortunate accident but as a direct result of a series of past decisions and actions undertaken quite purposefully. Sadly, they reflect both a history of disregard and the consequences of battles over the legitimacy, scope, professional authority, and political reach of public health.[7] A recent example is the use of tobacco settlement funds.

The various settlements in 1998 with a group of the major tobacco companies will provide $250 billion to the states over a 25-year period. These settlements were initially viewed as a colossal success for public health over one of its most important enemies. Although still in the middle years of this possible quarter-century windfall, state legislative and executive branch leaders have opted to use this money for a variety of purposes, some for health purposes but much for other ends. It was expected that approaches would vary from state to state, with most using some portion of the money to support tobacco cessation and prevention interventions. Early indications, however, are that as little as one-third of the settlement funds were earmarked for health programs and that the health share declined rapidly in the face of state budget deficits throughout the first and second decades of the century.

The tobacco company settlement can be viewed as a success story or as part of a full accounting of the massive failure of public health efforts in the battle against tobacco use. Why did it take 3 decades to change public perceptions and values to the point that settlement became inevitable? Without attention to the lessons of this saga and to strengthening the public health system, tobacco will be the first of many health hazards that are inadequately addressed and for which a negotiated settlement will eventually occur. If we look at the tobacco settlement as a signal of the failure of public health and evidence of a weak public health infrastructure, this windfall becomes, at best, a bittersweet victory. Perhaps the tobacco settlement windfall would best be directed toward averting the next tobacco-like settlement. Difficult questions arise, even in otherwise good times!

In any event, the settlement offered the possibility of a sustained increase in public health resources to the tune of about $10 billion annually for 25 years. Considering that only approximately $43 billion was expended for governmental public health activities in 2000, the tobacco funds represented a possible 25% increase. Additional funding to governmental public health agencies for bioterrorism preparedness on top of the tobacco settlement funds provided for a possible doubling of governmental public health activities in the early years of the 21st century. As we have seen, however, this was an illusion that never materialized.

These circumstances and other key issues and challenges facing the future of public health defy simple summarization. This chapter has examined several, including those offered by the achievements and limitations of public health practice in the 20th century and others offered by the IOM reports; other chapters presented many more. Which of these are most important remains a point of contention. It would be useful to have an official list that represents the consensus of policy makers and the public alike; however, because an official list is lacking, several general conclusions as to the critical challenges and obstacles facing the future of public health in the United States are offered here. They summarize some of the important themes of this text in describing why we need more effective public health efforts.

The Easy Problems Have Already Been Solved

Major successes have been achieved through public health efforts over the past 150 years, largely related to massive reductions in infectious diseases but also involving substantial declines in death rates for injuries and several major chronic diseases since about 1960. The list of current problems for public health includes the more difficult chronic diseases, new and emerging conditions, including bioterrorism, and broader social problems with health effects (teen pregnancy and violence are good examples) that have identifiable risk and contributing factors that can be addressed only through collective action. The days of command-and-control approaches to relatively simple infectious risks are behind us. In the past, environmental sanitation and engineering could collaborate with communicable disease control expertise to address important public health problems. The collaborations needed for violence prevention or bioterrorism preparedness require very different skills and relationships.

To a Hammer, the Entire World Looks Like a Nail

Behind the aphorism that to a hammer, the entire world looks like a nail is the perception that common education and work experiences foster common professional perspectives. The danger lies in believing that one's own professional tools are adequate to the task of dealing with all of the problems and needs that are served by the profession. Each profession has its own scientific base and jargon. Problems are given labels or diagnoses, using the profession's specialized language, so that the tools of the profession can be brought to bear on those problems. All too often, however, the problems come to be considered as the domain of that profession, and the potential contributions of other professions and disciplines are underappreciated. Although public health professionals are remarkably diverse in terms of their educational and experiential backgrounds, we can also fall into this trap. When we do, bridges to other partners are not built, and collaborations do not take place. As a result, problems that can be addressed only through collaborative, intersectoral approaches flourish unabated.

A Friend in Need Is a Friend Indeed

Finding the means to build such bridges can be difficult, but some key collaborations appear to be absolutely essential for the work of public health to succeed. Certainly, links between public health and medical care must be improved for both to prosper in a reforming health system. Links with businesses also represent another avenue for mutually successful collaborations. The key is to find major areas of common purpose. For medical care interests, the common denominator is that prevention saves money and rewards those who use it as an investment strategy. For business interests, the bottom line has to be improved, and businesses must accept the premise that improving health status in the community serves their bottom lines through healthier, more productive workers and healthier and wealthier consumers.

You Get What You Pay For

There is good cause to question the current national investment strategy as it relates to health. The excess capacity that has been established in the American health system is becoming increasingly unaffordable, and the results are nothing about which to write home. Still, the competition for additional dollars is intense among the major interests that dominate the health industry, and there is only minimal movement to alter the current balance between treatment and prevention strategies. With less than 5% of all health expenditures supporting public health's core functions and essential services and only about 1% supporting population-based prevention, even small shifts could reap substantial rewards. The argument that resources are limited and that there simply are not adequate resources to meet treatment, as well as prevention purposes, is uniquely American and quite inimical to the public's health. More disconcerting yet are the lost opportunities in securing and using recent tobacco settlement and bioterrorism preparedness funding to shore up a sagging public health infrastructure.

It's Not My Job?

The job description of public health has never been clear. As a result, public health has become quite proficient in delivering specific services, with less attention paid to mobilizing action toward those factors that most seriously affect community health status. Among traditional health-related factors, tobacco, alcohol, and diet are factors responsible for much of modern America's mortality (or lack thereof) and morbidity. Nonetheless, the resources supporting interventions directed toward these factors are minuscule. Similarly, the primary cause of America's relatively poor health outcomes, in comparison with other developed nations, as well as the most likely source for further health gains in the United States, resides in the huge and increasing gaps among racial and ethnic groups. The public health system, from national to state and local levels, must recognize these circumstances and move beyond them to advocate and build constituencies aggressively for efforts that target the most important of the traditional health risk factors and that promote social policies that will both minimize and equalize risks throughout the population. The task is as simple as following the golden rule and doing for others what we want done for ourselves because efforts to improve the health of others make everyone healthier. This does not constitute a new job description for public health in the United States, but rather a recommitment to an old, reasonably successful, and absolutely necessary one.

REFERENCES

1. Centers for Disease Control and Prevention. *Addressing Emerging Infectious Disease Threats: A Prevention Strategy for the United States*. Atlanta, GA: U.S. Public Health Service; 1994.
2. U.S. Department of Health and Human Services. *Healthy People 2020*. Available at www.healthypeople.gov. Accessed June 15, 2014.
3. McKinlay JB, Marceau LD. To boldly go.... *Am J Public Health*. 2000; *90*: 25–33.
4. Institute of Medicine. *The Future of Public Health*. Washington, DC: National Academy Press; 1988.
5. Institute of Medicine. *The Future of the Public's Health in the 21st Century*. Washington, DC: National Academy Press; 2003.
6. Institute of Medicine. *Who Will Keep the Public Healthy? Educating Public Health Professionals for the 21st Century*. Washington, DC: National Academy Press; 2003.
7. Fee E, Brown TM. The unfulfilled promise of public health: déjà vu all over again. *Health Aff*. 2002; *21*: 31–43.

Part II

Case Studies

The second part of this book consists of case studies that complement and supplement the topics covered in the 10 main chapters. The case studies are of varying length and complexity, but all address issues important to modern public health practice. Each has learning objectives, content, discussion questions, and references. Although the case studies were not designed to focus on or accompany a specific chapter of the textbook, many align well with one or more chapters.

Case Study 1 examines the chronology of public health events in Chicago, a topic that fits well with the sections of Chapter 1 presenting a brief history of public health in the United States. This case study also offers insights into the characteristics of the governmental health agencies described in Chapter 4 and the public health services available in communities in Chapters 5 and 8. Case Study 2 traces the history of the Centers for Disease Control and Prevention and also interfaces well with Chapters 1 and 4.

Chapter 2 examines measures of population health, a broad topic that can be supplemented by several different case studies, including Case Study 6 on outcome oriented perinatal surveillance, Case Study 8 on the aftermath of the Gulf oil spill, and Case Study 10 on the public health achievements of the first decade of the 21st century. Case Study 7 on the University of Illinois Hospital fits well with the examination in Chapter 3 of the U.S. health system. In addition to the case studies on Chicago's public health history and the Centers for Disease Control and Prevention, Chapter 4 covers the role of law in public health, a topic central to the story told in Case Study 5 (Ragsdale U.S. Supreme Court Case).

Chapter 5 covers community health needs assessments and community health improvement initiatives among other important topics. The story of a massive contaminated milk outbreak (Case Study 4) provides an opportunity to further explore and apply these concepts, as does Case Study 8 grounded in the Gulf oil spill aftermath. Elements of Case Study 8 also complement the program development sections of Chapter 8 and the emergency response topics in Chapter 9.

Chapter 6 examines issues related to the public health workforce, while Chapter 7 focuses on other key components of public health infrastructure. These topics permeate virtually all of the case studies included in this book.

Case studies on coalition building and program development (Case Study 11) and on mandatory premarital HIV testing (Case Study 3) parallel many of the themes included in Chapter 8, which emphasizes concepts and principles of public health program planning, development, and evaluation. A tabletop exercise case study (Case Study 9) offers a similar opportunity to appreciate the inner workings of public health emergency preparedness, the central topic of Chapter 9. Finally, the future challenges for public health described in Chapter 10 can be enhanced through the use of the case study previously mentioned on public health achievements in the first decade of the 21st century (Case Study 10).

In sum, the case studies provided in Part II offer a variety of options for instructors and students. The case study examples provided here may help stimulate course instructors to bring in or develop other case studies, including those based on their own experiences in public health practice. More than a few of those offered here are based on the actual public health practice experiences of the author.

History of Public Health in Chicago

The history of public health events in Chicago traces the evolution of public health responses and activities over the past 180 years in the United States. Chicago's public health history parallels that of many American urban centers, offering a lens through which the evolution of public health responses can be viewed.

LEARNING OBJECTIVES

Through review and discussion of this case study, students will be able to:

- Describe how public health activities and responses have evolved into their current form.

- Identify influences on public health activities and responses over the past 200 years.

- Describe past and present scientific, legal, political, ethical, media, and financial challenges facing public health organizations in large cities.

- Explain how and why large cities face unique public health challenges today.

SELECTED HISTORY OF PUBLIC HEALTH EVENTS IN CHICAGO, 1834–2014

1834 A temporary board of health was formed to fight the threat of cholera.

1835 The Chicago Board of Health was established by the state legislature to secure the general health of the inhabitants due to the threat of a cholera epidemic. Chicago, then a town, had an estimated 3,265 residents.

1837 Chicago was incorporated as a city of 4,170 residents. Three health commissioners and a health officer were named to inspect marketplaces, prepare death certificates, construct a pest house, visit persons suffering from infectious diseases in their homes, and board vessels in the harbor to check on the health of crew members.

1841 Vital statistics started in a limited way with collection of data (age, gender, disease) related to deaths; an ordinance requiring reports of death was passed but not enforced for several years.

1846	A committee of the Chicago Medical Society reported the mortality rates through 1850.
1848	The first cooperative effort of the medical profession and city officials was begun to prevent the spread of smallpox as physicians volunteered to vaccinate the poor without charge.
1849	Cholera was brought to Chicago by the emigrant boat *John Drew* from New Orleans, killing 1 in 36 of the entire population. A district health officer was appointed for each city block.
1851	A new city charter provided greater powers in health matters to the city council. In the mid-1850s, with the city free from smallpox and cholera, the powers of the Board of Health were reduced accordingly.
1855	Sewerage became an issue; the Board of Sewerage Commissioners was appointed, and the first sewers were constructed the following year. The quarantine placard was introduced with signs reading "Smallpox Here" after 30 died of the disease.
1857	The financial depression of 1857 caused the Board of Health to be viewed as a luxury; it was abolished, and its duties were transferred to the police department. A new permanent city hospital was completed at a cost of $75,000 (later taken over by Cook County Hospital as one of its earlier buildings).
1862	A smallpox outbreak caused the city council to appoint a health officer to work with the police department, but severely circumscribed tenure and duties rendered the position meaningless.
1867	A new Board of Health was established in response to the 1866 cholera outbreak, with authority independent of the city council and police department.
1868	A meat inspection was initiated at Union Stock Yards.
1869	The Board of Health required vaccination of all children.
1870	The first milk ordinance was instituted, making it illegal to sell skim milk unless so labeled.
1871	Help was given to refugees of the Chicago fire; homeless camps were inspected, and controls were initiated for food supply and epidemic prevention. Birth and death records were lost in the fire.
1872	In the aftermath of the Great Fire, the death rate increased 32.6% to 27.6 deaths per 1,000 persons. Smallpox attacked 2,382 and killed 655. Fatalities among children under 5 years old were the highest ever recorded. (For the period 1843 to 1872, children under 5 years old accounted for half of all deaths occurring in the city.)
1876	The health functions of city government were reorganized under a health department, and the health commissioner position was established.
1877	The health commissioner required the reporting of contagious diseases by physicians, a move opposed by many physicians.

1885   A cholera and typhoid epidemic killed 90,000 Chicagoans when a heavy storm washed sewage into Lake Michigan, the city's source of drinking water.

1888   The Chicago Visiting Nurse Association was founded.

1889   Drainage and plumbing regulations were issued, and five women inspectors of tenements were appointed.

1890   Garbage disposal was placed under the direction of a general sanitary officer in the health department.

1892   Full milk inspection started. Laws requiring reporting of communicable diseases existed; however, doctors argued that they should receive payments for reporting as they received under state law for reporting births. Without this reimbursement, many physicians refused to comply and were prosecuted.

1893   A bacteriological laboratory opened to conduct microscopic examinations of milk samples and to examine throat cultures for diphtheria. A "Boil the Water" crusade against typhoid was conducted.

1893/94 The last smallpox epidemic to cause great loss of life occurred (1,033 died in its second year). Vigorous vaccination efforts (1,084,500 given) resulted in a reduction of cases to seven in 1897. During this period, the health department was the first to proclaim the superiority of hermetically sealed glycerinated vaccine. Circulars distributed on hot weather care of babies were one of the first public education efforts. The health department began publishing a monthly statement of mortality.

1895   The first diphtheria antitoxin was issued, and a corps of antitoxin administrators was appointed. Daily analysis of the water supply was inaugurated.

1896   Medical school inspections were inaugurated—the second city in the United States to do so. Rules regulating the practice of midwifery were promulgated.

1899   A campaign against infant mortality enlisted support of a voluntary corps of 73 physicians.

1900   Sanitary engineers reversed the flow of the Chicago River to prevent a recurrence of epidemics, giving the city the world's only river that runs backward. The health department published a study reporting that the average span of life in Chicago more than doubled in a generation.

1901   An ordinance was passed prohibiting spitting in public places. The health department began publishing the state of the city's health every week in the newspapers; the monthly statement of mortality was discontinued.

1902   The Milk Commission of Chicago was established to ensure that pasteurized milk was made available for needy children; dairy inspections were started with the salaries of two dairy inspectors initially paid for by the Chicago Civic Federation. Fourth of July "Don'ts" were first promulgated to prevent accidents.

1903   A tuberculosis committee of the Visiting Nurse Association was established; it reorganized in 1906 as the Chicago Tuberculosis Institute.

1905   The 39th Street intercepting sewer opened, resulting in a marked decrease in typhoid deaths.

1906   The city council passed an ordinance providing for the licensing and control of restaurants.

1907   The Chicago Tuberculosis Institute opened dispensaries for the diagnosis and treatment of tuberculosis cases.

1908   A full communicable disease program was inaugurated, and 100 physicians were sent to congested districts during July and August to instruct mothers in baby care. Forty nurses were loaned to the health department by the Visiting Nurse Association of Chicago to help in a scarlet fever epidemic. They were so effective that the city council appropriated funds to hire the department's first nurses to work in maternal and child welfare and communicable and venereal diseases.

1909   Chicago became the first city in the United States to adopt a compulsory milk pasteurization ordinance. Public health nurses from the Board of Health, Visiting Nurse Association, and United Charities collaborated to become "finders of sick infants" and referred these babies and their mothers to tent camps where treatment was provided and hygiene classes were held.

1910   The Municipal Social Hygiene Clinic was established, and dispensaries were required to report venereal diseases. New milk standards were applied to ice cream. Health department nurses were assigned to conduct intensive follow up on babies in hospital wards where infant death rates were high; the Infant Welfare Society was organized as the successor to the Milk Commission.

1911   Common drinking cups and common roller towels were prohibited by ordinance.

1912   Sterilization of Chicago's water began, and within 4 years, the entire supply was being treated, causing a dramatic decline in the city's typhoid fever rate—from second highest among the 20 largest U.S. cities in 1881 to the lowest by 1917.

1915   The *Eastland*, a lake excursion boat docked at the Clark Street Bridge, rolled over while loaded with passengers, leading to the greatest loss of life (844 deaths) ever associated with a single shipwreck on the Great Lakes. Dental services were provided in Chicago public schools after a 3-year introductory pilot program was funded by a local philanthropist. The Municipal Tuberculosis Sanitarium opened.

1916   A policy was initiated to hospitalize all cases of infantile paralysis (polio) after 34 of 254 afflicted patients died.

1917   The Municipal Contagious Disease Hospital was established. New health ordinances ranged from requiring the reporting and treatment of venereal diseases to requiring the screening of residences, stables, and barns against fleas. Immunization against diphtheria with von Behring's toxin-antitoxin started in public schools and institutions.

1918   Influenza became a reportable disease with the pandemic of influenza reaching Chicago, causing 381 deaths on one day (October 17) alone.

1919   The health department won its first case in the prosecution of landlords for failure to provide sufficient heat to tenants.

1920   The right of the health department to quarantine carriers of contagion was upheld in the Superior Court of Cook County.

1922   A new health commissioner began a campaign against venereal disease, proposing education and distribution of prophylactic outfits in brothels; opposition from the medical profession was based more on moral than medical grounds.

1923   A committee was appointed on prenatal care in the first concerted effort to coordinate the activities of all agencies doing prenatal work in the city. Inspection of summer camps for children was inaugurated. Venereal disease clinics were established at the Cook County Jail and House of Correction.

1924   Venereal disease prevention literature was distributed to 500,000 homes in Chicago.

1925   The health department instituted a regular schedule of home visits by nurses during the first 6 months of an infant's life. Conferences were inaugurated for care of preschool children. Installation of sanitary types of drinking fountains was ordered.

1927   The health commissioner was forced to resign when the mayor directed that the health department include political literature with information about baby care to be distributed to all Chicago mothers.

1930   An intensive campaign against diphtheria resulted in 400,219 injections being given in 3 months.

1932   The staff of 300 nurses were carried throughout the city on buses to give diphtheria inoculations. Physicians were sent to the homes of mothers unable to take children to welfare stations for shots. After the campaign, cases dropped to 154 with 9 deaths compared with 1,266 cases with 68 deaths the previous year.

1933   There was an outbreak of amebic dysentery among out-of-town guests who came to the Century of Progress (1,409 cases and 98 deaths scattered in 43 states, the Territory of Hawaii, and three Canadian provinces) in the first recognized waterborne epidemic of the disease in a civilian population. The cause was traced to water contamination through faulty plumbing.

1934   A plumbing survey for cross connections in hotels and mercantile buildings was begun to prevent future amebic dysentery outbreaks. As a result of drinking from a contaminated water supply at the Union Stock Yards fire on May 19, 69 persons contracted typhoid fever, 11 of whom died.

1935   An ordinance was passed requiring that only Grade A milk and milk products could be sold in Chicago. A premature infant welfare program was initiated. A mother's milk station started operating to supply breast milk to premature, sick, or debilitated infants whose parents could not afford this expense.

1936   Summer brought 210 deaths from sunstroke and exhaustion compared with 11 from the same cause in 1935. With 1,000 premature infants under supervision, two additional premature stations opened, making 31 conferences available each week.

1937   Chicago public schools opened 3 weeks late because of a polio scare. The Chicago Syphilis Control Project was established, with the emphasis on breaking the chain of infection.

1942   The Chicago Intensive Treatment Center for venereal disease launched an effort so successful that it won a War Department commendation in 1943 and recorded a declining venereal disease rate after World War II demobilization, in contrast to soaring rates in other large cities.

1946   The Chicago/Cook County health survey was undertaken by the U.S. Public Health Service, including an audit of all city and county facilities conducted by outside experts. Various recommendations were made, including more food inspection staff, establishment of district health centers, restructuring of the Board of Health with an executive director and deputies in charge of engineering, preventive medicine, and district health services.

1947   The mental health section for the health department was approved.

1948   A federal grant of $46,270 was made available through the state to subsidize a psychiatric program. A comprehensive food ordinance was adopted by the city council.

1952   Chicago counted 1,203 cases of polio, including 82 deaths and hundreds of persons with paralysis. Frightened parents kept their youngsters out of movie theaters and swimming pools. Beaches closed. An insect and rodent control program started.

1955   Chicago was one of the first cities in the United States to introduce the Salk vaccine after it was pronounced safe and effective against the polio virus on April 12.

1956   With warning signs of an approaching polio epidemic, mass inoculations of the Salk vaccine were given in all parts of the city, with department staff working in vacant stores, garages, and street corners, from the backs of trucks, and in park field houses. Chicago took the lead among major American cities in introducing a water fluoridation program, which reduced tooth decay among children.

1957   The Nursing Home Section and Hospital Inspection Unit was initiated.

1958   A section for chronic illness was activated, with mental health as one of its activities.

1959	The First Community Mental Health Center started on the south side.
1960	The Bureau of Institutional Care consolidated nursing home and hospital inspection services.
1961	The Division of Adult Health and Aging began consolidating activities of chronic diseases, cardiovascular diseases, diabetes, cervical cancer, rheumatic heart fever, and nutrition. A lead poison survey began on Chicago's West Side.
1962	The mental health division, with more than 15 community-based mental health centers, was established in the health department.
1965	Family planning was initiated in a limited number of clinics.
1966	Testing for sickle cell was initiated; citywide lead poisoning screening and treatment began.
1968	Planning for Comprehensive Neighborhood Health Centers in four areas began in cooperation with the Chicago Model Cities program.
1970	The first Model Cities Neighborhood Health Center opened in Uptown. A record 1.2 million inoculations were provided for Chicago children in an immunization drive.
1972	Chicago became the first city in the nation to limit lead content in household paint to 0.06% to fight lead poisoning in children.
1973	Englewood Neighborhood Health Center opened. Forty hospitals were approved as trauma centers in accordance with state statute on emergency medical services.
1974	The Women, Infant, and Children supplemental nutrition program was initiated. A senior citizen clinic and new hypertension center opened, while plans were unveiled to phase out the Tuberculosis Sanitarium.
1975	The city council revised the municipal code to delineate the duties of the nine-member Board of Health as a policymaking body and the Department of Health as the agency administering health programs and enforcing regulations. Outpatient tuberculosis services were decentralized to five health centers. A citywide hypertension control program began, with more than 150,000 persons screened in the first 7 months. The Parents as Resources Program was established at selected clinics and health centers to promote parenting and early childhood stimulation. A 6-day milk dating ordinance was enacted requiring that all milk and Grade A milk products be stamped for a 6-day shelf life.
1976	The health department formed an interdisciplinary committee on child abuse with representatives from health, law enforcement, and welfare agencies. A maternal health clinic was established at Simpson School, a Board of Education alternative school for pregnant students. The largest immunization program in the city's history was launched to protect citizens from swine flu.

1977   The first official agreement between the health department and the state child welfare agency for interagency child protective staffing took place. Cooperative agreements were reached with perinatal centers and community hospitals to provide referral services, counseling, and staff consultation by public health nurses as a means to combat infant mortality. Chicago Department of Human Services staff members were trained as outreach workers to assist public health nurses in reaching newborns. An Infant Mortality Multidisciplinary Committee was established to review infant deaths and make recommendations to the health commissioner.

1979   The first Hispanic health commissioner was appointed. An integrated perinatal system of six perinatal networks was developed to meet guidelines established by the Chicago Maternal and Child Health Advisory Committee.

1981   The Chicago Alcohol Treatment Center came under the jurisdiction of the health department only to be closed several years later and its funding used to support community-based providers of substance abuse treatment services. A refugee health program was initiated.

1983   A Chicago Area AIDS Task Force was established and the health department created an AIDS Activity Office. For the first time since infant deaths were recorded in Chicago, fewer than 1,000 infants died before reaching their first birthday.

1984   The first African American health commissioner was appointed. An ordinance made Chicago the first city in the nation to ban the sale of leaded gasoline, although implementation of the ordinance was delayed by federal regulations. The Partnerships in Health Program was initiated with hospitals to assure continuity of care for health department patients. The health department opened five Good Health Places in cooperation with community organizations.

1985   The health department sponsored the city's first major pastoral conference on religion and health. The Lead Poisoning Screening Program surpassed the one-million level in screenings.

1986   The infant mortality reduction strategic plan was developed.

1987   The first child lead poisoning death in nearly a decade resulted in the establishment of the Mayor's Task Force on Lead Poisoning.

1988   Chicago's first Clean Indoor Air Ordinance was passed by the city council, restricting smoking in restaurants, workplaces, and public spaces.

1989   The health department coordinated the development of the Chicago AIDS Strategic Plan through a multidisciplinary advisory council of 125 individuals.

1990   The Chicago/Cook County Health Care Summit produced a plan to improve local delivery of health services, calling for ambulatory care reforms, restructuring of inpatient care, and changes in system financing. As a result, the Chicago and

	Cook County Ambulatory Care Council was established to assess health needs and undertake initiatives.
1991	The Office of Epidemiology was established in the health department.
1993	The first woman and nonphysician health commissioner was appointed and later taken into custody for violating a court order to conduct lead testing on students who were viewed as older than the populations most at risk for lead poisoning.
1995	Extreme heat conditions in Chicago during July resulted in 514 heat-related deaths. The Violence Prevention Office was established.
1997	The city council passed the Managed Care Consumer Protection ordinance, calling for the health department to create an Office of Managed Care—the nation's first municipal effort to monitor the managed care industry.
1998	The health department coordinated the development of the Chicago Violence Prevention Strategic Plan, developed by more than 150 participants. The Chicago Turning Point Partnership convened to develop a plan to strengthen the public health infrastructure in Chicago.
1999	The Office of Lesbian and Gay Health was established in the health department.
2001	The health department established a bioterrorism preparedness unit.
2002	The health department received a federal grant for bioterrorism preparedness and response. The Northern Illinois Public Health Consortium, an organization dedicated to increasing the capacity of local health departments in northeastern Illinois to respond to public health threats, was incorporated.
2003	The Chicago Center for Community Partnerships was established to strengthen the health department's collaborations with Chicago neighborhoods. Chicago participated in a national bioterrorism response exercise involving city, state, and federal government top officials.
2006	The health department established the Office of Chronic Disease. City agencies came together to fight obesity through the Interagency Departmental Task Force on Childhood Obesity, led by the health department.
2008	A stronger Clean Indoor Air Ordinance took effect, prohibiting smoking in virtually all enclosed public places and enclosed places of employment.
2009	Thousands of Chicagoans were infected with influenza A (H1N1, also referred to as swine flu), with more than 1,000 hospitalized and 150 needing ICU care. The health department distributed more than 1.1 million doses of H1N1 vaccine to health providers throughout Chicago and administered 100,000 doses of the vaccine in mass immunization clinics. Responsibility for vital statistics was turned over to Cook County.

2010   The health department established a social media presence via Facebook and Twitter.

2011   Healthy Chicago, the city's first comprehensive public health priorities agenda, was released, to be implemented through an interagency council of 15 city agencies. The health department established the Office of Adolescent and School Health. New Board of Health day care center guidelines took effect, addressing sweetened beverages, physical activity, and screen time in an effort to reduce childhood obesity.

2012   The health department coordinated public health preparedness activities related to the North American Treaty Organization Summit held in the city. Eighteen public health data sets were made available on the health department's website for easy access by policymakers, researchers, and community members. The LGBT Action Plan was released in partnership with Chicago's lesbian, gay, bisexual, and transgendered communities. Seven primary care centers were transitioned to Federally Qualified Health Centers and 12 mental health centers were consolidated into six in order to assure quality of care. A Mobile Food Dispenser Produce Business License ordinance was enacted to encourage fresh, healthy food carts to operate across the city, particularly in underserved areas.

2014   The Chicago Department of Public Health became one of the first local health departments in the United States to be accredited by the new Public Health Accreditation Board.

QUESTIONS FOR DISCUSSION

1. Which influences were most responsible for the developments delineated in this chronology?
2. Does this history suggest that public health functions have changed over time as well?

ADDITIONAL RESOURCES

1. Chicago Department of Health. *150 Years of Municipal Health Care in the City of Chicago: Board of Health, Department of Health 1835–1985*. Chicago, IL: Chicago Department of Health; 1985.

2. Illinois Department of Public Health. Medicine in Chicago: 1850–1950; chapter in *The Social and Scientific Development of a City*; TN Bonner. *The Rise and Fall of Disease in Illinois*. Springfield: Illinois Department of Public Health; 1927.

3. Chicago Department of Public Health. *Healthy Chicago: Historical Highlights of Public Health in Chicago 1834–2012*. Chicago, IL: Office of Policy, Planning and Legislative Affairs, Chicago Department of Public Health; 2012.

Centers for Disease Control and Prevention

This case study examines one of the world's best known public health organizations, although hardly one of the oldest. As the Centers for Disease Control and Prevention approaches its 70th birthday, its story describes many of the public health threats and challenges facing the United States since the mid-20th century.

LEARNING OBJECTIVES

Through review and discussion of this case study, students will be able to:

- Identify the goals and aspirations that have guided the Centers for Disease Control and Prevention (CDC) since its establishment in 1946.

- Describe the major accomplishments of the CDC over the past 7 decades.

- Describe the strengths and weaknesses of the CDC in its role as the premier public health agency in the United States.

HISTORY OF THE CENTERS FOR DISEASE CONTROL AND PREVENTION[1]

The Centers for Disease Control and Prevention (CDC), an institution synonymous around the world with public health, was 69 years old on July 1, 2015. The Communicable Disease Center was organized in Atlanta, Georgia, on July 1, 1946; its founder, Dr. Joseph W. Mountin, was a visionary public health leader who had high hopes for this small and comparatively insignificant branch of the Public Health Service (PHS). It occupied only one floor of the Volunteer Building on Peachtree Street and had fewer than 400 employees, most of whom were engineers and entomologists. Until the previous day, they had worked for Malaria Control in War Areas, the predecessor of the CDC, which had successfully kept the southeastern states malaria free during World War II and, for approximately 1 year, from murine typhus fever. The new institution would expand its interests to include all communicable diseases and would be the servant of the states, providing practical help whenever called.

Distinguished scientists soon filled the CDC's laboratories, and many states and foreign countries sent their public health staffs to Atlanta for training. Any tropical disease with an insect vector and all those of zoological origin came within its purview. Dr. Mountin was not satisfied with this progress, and he impatiently pushed the staff to do more. He reminded them that except for tuberculosis and venereal disease, which had separate units in Washington, DC, the CDC was responsible for any communicable disease. To survive, it had to become a center for epidemiology.

Medical epidemiologists were scarce, and it was not until 1949 that Dr. Alexander Langmuir arrived to head the epidemiology branch. He saw the CDC as "the promised land," full of possibilities. Within months, he launched the first-ever disease surveillance program, which confirmed his suspicion that malaria, on which the CDC spent the largest portion of its budget, had long since disappeared. Subsequently, disease surveillance became the cornerstone on which the CDC's mission of service to the states was built and in time changed the practice of public health.

The outbreak of the Korean War in 1950 was the impetus for creating the CDC's Epidemic Intelligence Service. The threat of biological warfare loomed, and Dr. Langmuir, the most knowledgeable person in the PHS about this arcane subject, saw an opportunity to train epidemiologists who would guard against ordinary threats to public health while watching out for alien germs. The first class of Epidemic Intelligence Service officers arrived in Atlanta for training in 1951 and pledged to go wherever they were called for the next 2 years. These "disease detectives" quickly gained fame for "shoe-leather epidemiology" through which they ferreted out the cause of disease outbreaks.

The survival of the CDC as an institution was not at all certain in the 1950s. In 1947, Emory University gave land on Clifton Road for a headquarters, but construction did not begin for more than a decade. The PHS was so intent on research and the rapid growth of the National Institutes of Health that it showed little interest in what happened in Atlanta. Congress, despite the long delay in appropriating money for new buildings, was much more receptive to the CDC's pleas for support than either the PHS or the Bureau of the Budget.

Two major health crises in the mid-1950s established the CDC's credibility and ensured its survival. In 1955, when poliomyelitis appeared in children who had received the recently approved Salk vaccine, the national inoculation program was stopped. The cases were traced to contaminated vaccine from a laboratory in California; the problem was corrected, and the inoculation program, at least for first and second graders, was resumed. The resistance of these 6 and 7 year olds to polio, compared with that of older children, proved the effectiveness of the vaccine. Two years later, surveillance was used again to trace the course of a massive influenza epidemic. From the data gathered in 1957 and subsequent years, the national guidelines for influenza vaccine were developed.

The CDC grew by acquisition. The venereal disease program came to Atlanta in 1957 and with it the first Public Health Advisors, nonscience college graduates destined to play an important role in making the CDC's disease-control programs work. The tuberculosis program moved in 1960, immunization practices and the *Morbidity and Mortality Weekly Report* (MMWR) in 1961. The Foreign Quarantine Service, one of the oldest and most prestigious units of the PHS, came in 1967; many of its positions were soon switched to other uses as better ways of doing the work of quarantine, primarily through overseas surveillance. The long-established nutrition program also moved to the CDC, as well as the National Institute for Occupational Safety and Health, and work of already established units increased. Immunization tackled measles and rubella control; epidemiology added family planning and surveillance of chronic diseases. When the CDC joined the international malaria eradication program and accepted responsibility for protecting the earth from moon germs and vice versa, the CDC's mission stretched overseas and into space.

The CDC played a key role in one of the greatest triumphs of public health: the eradication of smallpox. In 1962, it established a smallpox surveillance unit and a year later tested a newly developed jet gun and vaccine in the Pacific island nation of Tonga. After refining vaccination techniques in Brazil, the CDC began work in Central and West Africa in 1966. When millions of people there had been vaccinated, the CDC used surveillance to speed the work along. The World Health Organization used this "eradication escalation" technique elsewhere with such success that global eradication of smallpox was achieved by 1977. The United States spent only $32 million on the project, about the cost of keeping smallpox at bay for 2.5 months.

The CDC also achieved notable success at home tracking new and mysterious disease outbreaks. In the mid-1970s and early 1980s, it found the cause of Legionnaires' disease and toxic-shock syndrome. A fatal disease, subsequently named AIDS, was first mentioned in the June 5, 1981, issue of MMWR. Since then, MMWR has published numerous follow-up articles about AIDS, and one of the largest portions of the CDC's budget and staff is assigned to address this disease.

Although the CDC succeeded more often than it failed, it did not escape criticism. For example, television and press reports about the Tuskegee study on long-term effects of untreated syphilis in black men created a storm of protest in 1972. This study had been initiated by the PHS and other organizations in 1932 and was transferred to the CDC in 1957. Although the effectiveness of penicillin as a therapy for syphilis had been established during the late 1940s, participants in this study remained untreated until the study was brought to public attention. The CDC also was criticized because of the 1976 effort to vaccinate the U.S. population against swine flu, the infamous killer of 1918–1919. When some vaccinees developed Guillain-Barré syndrome, the campaign was stopped immediately; the epidemic never occurred.

As the scope of the CDC's activities expanded far beyond communicable diseases, its name had to be changed. In 1970, it became the Center for Disease Control, and in 1981, after extensive reorganization, Center became Centers. The words "and Prevention" were added in 1992, but by law, the well-known three-letter acronym was retained. In health emergencies, the CDC means an answer to SOS calls from anywhere in the world, such as the recent one from Zaire where Ebola fever raged.

NEW RESPONSIBILITIES BRING NEW CHALLENGES[2]

The growing momentum toward expanding the CDC's responsibilities beyond infectious diseases gained strength during the 1980s. Tremendous advances in controlling infectious diseases had dramatically reduced illness and death from many long-standing health threats. In addition, the detrimental effects of chronic and other noncommunicable diseases on the nation's health were rapidly increasing. Programs to address cancer, heart disease, diabetes, and other leading killers became central to the CDC's focus. Nevertheless, for much of this decade, a newly emerging infectious disease would demand the skills and talents of persons across the agency. These new responsibilities led to additional funding, programs, staff, and partnerships for the growing agency while introducing a host of new challenges.

Emergence of AIDS Brings Unprecedented Public Health Conflict

The formidable challenges presented by the CDC's broadening responsibilities underscored the importance of strictly adhering to science in presenting findings and developing policy. This lesson would prove even more critical as a new infectious disease began emerging in young, homosexual men in the United States, challenging the public health community in unforeseen ways and eventually changing world health. Fully entrenched by the time it was recognized in 1981, the disease, eventually given the name AIDS, reintroduced the public to fear of infectious diseases and divided the country across social, religious, and political lines.

Before AIDS, public fear of infectious diseases had largely subsided because of the availability and widespread use of vaccines and antibiotics. Many believed most infectious diseases were curable and no longer life threatening, affording a new level of health not enjoyed by previous generations. AIDS abruptly corrected this misperception, emerging as a new health threat with devastating consequences and a host of medical, ethical, legal, and economic implications.

Developing Evidence-Based Guidelines

Not only was the new condition baffling, the myriad of associated diseases, termed *opportunistic infections* because they were usually only seen in persons with drug-suppressed or otherwise severely compromised immune systems, were unfamiliar to most physicians and scientists; however, within 1 year of the first case reports, a case definition had been developed and all major routes of transmission had been identified. In March 1983, the CDC published the first set of guidelines for preventing the disease. Based on the best available science at the time, these recommendations proved essentially correct and have not been revised significantly.

In 1984, the cause of the disease was determined to be a previously unrecognized retrovirus, first called human T-lymphotropic virus type III/lymphadenopathy-associated virus (HTLV-III/LAV) and later renamed human immunodeficiency virus (HIV). In March 1985, a test to detect antibodies to the virus was licensed by the Food and Drug Administration (FDA) for use in screening donated blood and plasma. Although the test was not approved for individual testing, public health officials recognized that many at-risk persons would seek testing at blood banks to learn their infection status. By this time, sufficient funds had been authorized by Congress to enable the CDC to begin funding AIDS prevention activities in state and local health departments (LHDs). Through cooperative agreements, the CDC awarded funds to 55 state and LHDs to establish alternate testing sites for at-risk persons to obtain antibody tests free of charge outside the blood bank setting. Such sites were established both to decrease potential false-negative donations and to ensure that persons wishing to be tested would receive appropriate pre- and posttest counseling and referrals. The use of the antibody test for individual testing was approved by the FDA in 1986. The ability to test persons for the virus offered new opportunities for prevention and for treatment to possibly delay the onset of the disease. Unfortunately, this medical advancement also unleashed a new set of fears among an already stigmatized population, especially regarding increased discriminatory actions related to education, employment, health care, and insurance.

Scientifically, these early years of AIDS were characterized by unprecedented progress toward understanding a new, highly complex infectious disease. In 1985, the first AIDS conference was held, and the World Health Organization formed a network of AIDS collaborating centers. By the end of 1986, the CDC had published nearly 100 MMWR reports related to AIDS. These reports included recommendations to prevent transmission of the virus through transfusions, transplants, patient care, and perinatal exposure; workplace and school-based guidelines; and critical reports from state and LHDs outlining the epidemic's effect in their areas. The CDC's AIDS surveillance programs were among the most comprehensive disease-tracking measures ever undertaken. These programs yielded data that highlighted growing epidemics outside of major metropolitan areas and among minority populations, allowing for more targeted prevention measures and funding.

Fear Affects Public Policy

Despite solid scientific advances, no epidemic in history has engendered a greater level of controversy. Divisive views over the epidemic's earliest and most severely affected populations, homosexual/bisexual men and intravenous drug users, undoubtedly hindered progress on many fronts, including risk communication and funding for prevention and research. Some in Congress claimed that AIDS spending was exorbitant, disproportional to the magnitude of the problem, whereas others argued that inadequate funding was slowing research on testing, treatment, and vaccine development. The public also became involved in these disputes, disagreeing on transmission risks, populations that should be tested, and restrictions on infected persons. The media fueled their interests. In describing results from a 1985 poll of more than 2,000 persons, *The New York Times* reported that "51 percent of the respondents supported a quarantine of acquired immune deficiency syndrome patients, 48 percent would approve identity cards for those who have taken tests indicating the presence of AIDS antibodies, and 15 percent supported tattooing those with AIDS."

Although these arguments were vocalized as focusing on rights of the public versus rights of AIDS patients, in reality they were driven by fear. The medical and scientific community had difficulty communicating the risks associated with this new disease with the same level of certainty demanded by the public. Studies conducted among family members of AIDS patients had provided strong evidence of the lack of transmission from casual contact; however, many persons, including lawmakers, believed otherwise and were not readily dissuaded.

In particular, school attendance by children with AIDS was the subject of intense debate. The CDC's 1985 recommendations on education and foster care for children with HIV/AIDS stated that decisions regarding the type of education and care setting for infected children should be made on an individual basis but that "for most infected school-aged children, the benefits of an unrestricted setting would outweigh the risks of their acquiring potentially harmful infections in the setting and the apparent nonexistent risk of transmission of HTLV-III/LAV." Soon after the release of these guidelines in late August 1985, *The Washington Post* ran an op-ed piece titled, "Worry about the Survival of Society First; Then AIDS Victims' Rights," which was picked up by newspapers across the country. Playing to the public's fear and skepticism, the editorial argued that many of the laws that had been enacted to protect AIDS patients from discrimination were misguided and cited the CDC's recent guidelines as remiss.

In many areas of the country, these recommendations were met with staunch opposition. In Florida, the parents of three HIV-infected hemophilic sons, Ricky, Robert, and Randy Ray, were plaintiffs in a federal lawsuit against their local school board to allow their children to attend public school. A week after the court's ruling in favor of the Rays, their home was burned. In Indiana, the experiences endured by a young man named Ryan White would ultimately change public opinion on AIDS throughout the world and lead to specifically designated federal resources for AIDS patients through the 1990 Ryan White Comprehensive AIDS Resources Emergency Act.

At the CDC, measures to expand surveillance and case reporting and to develop new prevention guidelines required dedicated consensus building that went beyond the medical and scientific community to include affected persons, special interest and political groups, and the public. Throughout these processes, the CDC worked to ensure that these new recommendations and guidelines reflected the best available science, a commitment that has served public health well. For example, the CDC's 1988 recommendations for preventing HIV transmission in healthcare settings recommended that blood and certain body fluids from every single patient be viewed as potentially infectious for HIV or other bloodborne pathogens. These guidelines became known as "universal blood and body fluid precautions" or "universal precautions" and led to permanent changes in healthcare practices throughout the world.

Strengthening State and Local Public Health Infrastructures

By the mid-1980s, both funding and political support were available to launch widespread public information campaigns, viewed as critical in stemming the epidemic and enabling those already infected to receive treatment and other services. The CDC's National AIDS Hotline was started in 1983 to enhance surveillance for the disease, but its role quickly expanded to address the urgent need for disseminating accurate and timely information. In 1987, the CDC established the National AIDS Clearinghouse to distribute printed materials on AIDS. The same year, the CDC launched America Responds to AIDS, a substantial, nationwide public information campaign that had been developed through extensive formative research. Over the next 4 years, five separate phases of informational materials were developed and released to the general public, ranging from basic information on the disease to specific information for different risk groups. The largest of these came in 1988, when more than 107 million copies of the brochure "Understanding AIDS" were delivered to homes and residential post office boxes in the United States. A Spanish version also was distributed in Puerto Rico and other predominantly Spanish-speaking areas. The brochure, developed by the CDC in consultation with Surgeon General C. Everett Koop, other health experts, and public citizens, marked the first time the federal government had attempted to contact every resident directly by mail regarding a public health problem. Koop's open stance against smoking had made him a well-recognized public health official, and his commitment to educating the public on HIV/AIDS made him a highly effective and credible spokesperson in this effort.

In addition to expanded funding for AIDS surveillance and prevention activities at state and LHDs, the CDC began funding national and regional minority organizations, community-based organizations, and the faith-based community for these activities in 1988 to 1989. This increased funding for extramural activities is reflected in the CDC's budget for those years, which nearly tripled from fiscal years 1983 to 1989 without a commensurate increase in full-time employees. The systems and services developed and implemented in response to the AIDS epidemic helped build and maintain public health infrastructures at multiple levels and would improve capabilities and serve as a model for other disease detection and prevention measures.

During 1981 to 1989, more than 100,000 cases of AIDS in the United States were reported to the CDC, approximately one-third of them in 1989 alone. Although cases were reported from all 50 states, the District of Columbia, and four U.S. territories, two-thirds of the cases were reported from five states: New York, New Jersey, Florida, Texas, and California. In addition, although the epidemic had spread beyond the earliest risk groups of homosexual/bisexual men and intravenous drug users, these groups continued to account for nearly 90% of cases.

Today, the epidemic's global effect is staggering, with nearly 40 million persons living with HIV throughout the world in 2006. The fear of the disease that so adversely affected the U.S. response during the early years of the epidemic has largely subsided in this country, dissolving much of the resistance to new policies and procedures and enabling better acceptance and delivery of new prevention and treatment strategies. A clear example of this change is reflected in the CDC's new HIV testing recommendations. Published in September 2006, these evidence-based recommendations call for nearly universal testing of patients in healthcare settings, a strategy that would not have been possible to put forward as recently as a decade ago. In many of the world's most heavily affected regions, however, fear and lack of education about the disease continue to impede prevention measures and stigmatize infected persons. As new funding and partners are united globally to address the pandemic, primary prevention measures must first focus on ending the fear.

An Expanded Agency

Change, expansion, and growing domestic and international visibility characterized the CDC's recent decades. Exacting science and honest risk communication proved to be the agency's most effective prevention tools. Lessons learned from past successes and challenges will serve the CDC well as its roles and responsibilities toward protecting the nation's health continue to expand.

Seventy years ago the CDC's agenda was noncontroversial (hardly anyone objected to the pursuit of germs), and Atlanta was a backwater. Today, the CDC's programs are often tied to economic, political, and social issues, and Atlanta is as near Washington as the tap of a keyboard.

QUESTIONS FOR DISCUSSION

1. To what extent has the Centers for Disease Control and Prevention (CDC) achieved the aspirations of Dr. Joseph Mountin, its founding director?
2. At which points in its history have political and bureaucratic obstacles limited the effectiveness of the CDC?
3. Which role does the CDC play with respect to the national network of state and local public health agencies?

REFERENCES

1. Reprinted in part and adapted from the Centers for Disease Control and Prevention. History of CDC. *MMWR*. 1996; *45*: 426–430.
2. Reprinted in part and adapted from Mason JO. CDC's 60th anniversary: director's perspective. *MMWR*. 2006; *55*: 1354–1359.

Mandatory Premarital Screening for Antibody to the Human Immunodeficiency Virus

This case study was adapted and expanded by Bernard Turnock from one developed in 1987 for the Centers for Disease Control and Prevention by Lyle Peterson, Guthrie Birkhead, and Richard Dicker. Dr. Turnock served as director of the Illinois Department of Public Health from 1985 to 1990 when the events described in this case study occurred in Illinois. Discussion questions are embedded in the scenario as it unfolds.

LEARNING OBJECTIVES

Through review and discussion of this case study, students will be able to:

- Define and perform calculations of sensitivity, specificity, predictive-value positive, and predictive-value negative.
- Describe the relationship between prevalence and predictive value.
- Discuss the trade-offs between sensitivity and specificity.
- List the principles of a good screening program.
- Identify political and policy implications of the use of screening tests in populations with different levels of prevalence.

SCENARIO

In December 1982, a report in the *Morbidity and Mortality Weekly Report* described three persons who had developed AIDS but who had neither of the previously known risk factors for the disease: homosexual/bisexual activity with numerous partners and intravenous drug use. These three persons had previously received whole-blood transfusions. By 1983, widespread recognition of the problem of transfusion-related AIDS led to controversial recommendations that persons in known high-risk groups voluntarily defer from donating blood. In June 1984, after the discovery of HIV, five companies were licensed to produce enzyme-linked immunosorbent assay (EIA, then called ELISA) test kits for detecting HIV antibody. A Food and Drug Administration (FDA) spokesman stated that "getting this test out to the blood banks is our

No. 1 priority...." Blood bank directors anxiously awaited the availability of the first test kit for screening blood, which was approved by the FDA in early March 1985.

In the prelicensure evaluation, sensitivity and specificity of the test kits were estimated using blood samples from four groups: those with AIDS by Centers for Disease Control and Prevention criteria, those with other symptoms and signs of HIV infection, those with various autoimmune disorders and neoplastic diseases that could give a false-positive test result, and presumably healthy blood and plasma donors. Numerous complex issues were discussed even before licensure. Among them were understanding the magnitude of the problem of false-positive test results and determining whether test-positive blood donors should be notified.

It is now March 1985. The first HIV antibody test kits will arrive in blood banks in the state in a few hours. Meeting to discuss the appropriate use of this test are the state health director, the state epidemiologist, the medical director of the regional blood bank, and the director of the State Department of Alcohol and Substance Abuse.

To help in the discussions, the group reviews the prelicensure information regarding the sensitivity and specificity of test kit A. The information indicates that the sensitivity of test kit A is 95% (0.95), and the specificity is 98% (0.98). These and related measures are defined in Table CS 3-1.

Table CS 3-1 Relationship of Antibody Status to Test Results: Definitions for Sensitivity, Specificity, Predictive-Value Positive, and Predictive-Value Negative

		Actual Antibody Status		
		Present	Absent	Total
Test result	Positive	True positive (A)	False positive (B)	All positive tests (A + B)
	Negative	False negative (C)	True negative (D)	All negative tests (C + D)
	Total	All with antibody (A + C)	All without antibody (B + D)	Total (A + B + C + D)

- Sensitivity: the probability that the test result will be positive when administered to persons who actually have the antibody. Sensitivity = true positives/all with antibody. Algebraically, sensitivity = A/(A + C).
- Specificity: the probability that the test result will be negative when administered to persons who are actually without the antibody. Specificity = true negatives/all without antibody. Algebraically, specificity = D/(B + D).
- Predictive-value positive (PVP): the probability that a person with a positive screening test result actually has the antibody. PVP = true positives/all with positive test. Algebraically, PVP = A/(A + B).
- Predictive-value negative (PVN): the probability that a person with a negative screening test result actually does not have the antibody. PVN = true negatives/all with negative test. Algebraically, PVN = D/(C + D).

Question 1: With this information, by constructing a 2-by-2 table, calculate the predictive-value positive and predictive-value negative of the EIA in a hypothetical population of 1,000,000 blood donors. Using a separate 2-by-2 table, calculate predictive-value positive and predictive-value negative for a population of 1,000 drug users. Assume that the actual prevalence of HIV antibody among blood donors is 0.04% (0.0004) and that of intravenous drug users is 10% (0.10).

The blood bank medical director wants assistance in evaluating the EIA as a test for screening donor blood in the state. In particular, she is concerned about the possibility that some antibody-positive units will be missed by the test, and she wonders about false-positive test results because she is under pressure to develop a notification procedure for EIA-positive donors.

Question 2: Do you think that the EIA is a good screening test for the blood bank? What would you recommend to the blood bank medical director about notification of EIA-positive blood donors?

The director of the Department of Alcohol and Substance Abuse has noticed a dramatic increase in AIDS among clients in his intravenous drug abuse treatment programs. For planning purposes, he wants to conduct a voluntary HIV antibody seroprevalence survey of intravenous drug abuse clients and would like to assess the feasibility of using the test results as part of behavior modification counseling.

Question 3: Do you think that the EIA performs well enough to justify informing test-positive clients in the drug abuse clinics that they are positive for HIV?

Question 4: If sensitivity and specificity remain constant, what is the relationship of prevalence to predictive-value positive and predictive-value negative?

EIA results are recorded as optical-density (OD) ratios. The OD ratio is the ratio of absorbance of the tested sample to the absorbance of the control sample. The greater the OD ratio, the more "positive" the test result. The EIA, as with most other screening tests, is not perfect; there is some overlap of OD ratios of samples that are actually antibody positive and those that are actually antibody negative. Establishing the cutoff value to define a positive test result from a negative one can be somewhat arbitrary. Suppose that the test manufacturer initially considered that an OD ratio of 2.0 or higher would be considered positive.

Question 5: In terms of sensitivity and specificity, what happens if you raise the cutoff from 2.0 to 3.0?

Question 6: In terms of sensitivity and specificity, what happens if you lower the cutoff from 2.0 to 1.0?

Question 7: From what you know now, what is the relationship between sensitivity and specificity of a screening test?

Question 8: If the scenario above described HIV antibody test results for normal and persons with HIV/AIDS, where might the blood bank medical director and the head of drug treatment want the cutoff point to be for each program? Who would likely want a lower cutoff value? Why?

The blood bank medical director is concerned that, because of the low predictive-value positive of the EIA in the blood donor population, the blood bank personnel cannot properly inform those who are EIA positive of their actual antibody status. For this reason, she wishes to evaluate the Western blot test as a confirmatory test for HIV antibody. The Western blot test identifies antibodies to specific proteins associated with HIV. The Western blot is the most widely used secondary test to detect HIV antibody because its specificity exceeds 99.99%; however, it is not used as a primary screening test because it is expensive and technically difficult to perform. Its sensitivity is thought to be lower than that of the EIA.

Because the Western blot test is not yet generally available, the blood bank medical director is wondering whether the initial EIA-positive results can be confirmed by repeating the EIA and by considering persons to have the antibody only if results of both tests are positive. The state epidemiologist suggests that they compare the performance of the repeat EIA and the Western blot as confirmatory tests. To do this, they will use the earlier hypothetical sample of 1,000,000 blood donors. They assume that serum specimens that are initially positive by EIA are then split into two portions; a repeat EIA is performed on one portion and a Western blot test on the other portion.

Question 9: What is the actual antibody prevalence in the population of persons whose blood samples will undergo a second test?

Question 10: Calculate the predictive-value positive of the two sequences of tests: EIA-EIA and EIA-Western blot. Assume that the sensitivity and specificity of the EIA are 95% and 98%, respectively. Assume that the sensitivity and specificity of the Western blot are 80% and 99.99%, respectively. Also assume that the tests are independent, even though they may not be (e.g., those with cross-reactive proteins are likely to cross react each time).

Question 11: Why does the predictive-value positive increase so dramatically with the addition of a second test? Why is the predictive-value positive higher for the EIA-Western blot sequence than for the EIA-EIA sequence?

The combination of EIA and Western blot testing is quickly implemented by blood donation centers, and the number of new AIDS cases attributed to blood donations declines rapidly. The use of these screening tests for the purpose of safeguarding the blood supply appears to be very successful.

AIDS remains a major public health concern as the number of new cases, especially among men having sex with men and intravenous drug users, continues to grow in Illinois and elsewhere. Despite the growth of the epidemic, there is little political activity in the way of new laws to deal with AIDS in 1985 and 1986. Only a few legislative proposals are introduced into the state legislature during that period. In early 1987, however, more than 60 legislative proposals are introduced into the state legislature. About three-fourths of these call for testing various subgroups in the population, including food handlers, teachers, public safety personnel, and marriage license applicants.

Question 12: What might have happened in 1986/1987 to prompt increased political and legislative attention to the AIDS epidemic? Why do you think so many proposals focused on testing various subgroups in the population?

It is now 1987 and the governor has asked the state health director to evaluate a proposed premarital HIV-antibody screening program. A bill to establish the program is to be voted on by the state legislature tomorrow. It will amend a long-standing state law requiring marriage license applicants to submit information from a physician that they are free from transmissible syphilis. An estimated 200,000 people will get married in the state in the next year. The proposed legislation requires that each prospective bride and groom submit a blood sample for EIA testing. Samples that test positive by EIA will undergo confirmatory Western blot testing.

The legislation describes the goal of the screening program to decrease inadvertent perinatal or sexual HIV transmission by determining who among those to be married are likely infected with the virus.

Question 13: Which criteria are used in evaluating mass screening programs? Which of these criteria would you consider to be most important in evaluating this proposed screening program?

Table CS 3-2 shows the possible results of the testing, assuming that persons getting married have the same actual HIV antibody prevalence as blood donors (0.04%). In 1987, the sensitivity and specificity of the improved EIA test kit A available at the time were 97% and 99.8%, respectively. The Western blot sensitivity and specificity were 95% and 99.99%, respectively.

Question 14: Compute the cost of the screening program. Assume a cost of $90.00 for every initial EIA test ($30.00 laboratory fee and $60.00 healthcare provider visit) and an additional $100.00 for EIA-positive persons who will need additional testing. What is the cost of the screening program in the next year? What is the cost per identified antibody-positive person?

These results do not fully reflect some of the qualitative effects of what took place in Illinois in 1988 to 1989. As noted previously here, the prevalence rate for premarital tests in Illinois was found to be about one-half of that used in the earlier example (2 per 10,000). The research literature on HIV testing identifies an important additional consideration:

Table CS 3-2   Case Study Test Results

		Actual Antibody Status		
		Present	Absent	Total
Test result	Positive	78	400	478
	Negative	2	199,520	199,522
	Total	80	199,920	200,000

Note: 478 positive tests to undergo Western blot testing.
Follow-Up Western Blot Test

		Actual Antibody Status		
		Present	Absent	Total
Test result	Positive	74	0	74
	Negative	4	400	404
	Total	78	400	478

Note: With sequential tests, sensitivity = 92% (74/80); specificity = 100% (199,920/199,920); predictive-value positive = 100% (74/74).

the background false-positivity rate that occurs, even when serial testing protocols are used. For example, it may be that 1 person per 10,000 will have a falsely positive result, even after serial tests are performed. That may not be a serious problem when testing is performed on populations in which the prevalence is high, such as those attending testing and counseling centers (where the prevalence is greater than 300 per 10,000). In this situation, more than 99% of positive tests would occur to people who really had the antibody, but in a population with a prevalence of 4 per 10,000, one-fourth of those who test positive would not actually carry the antibody. In a population with a prevalence of 2 per 10,000, approximately half would not actually carry the antibody; however, they would be given the same information ("you are positive") as those who actually were positive, and they might make important life decisions (to marry, to have children, to continue with a pregnancy, etc.) based on information that has a 25% probability (at 4 per 10,000 prevalence) or 50% probability (at 2 per 10,000 prevalence) to be incorrect.

> *Question 15: What is your final recommendation to the governor? What are the three strongest arguments in support of your recommendation?*

Despite the opposition of the public health and medical community (among many others), a law is enacted that requires all marriage license applicants to submit evidence of having been tested for HIV antibodies. This law is part of a package of 17 bills addressing a wide variety of AIDS issues that was considered the most comprehensive AIDS legislative package in the nation. Virtually all of the bills included in this package were supported by public health advocates and officials, except for the one that would require all marriage license applicants to provide evidence of having been tested for HIV antibody. That particular provision took effect on January 1, 1988, and continued through August 1989.

Question 16: Review the data summarized in Table CS 3-3. Does the information from this experience support your initial recommendations and arguments? Are there other factors that you would not have predicted that eventually may have contributed to the legislature's and governor's decision to repeal this law?

Table CS 3-3   Twenty-Month Experience with Illinois Premarital HIV Testing Law

56 positives out of 260,000 tests (2 per 10,000) for comparison purposes (at that time)
- 1,530 per 10,000—intravenous drug users
- 318 per 10,000—counseling/testing sites
- 11 per 10,000—military recruits
- 9 per 10,000—women of childbearing age
- 3 per 10,000—blood donors statewide
- 4 per 10,000—blood donors, Cook and collar counties
- 2 per 10,000—marriage license applicants

37 males, 19 females

26 white, 23 black, 6 Hispanic

23 from Cook County, 17 from collar counties, 14 from down-state Illinois
- 2 per 10,000 Cook County
- 3 per 10,000 DuPage County
- 4 per 10,000 Lake County
- 7 per 10,000 Will County

28 reported risk factors (10 sexual contact, 14 intravenous drug use, 4 transfusion)

Marriage licenses issued by year:
- 1987—99,000
- 1988—77,000 (premarital HIV testing law in effect all year)
- 1989—87,000 (premarital HIV testing law in effect 8 months of year)
- 1990—100,000

Number of marriage licenses issued to Illinois residents in selected counties of bordering states, 1987 versus 1988:
- Scott County (Iowa) 240 versus 560
- Lake County (Indiana) 210 versus 1,000
- Kenosha County (Wisconsin) 110 versus 1,210
- Paducah County (Kentucky) 320 versus 1,710

Data from Turnock RJ, Lokar K, unpublished data

Question 17: It is now the current year and a new bill has been introduced into the state legislature that would require all elementary and secondary school teachers in the state to provide evidence of having been tested for HIV antibody as a requirement for securing teacher certification. All teachers must be certified in order to be hired or continued by a school district, public or private. Because of your expertise in HIV screening tests, the governor has asked you to write a memo outlining whether he should sign this bill into law if it reaches his desk.

ADDITIONAL RESOURCES

1. McKilip J. The effect of mandatory premarital HIV testing on marriage: the case of Illinois. *Am J Public Health*. 1991; *81*: 650–653.
2. Peterson LR, White CR. The premarital screening study group: premarital screening for antibodies to human immunodeficiency virus in the United States. *Am J Public Health*. 1990; *80*: 1087–1090.
3. Turnock BJ, Kelly CJ. Mandatory premarital testing for human immunodeficiency virus: the Illinois experience. *JAMA*. 1989; *261*: 3415–3418.

Massive Outbreak of Antimicrobial-Resistant Salmonellosis Traced to Contaminated Milk

Protecting the public from foodborne illnesses has become increasingly complex in recent decades as a result of advances in food technology, competitive forces within the food service industry, and declining resources for governmental public health agencies. Yet the public's expectation of a safe food supply has never been higher. State and local governmental public health agencies, in particular, face new challenges in assuring the highest level of public protection. Food safety efforts now utilize a "multiple barrier" strategy rather than relying on controls imposed at any single stage in the production, distribution, and use cycle. Coordination and communication among food producers, retailers, food service establishments, consumers, and government regulators are essential both to prevent and control foodborne outbreaks. This case study, based on actual events but depicting fictionalized identities for the individuals and organizations involved, underscores several important aspects and influences of leadership, organizational structure, resources, and workforce in everyday public health practice.

LEARNING OBJECTIVES

Through review and discussion of this case study, students will be able to:

- Describe how communicable disease reports are investigated by local and state public health agencies.

- Describe the scientific, legal, political, ethical, media, and financial implications of large-scale disease outbreaks related to contaminated food.

- Explain how and why perceived breakdowns in public health protection often result in reform and improvements.

SCENARIO

On a rainy April day in the mid 1980s, Mindy Williams, the Pottowottomi County Department of Health communicable disease investigator, was following up on four reports of *Salmonella* infections called in to her office by staff at Pottowottomi Memorial Hospital.

Pottowottomi County is a largely rural county about 40 miles from Chicago, the state's major urban center. All four cases were students at the local community college who became ill over the previous weekend, causing them to visit the college health service clinic complaining of fever, diarrhea, and vomiting. Stool samples were taken and sent to the hospital lab. Williams interviewed the students and identified a common meal approximately 36 hours before the students began exhibiting symptoms. Their food histories suggested that roast beef served at a soccer club banquet may have been involved. Inspection of the kitchen and food handlers turned up no new information. None of the food from that common meal was available for testing. The county health department staff reemphasized proper food preparation and handling practices for the college kitchen staff and forwarded their reports and results to the Illinois Department of Public Health in Springfield.

In a seemingly unrelated incident later that week, a woman from the blue collar suburb of Goshen, about 15 miles from Chicago, became ill with gastroenteritis, making her sick enough to visit her family physician. Goshen is located in Cook County but has its own municipal health department. Stool cultures were confirmed positive for *Salmonella*. No other family members were ill, and there was nothing unusual or suggestive in the woman's recent history. In the days preceding her symptoms, the woman had been about her regular routine of carpooling her children to baseball games and swimming lessons and shopping at her neighborhood supermarket.

During this same week, in two other suburbs of Chicago, each served by a different county-based local health department, two unrelated families began to experience flu-like symptoms that spread among the family members. Both families consulted their family doctors and were advised to rest and switch to clear liquid diets. Later that week, stool cultures were taken from the mother of one of those families and a toddler from the other. Both cultures were positive for *Salmonella* and were reported to their respective local health departments.

No additional investigations were initiated by the local health agencies in any of these April occurrences as *Salmonella* infections are not uncommon and each of these occurrences was viewed as a routine, isolated situation.

Four months later, in August, four local health departments serving counties northwest of Chicago and the Chicago Department of Health (its official name at that time) were coordinating efforts with state health department staff to investigate a large outbreak of salmonellosis affecting some 70 confirmed cases. Detailed food and product histories revealed no clear factors in common, although a suspicious but insignificant association with shopping at the Heartland Supermarket chain was noted. No particular food product was associated with these illnesses. Chuck Imperato, the communicable disease epidemiologist in the state health department's infectious disease control unit (which reported to the deputy director for health protection), recommended that state food investigators inspect the supermarket facilities in that region and that the state health department's dairy inspectors inspect the dairy plant that provided milk to the supermarket chain. The food and dairy inspectors worked in the state health department's food, drugs, and dairy unit, which reported to the deputy director for health regulations. These inspections were performed but resulted in no new information and the investigation was closed.

On March 20 of the following year, approximately 41,000 gallons of 2% milk carrying a March 29 expiration date were produced at Heartland Dairy in the west suburbs of Chicago. Within 24 hours, virtually all of the milk was shipped to stores and placed on shelves ready for sale throughout the metropolitan area.

On March 29, a Friday, the state health department began receiving "cluster reports" through its regional office and from several local health departments that hospitals in three separate counties were reporting an increase in *Salmonella* cases. One hospital reported that it had isolated a strain of *Salmonella* typhimurium similar to the unusual antimicrobial resistance pattern associated with the outbreak that had occurred in August of the previous year. By 4:30 p.m. a total of 16 cases of *Salmonella* Group B had been reported. Early verbal reports from victims suggested a possible link with Heartland 2% milk. Based on these early reports, Chuck Imperato at the state health agency suggested consideration of a voluntary withdrawal of the 2% milk products. After extensive discussion of this option with Mack Miller, director of the Food, Drug, and Dairy Program, and with Imperato's supervisor, Dr. Sally Harding, it was agreed that not enough evidence had been developed to support this action. Miller alerted his supervisor, Dr. Frank McCarthy, of the developments. During the evening hours, Harding advised the state health department laboratory staff to stand ready over the weekend to receive products that might be pulled off store shelves as well as samples from ill individuals. Harding also called the enteric branch at the Centers for Disease Control and Prevention (CDC) to request on-site assistance with what appeared to be a large-scale outbreak in the making.

On Saturday, March 30, the lab began receiving unopened product from stores, as well as opened samples that would be tested by both the health department and the producer. CDC staff member Dr. Jack Greider arrived and began working with state staff to design a case-control study. The running total of suspected cases had now climbed to 35. Also on March 30, Heartland Dairy was producing more 2% milk with an expiration date of April 8.

By Sunday, March 31, suspected cases had reached 100, with some 50 already confirmed as *Salmonella*. Lab culturing of suspected product was initiated, with the results due in 72 hours, and case-control studies began to pair control groups with ill patients to identify the common exposures. Mack Miller contacted the Food and Drug Administration (FDA) regional office in Chicago to alert them to developments to date.

At about this time, the April 8 batch of 2% milk was shipped to stores and placed on shelves for sale throughout the metropolitan area.

On Monday, April 1, the state health director phoned the milk producer with the news that the case-control study had implicated their 2% product shelf-dated March 29 and that this information would soon be made public. The announcement was made and the product was voluntarily recalled by Heartland. With milk products now implicated, FDA staff joined the investigation team with state and federal public health personnel. An extensive media campaign sought to alert consumers to discard any of the implicated 2% milk in their refrigerators. For the next few days, regular media updates were provided as the investigation continued. During one of the media briefing sessions on April 1, *The Chicago Sun-Times* government reporter Lois Lane inquired whether the current outbreak was related to the one that had occurred in August of the previous year. By 6:00 p.m., the case count exceeded 250.

The actual on-site investigation of the dairy plant began on April 2. Cases had now reached 300. On Wednesday, April 3, with the case count now exceeding 350, the milk products were found to be presumptively positive for *Salmonella*. A cross connection was found at the dairy during the on-site investigation and was corrected immediately.

As the investigation continued the next day (April 4), confirmed positive results were reported on the 2% milk product being tested, identifying the same microorganism that was implicated from patient stool samples. As Heartland's dairy received much of its raw milk from outside the state, neighboring states were asked to sample raw dairy products. Later that day, active surveillance efforts provided some evidence that no new infections were occurring, even though the total number of cases related to the outbreak was steadily climbing as additional reports were forwarded to the state. At the time, it appeared that the outbreak was subsiding and that control issues would soon become less important than investigation issues for the rest of the outbreak.

Friday, April 5, was Good Friday. The investigating team from the federal and state health agencies did not have a high level of confidence that the cross connection was the ultimate cause, and the state health director determined that no public announcement would be made at that time regarding the cause of the outbreak. A meeting was scheduled for Monday to review findings further before any public release. Activity over the Easter weekend was limited.

On Monday, April 8, the investigating team met to review the violations found by the on-site investigation at the dairy plant. The team reached consensus not to announce the cross connection as the definitive cause. During the afternoon hours, new reports were received of illnesses possibly related to other milk products produced by the dairy. Further lab confirmations came in of *Salmonella* found in unopened product. The dairy continued to operate, producing skim milk with a April 17 expiration date.

On Tuesday, April 9, the team recommended and the state health director agreed to seek closing the dairy plant. Lawyers from the health department communicated the decision to the president and chief executive officer of Heartland Industries. Heartland complied with the request to close the dairy plant and to remove all liquid milk products from retail food store shelves in the face of increasing reports of illness. The dairy plant was not in production on April 9 as this was to be a "down day" for a regularly scheduled cleaning of the plant's production facilities. Skim milk produced the previous day was removed from shelves after being on sale for 12 hours or less. The investigating team reentered the plant. Prior to this time, all positive results were derived from products that had left the plant and were subsequently returned in either opened or sealed condition.

Beginning on Wednesday, April 10, the investigation expanded considerably. Public and media messages reminded consumers that all products made at the plant were to be taken off the shelves and out of consumers' refrigerators until their safety could be proven. On Monday, April 15, milk products with an April 17 shelf date were found to contain *Salmonella*. Lois Lane inquired why the state health director himself was not available for the daily public briefings. The state health director, a lawyer with an impressive background in substance abuse prevention and control, had been in daily contact with his staff while at his time-share vacation home in Mexico. Within a few hours of the Lois Lane inquiry, the governor fired the state health director for vacationing amidst an uncontrolled outbreak, pledging to replace him with a qualified public health physician.

Over the course of the next weeks and months, an exhaustive and extensive investigation of the dairy production plant was undertaken. The investigation resulted in the conclusion that a persistence of bacterial growth within the dairy plant, possibly related to the cross connection, resulted in the periodic seeding of milk products with *Salmonella*. In addition, samples from previous *Salmonella* outbreaks throughout Illinois and the nation were examined to identify any that might have the same "fingerprints." That fingerprinting eventually linked the smaller April and August outbreaks from the previous year with the massive outbreak beginning in March. All told, more than 20,000 confirmed cases of salmonellosis and an estimated 200,000 total actual cases resulted from these outbreaks.

Changes in the leadership, organization, and financing of the public health protection responsibilities at the state health department ensued. The dairy plant has yet to produce another gallon of milk and has remained closed to this day.

Some perceive that this outbreak represents a breakdown in public health protection from basic licensing, periodic inspections, and ongoing surveillance to rapid and decisive decision making and effective crisis communication and management. In part, the extensive changes made in the aftermath of this outbreak support these assertions. Immediate attention and considerable state resources were devoted to:

- Assure that public health professionals were put into key decision-making roles within the state health agency
- Remove any existing ambiguities as to the department's ability to act quickly and decisively in public health emergency situations
- Provide adequate staffing and resources for health protection activities
- Improve the statutory and regulatory framework for public health action
- Improve the programmatic framework for health protection at the state and local levels

The public, media, and political attention paid to the state health agency during this crisis quickly resulted in increased funding for the state public health agency, even benefiting programs other than those focusing on public health protection. For example, a massive infant mortality reduction program was proposed by the governor the following year and enacted with virtually unanimous support from the state legislature. One of the key questions for public health that emerges from this case study is why it takes a crisis or meltdown for gains such as these to be realized.

QUESTIONS FOR DISCUSSION

The definitive source of the bacterial contamination at the dairy plant was not the only unresolved question from this case and its investigation. Questions arose during the course of this emergency situation and its handling from many different sources and focused on even more basic public health responsibilities and expectations of government.

1. What does this case study tell us about the relationships among local, state, and federal public health agencies for the control of infectious diseases in general and for the prevention and control of foodborne illnesses in particular? Are these relationships portrayed similarly in the corresponding article in the *Journal of the American Medical Association* (JAMA)[1] and in the back story presented in the case study?

2. Were the proper actions taken at the proper time to maximally protect the public during this outbreak? At which point(s) did public health leadership fail to take appropriate action or succeed in seizing the initiative? Did the professional qualifications of the state health agency leadership matter in this case study? Are these issues apparent anywhere in the JAMA article?[1]

3. Do you believe that the organizational placement of the infectious disease control and food sanitation units within the state health agency affected decision making in this case study? Why or why not? At which point(s) were the state health department's organizational structures a barrier or a catalyst for effective crisis management?

4. At which point(s) were the state health department's links to local health departments and federal public health resources effective or ineffective in containing the crisis?

5. At which point(s) were activities to work with and through the media useful or harmful to outbreak control efforts?

6. Do you think there may be reasonable explanations to questions such as why the cross connection was not found on previous inspections of the dairy plant, why the massive outbreak was not immediately linked to the previous year's smaller outbreaks, and why the second wave of illnesses was not detected more quickly (was this possibly the result of overly passive surveillance, or the Easter weekend)?

REFERENCES

1. Ryan CA, Nickels MK, Hargrett-Bean NT, et al. Massive outbreak of antimicrobial-resistant salmonellosis traced to pasteurized milk. *JAMA*. 1987; *258*: 3269–3274.

Ragsdale U.S. Supreme Court Case

This case study, based on actual events, combines issues of constitutional and public health law with ethical, moral, political, and media considerations, leading to a near opportunity for the Supreme Court of the United States to overturn its landmark 1973 decision in Roe v. Wade.

LEARNING OBJECTIVES

Through review and discussion of this case study, students will be able to:

- Identify and explain the various categories of law encountered in public health practice, including constitutional, statutory, judicial, and administrative law.

- Describe the tension and conflict between protecting public health and safety and ensuring the civil rights of individuals.

- Explain the scientific, legal, ethical, political, and media issues related to the regulation of abortion services.

- Identify abortion services policy issues that affect health disparities and health equity.

SCENARIO

It had been more than 10 years since the Better Government Association and investigative reporter Pam Zekman's series on television and in *The Chicago Sun-Times* spotlighting unethical and substandard practices of outpatient abortion providers in the Chicago area. Zekman's investigation highlighted 12 women who suffered fatal infections or bled to death after an abortion procedure and dozens more who were seriously affected. Abortions were performed on women who were not pregnant, and several clinics used unlicensed and unqualified physicians and other health personnel. Some clinics falsified records for preoperative tests that were never performed and for complications that were not recorded on patient charts. Patients were operated on before anesthesia took effect, and others were moved out of recovery rooms before they were stable in order to make room for additional procedures. Several abortion clinics allegedly gave kickbacks for referrals received.

The proliferation of unregulated abortion services outside hospitals was one of the unintended results of the *Roe v. Wade* Supreme Court decision in 1973. State and local governments became reluctant to impose restrictions on abortion providers in view of the risk of these laws and regulations being challenged and overturned in federal courts. Many abortion providers offered high-quality services, but others did not.

The Zekman media exposé led to an immediate public outcry and rapid attention by the state legislature. Among other reforms, abortion clinics that did not provide other outpatient surgical services were explicitly brought under the jurisdiction of an existing state law that licensed ambulatory surgical treatment centers (ASTCs). Some ASTCs had already been performing abortions in addition to other outpatient surgical procedures, and some facilities doing only abortions had sought to be licensed as ASTCs anyway. At the time, ASTCs were a rapidly growing segment of the healthcare industry as many surgical procedures were being moved outside hospitals.

Dr. Richard Ragsdale's abortion clinic in Rockford, one of the few in Illinois outside Chicago, served a large geographic area in a predominantly rural part of the state more than 100 miles north and west of Chicago. At the time, about 40% of all abortions performed in the state took place in ASTCs, and about 50% of licensed ASTCs performed abortion procedures. With no other abortion clinics in the region, Dr. Ragsdale's ASTC, fully licensed by the state health agency for the past 12 years, saw its patient volume and reputation grow. The clinic's landlord, however, refused to renew Ragsdale's lease so that the facility could be remodeled to serve physicians associated with a large neighboring hospital. Dr. Ragsdale searched for a new location for his ASTC. After finding a suitable site, he submitted the necessary paperwork to the state and fully expected that his request would be routinely approved. Instead, he was advised that the state's certificate of need program required that there be public hearings to consider the need for this new facility.

The public hearings attracted large numbers of vocal anti-abortion organizations and individuals. The media attention and public controversy resulted in Ragsdale's new potential landlord withdrawing the lease offer. Ragsdale considered other sites but learned that his new facility would have to meet the full set of regulations for ASTCs, whereas his old facility had been grandfathered in as it was in operation before some of the stricter facility regulations became effective. Ragsdale determined that full compliance with the ASTC regulations at a new facility would increase the average annual cost to his patients by about $45 per patient. This led Dr. Ragsdale and the ACLU to challenge the state laws requiring certificate of need approval and licensing of abortion clinics, charging that these laws imposed an unnecessary and unconstitutional barrier to a woman's right to access first- and second-trimester abortion services, thereby violating the right to privacy provisions guaranteed in the 14th Amendment to the U.S. Constitution, the basic principle at the core of the *Roe v. Wade* decision.

A federal district court found in favor of Dr. Ragsdale and issued a preliminary injunction enjoining the state health department from enforcing health and safety regulations for abortion procedures performed within ASTCs, although the state could enforce health and safety regulations for other surgical procedures performed in those same facilities. In effect, the state could not regulate abortions in licensed ASTCs, and they could not regulate facilities that only performed abortions, whether licensed or not. The state health department appealed the decision, but the 19th Circuit U.S. Appeals Court upheld the decision of the lower court. With Neil Hartigan, the state's popular attorney general representing the state health department (the attorney general was widely regarded as his party's leading candidate to run against the incumbent governor in the following year's general election), the appeals court decision was then appealed to the U.S. Supreme Court.

The composition of the U.S. Supreme Court had changed significantly since 1973 when the *Roe v. Wade* case was decided. In the interval, the court had become increasingly conservative in its handling of cases involving civil rights, and there were fears that the court may even act to reverse the *Roe v. Wade* decision if an appropriate case came onto its docket. In mid-July, the Supreme Court handed down a decision that signaled a new direction, subtly opening the door for states to regulate some first- and second-trimester abortions to ensure the health and safety of pregnant women. On the same day, the court announced its acceptance of the appeal of the Ragsdale case.

Immediately, the Ragsdale case was widely viewed as one the Supreme Court would likely use to overturn the landmark *Roe v. Wade* ruling that legalized abortion in the United States. The main issue in the Ragsdale case was whether the state of Illinois could constitutionally license and regulate outpatient surgical facilities in which abortions were performed in the same manner that the state regulated other outpatient surgical procedures performed in these facilities. At question was whether the state had the constitutional authority to license, regulate, and set standards for ASTCs that performed abortions. Lower courts had ruled that these regulations unduly limited access to abortions, while the state argued that licensing regulations were necessary to protect the health and safety of women obtaining abortions at these facilities. If the Supreme Court were to decide that states did have such authority, then it might also use this case to revisit the *Roe v. Wade* decision and determine that states also had the authority to legally ban abortions entirely.

Neither party in this case wished to provide the Supreme Court with a vehicle to overturn *Roe v. Wade*, and the case was settled less than a week before oral arguments were to be heard before the Supreme Court. The settlement reinstated the state's authority to regulate outpatient facilities performing abortions, using a medically appropriate but less burdensome set of licensing regulations.

QUESTIONS FOR DISCUSSION

1. Which categories of law are involved in this case study? Which of these was most responsible for the initiation of Dr. Ragsdale's legal challenge? Which categories of law were involved in the settlement agreement for the case?

2. Who are the stakeholders in this case study and what are their interests and agendas?

3. If state laws and regulations were the focus of the legal challenge, why was the case initially heard before a federal district court?

4. Which legal, ethical, political, moral, religious, and constitutional issues emerged in this case study?

5. What role did the location of Dr. Ragsdale's clinic (in Rockford surrounded by a largely rural area) play in these events?

6. Should the state health officials have appealed the various lower and appellate court decisions?

7. Why would Dr. Ragsdale and the ACLU agree to a settlement after favorable decisions in the lower courts?

8. Why would the state health officials settle the case if they believed that the U.S. Supreme Court would restore their authority to regulate abortion clinics?

9. Did the different perspectives of the two parties make a settlement more likely or less likely? Why?

10. Were there any ultimate "winners" in this case study?

Outcome Oriented Perinatal Surveillance

This case study, based on actual events with fictionalized names, examines various influences on infant and neonatal mortality and how outcome data can be used to enhance the regulation of maternity and newborn care in hospitals.

LEARNING OBJECTIVES

Through review and discussion of this case study, students will be able to:

- Explain how risk-adjusted measures of health status can be applied to analyze health outcomes and to establish and monitor standards of care.
- Explain the concept of standardized mortality ratios.
- Explain the major determinants of neonatal mortality in terms of "better babies or better care."

SCENARIO

Mike Mangan's job with the city health department required travel via public transportation throughout the five boroughs that comprise New York City, exposing him to several interesting lessons. Most lack relevance to this story, but one important lesson was always to know where you are going and how you plan to get there. And even if you get off track and maybe even get lost, always keep the end in mind.

This keep-your-eyes-on-the-prize principle, however, frequently got in the way of doing the job young Dr. Mangan was traveling through-out New York City to do in the mid-1970s. That job was to visit hospitals large and small to assess their compliance with the city's licensing regulations for maternity and newborn care units. It is well recognized that New York City has a long and glorious history when it comes to maternity and newborn care, and the city health department took its responsibilities seriously. Each inspection team consisted of a physician, two public health nurses, and a public health social worker. Teams would spend a full day at most hospitals (2 to 3 days for the larger hospitals) meeting with administrators and professional staff, inspecting the physical facilities, reviewing policy and procedure manuals, talking to patients and their families, and examining countless patient records.

Each inspection would end with an exit conference that invariably included confrontational moments when the hospital staff would challenge the findings and/or dispute the recommendations of the review team. The most difficult interchanges often involved whether the licensing standards and regulations really equated with quality care and better outcomes. Although the inspection teams used state-of-the-art standards from the American College of Obstetricians and Gynecologists, American Academy of Pediatrics, and the National Committee on Perinatal Health, these confrontations virtually always arose.

Health department inspection teams commonly heard challenges such as these: So what if the bassinets in the nursery are 6 inches closer to one another than they should be, or if the only hand-washing sink in the room is not foot operated, or if the corridors are not as wide as the fire marshal required, or if two small nursery rooms have to share a registered nurse rather than each having one, or if the procedure manuals have not been updated in the past 3 years? Show me how these situations resulted in moms and babies dying—go check the records and see for yourselves! And Dr. Mangan and his team did, and found that outcomes were often much better than they feared and expected.

New York City was so well respected for the quality of its maternity and newborn care in the 1970s that delegations of public health and medical professionals would come from other parts of the United States or the world to see how it was done in the Big Apple. Dr. Mangan especially remembers one delegation as it was from his own hometown, Chicago. The Chicago health commissioner, director of maternal and child health (MCH), chairman of the city's MCH advisory committee, and two topnotch neonatologists came as part of the Chicago delegation. Basically, they wanted to know why New York City's outcomes for newborns were so much better than those of babies born in Chicago.

Dr. Mangan's boss told him to look into the data for the two cities and the inspection reports his team had been conducting on maternity and newborn units in New York City to see if he could shed some light as to what New York City was doing right to make this happen. The New York City health department leaders wanted to be able to explain to their visiting counterparts why perinatal care in New York City was so much better than that in Chicago.

At the time (circa 1977), a few researchers were just beginning to advance a concept that characterizes the two main pathways for differences in neonatal outcomes in simple terms: "better babies or better care." Did New York City have better outcomes because of better care (as the delegation from Chicago assumed), or were the differences actually due to better babies (a controversial topic even in those days)?

Long explanation made short, Dr. Mangan found that the birth weight distribution (i.e., the proportion of babies born in different birth weight categories) differed substantially between the two cities. Chicago had a much higher proportion of its babies born in the low birth weight (<2500 grams) and very low birth weight (<1500 grams, the very smallest) categories than did New York City. On the other hand, he found that, for babies in similar birth weight categories, outcomes were noticeably better for Chicago babies in virtually all weight categories. This finding suggested that perinatal care may actually have been better in Chicago than in New York City!

About 5 years and a few job changes later, Dr. Mangan found himself working back in his hometown for the Chicago Department of Health but with part of history repeating itself in terms of challenges and complaints advanced by hospital medical staff and administrators in Chicago. They argued that the city health department's maternity and newborn inspections were too focused on things that did not matter for quality or outcomes. Through an extensive series of meetings with these medical professionals and hospital administrators, the Chicago Department of Health collaboratively examined the evidence and rationale supporting the existing regulations. This led the city health department to propose a strategy for licensing and regulating maternity and newborn units that would focus on outcomes instead of indicators of structure and process. The Outcome Oriented Perinatal Surveillance System (OOPSS) was the result.[1] The approach in OOPSS was to use standardized mortality ratios, rather than crude death rates, as a tool to identify hospitals with outcomes that required additional investigation and to reduce the inspection burden (inspect less frequently, approve reasonable waiver requests for technical violations of structure and process standards) for those hospitals with more favorable outcomes. Incorporating outcome standards into perinatal regulations was a win-win proposition for both hospitals and health department inspection teams. Keeping the end in mind, in this case perinatal outcomes resonated with Mike Mangan based on his public health practice education in New York City.

QUESTIONS FOR DISCUSSION

1. Using the health problem analysis framework, illustrate how infant (and specifically neonatal) mortality rates are affected by "better babies or better care."
2. What is the public health "science" underlying the Outcome Oriented Perinatal Surveillance System?
3. Why are structure and process standards not equal to quality care and better outcomes?
4. Which aspects of perinatal networks and perinatal systems influence the outcomes for referral hospitals? For community hospitals? Which level of hospitals likely merits the closest scrutiny?
5. Which aspects of outcome-oriented regulatory systems place the regulators at risk? How?

6. Which strategies are useful for gaining buy-in for new regulatory strategies?
7. Does this case study reflect evidence-based public health? Why or why not? If it does, which types of evidence (Evidence of what? Etiology/causation? Or effectiveness? Or adaptability of an intervention?) appear in this case study? Cite specific examples and explain how each fits into one of these categories.
8. Which role, if any, do health disparities play in this case study?

REFERENCES

1. Turnock BJ, Masterson JW. Incorporating outcome standards into perinatal regulations. *Pub Hlth Reports*. 1986; *101*: 59–67.

University of Illinois Hospital

In this case study based on actual events, a state university attempts to unload its hospital facility yet maintain its teaching programs through a series of affiliation agreements with other influential institutions. The reactions of stakeholders, both pro and con, and the influence of an impartial impact assessment play out in media and political arenas.

LEARNING OBJECTIVES

Through review and discussion of this case study, students will be able to:

- Describe the agendas and relationships of the players and stakeholders in a local health system.

- Examine the social, political, economic, and media dimensions of health system change.

- Identify strategies for injecting a public health perspective into local health system change.

SCENARIO

In 1989, the University of Illinois made a move to get out of the hospital business after concluding that hospital operating deficits were out of control. The plan, advanced by the university president and discussed privately with the Board of Trustees before becoming public, involved a series of affiliation agreements.

Basically, the university would lease its relatively new hospital facility to Cook County, obviating the need for the county to build a replacement facility for its aging physical plant. Cook County Hospital had long been an important teaching site for the state university due to its close proximity (located only 2 blocks away). The university's College of Medicine would then affiliate with Michael Reese Hospital Medical Center (some 5 miles away) to serve as the primary location for the university's medical education and training activities and with the new Cook County Hospital for some as yet unspecified activities.

These proposed arrangements were hardly welcome news to faculty, students, and employees at University Hospital, to the professional staff and other workers at the existing county hospital, and to several neighboring institutions such as Rush University Medical Center, which is located within a few blocks of both the University of Illinois Hospital and Cook County Hospital. These complex affiliation agreements required approval by various state and county legislative bodies in addition to the boards of the various institutions. The proposed agreements portended significant changes for the provision of medical education and healthcare services in Chicago as well as other parts of Cook County.

Elected officials and other decision makers, affected parties, and the public raised wide-ranging and important questions as to the various possible effects of the proposed changes on the institutions involved, the quality of medical education, the access to appropriate healthcare services for the medically indigent, the economic and community development on Chicago's Near West Side, and the future of the employees affected. At one of the public hearings on these affiliations at which University of Illinois's president was under great fire, the state public health director proposed to the university president that the state health department perform an assessment of the impact of the proposed affiliations on access to health services in Chicago and Cook County. Such an impact assessment could inform some of the questions being posed and serve the public interest.

The state university president agreed but demanded that this study be completed within 30 days in order for the university's Board of Trustees to be able to vote on the affiliations at its next scheduled meeting. Through the concerted efforts of policy and planning staff at the Illinois Department of Public Health and the Chicago Department of Health, this task was completed on time and included input from several community forums and public hearings as well as written testimony from stakeholders and the public.

The health impact study assessed the communities and populations most affected, key metrics for the hospitals involved, implications for both inpatient and ambulatory care services, and the effect on selected specialized tertiary-level services (such as trauma, burn, perinatal, and transplantation services). A comprehensive financial analysis of the implications of the proposed affiliation agreements was also completed. The final report identified 48 findings and advanced two major conclusions and an additional integrative recommendation. The report concluded that the proposed affiliation agreements would not reduce access to healthcare services in Chicago if 11 critical conditions were met. The report also concluded that implementation of the proposed affiliations would result in considerable savings to county and state government as well as to the institutions involved. The report recommended that $25 million of that savings be set aside annually to increase access to health care through the development of expanded primary care networks currently operated by the city of Chicago and Cook County. Should this occur, this unique opportunity would actually result in greater access than previously existed.

The series of steps that needed to be taken together in order for the proposed affiliations to do no harm, as well as the recommendation to infuse savings from the affiliations into expanding access to primary care, received widespread media and political coverage. Those steps are as follows:

1. The affiliation agreement with Michael Reese Hospital should not go forward ahead of the agreement with Cook County.
2. Implementation of the agreements must not disrupt services to vulnerable populations.
3. University of Illinois faculty and residents must provide services at both Michael Reese and Cook County Hospitals in a flexible two-hospital system.
4. Inpatient bed capacity must be increased in obstetrics, pediatrics, and neonatal intensive care in order to offset the loss of these services by Cook County moving its hospital services into the old University Hospital.
5. Michael Reese Hospital must replace the University Hospital as a Perinatal Referral Center and assume responsibility for University of Illinois Hospital's perinatal network.
6. Michael Reese Hospital must remain in the Chicago trauma network as a Trauma Center.
7. Michael Reese Hospital must continue University Hospital's transplantation services.
8. University Hospital employees must be guaranteed employment after the affiliations are in place.
9. State of Illinois public aid contracts must be revised so that patient days are allotted consistent with physician redeployments as a result of these agreements.
10. Two new ambulatory care centers must be built on Chicago's south and west sides.
11. Decentralization of county inpatient services must be accompanied by decentralization of outpatient services.
12. Twenty-five million dollars annually from the projected savings from these affiliation agreements should be reinvested in increasing access to health care for Chicago and Cook County's poor and medically indigent populations.

The safeguards in this policy framework were quickly and vigorously endorsed by both Chicago newspapers, shifting the public policy debate for the first time to the community-wide effects of the proposed affiliation agreements. The impact report was received as neither a rubber stamp for nor as a roadblock to the proposed affiliations. It did, however, raise the bar for the discussions from one of pursuing narrow institutional self-interests to one of seizing a truly unique opportunity. In the end, the impact report offered a context that allowed the effects on public health to trump the effects on private interests and institutional agendas. With these heightened expectations on the table, the affiliation agreements soon imploded. The University of Illinois kept its hospital but fired its vice chancellor for health services and reassigned the dean of the medical college. The county eventually constructed an expensive new facility to replace its aging physical plant, leaving Rush Medical Center free to focus on nonindigent patients. And access to health care in Chicago was no better or worse than it was before. The public policy agenda articulated by the impact study became the basis for better coordination of ambulatory care services between the Chicago Health Department and the Cook County Hospital system in a new Ambulatory Services Council and a year later in the Chicago and Cook County Health Care Summit.

QUESTIONS FOR DISCUSSION

1. Which components of Chicago's health system are involved in this case study? How do each of these influence health at the individual or population levels?
2. Who are the major stakeholders in this case study? What are their main interests and agendas? How are these threatened or advanced by the agenda of the state university?
3. Which role did the state public health agency play in this case study? Whose interests and agendas did it threaten or advance?
4. How could the health impact study change the nature of the public policy debate? Would it likely change the outcome of that debate? Why or why not?
5. What were the negative results of these events? What were the positive results? Did the positives outweigh the negatives?

Gulf Oil Spill Aftermath

This case study, developed by Emily Ahonen PhD, MPH, explores the issues that occurred in the immediate aftermath of the Gulf oil spill disaster, offering an opportunity to focus on health and well-being and how they are protected, measured, and improved in communities experiencing massive environmental and social disruptions. The case is based on real events, places, and factual information, but the specific situations and individuals described are fictional.

LEARNING OBJECTIVES

Through review and discussion of this case study, students will be able to:

- Describe the human health and well-being effects of a massive oil spill in the Gulf of Mexico.

- Discuss challenges to public health work in disaster situations.

- Identify aspects of public health communication that should be considered by characters in this case.

- Delineate the health protection needs of response workers and volunteers.

- Develop measures of community health that can be integrated into community health needs assessments and community health improvement initiatives in coastal communities affected by a massive oil spill.

- Compare and contrast the health systems in different states, including the state–local public health network, and the implications of any differences on public health activities and population health status.

- Identify barriers that might limit the effectiveness of a community-wide intervention.

- Describe problems and issues that can occur among federal, state, and local health agencies and the responsible parties in responding to a massive oil spill or similar disaster.

- Describe information gaps that limit our understanding of the specific health effects of oil spills.

BACKGROUND

The Deepwater Horizon (DWH), a semi-submersible drilling rig operating in 5,000 feet of water just beyond the Outer Continental Shelf in the Gulf of Mexico, suffered a series of safety, regulatory, and over-sight problems and exploded on April 20, 2010, burning for 36 hours before sinking. Initially, 11 rig workers were killed and 16 were seriously injured. Stopping the flow of oil into the Gulf waters and containing the spilled oil proved extraordinarily difficult, in part because technology developments in containment and cleanup had not kept pace with the progression of production techniques.[1] Nine days after the disaster, it was deemed a Spill of National Significance,[2] the largest ever in U.S. history. Oil leaked into the Gulf until August, and response and remediation continued for months, organized under the National Oil and Hazard-ous Substances Pollution Contingency Plan (shortened to the National Contingency Plan, or NCP).[3] This plan provides for a unified command structure that includes a standing National Response Team, with repre-sentatives from federal agencies, and a Regional Response Team com-posed of regional representatives from each of the federal agencies, led by a Federal On-scene Coordinator. The NCP also includes the Respon-sible Party (in this case, British Petroleum), who is to carry out and pay for response. After the spill was declared one of national significance, resources were coordinated by a National Incident Command. Because it occurred in coastal waters, the U.S. Coast Guard led the incident com-mand.[4] This structure differs from that applied to other disasters under the National Response Framework, where response is state directed and partially federally funded under the Stafford Act. Some confusion appears to have existed about which of these two plans was to be used during the DWH incident and also about delineation of leadership when the spill was deemed nationally significant; how to approach the inclusion of the Responsible Party in response efforts was also a contentious issue.[1]

Although the depth of the waters in which the drill and rig were situated complicates estimates, millions of barrels of oil spilled into the waters.[5] In an effort to mitigate the effects of that volume of oil, controlled burns and more than one million gallons of dispersant were added to the mix of chemicals in the air and waters of the Gulf region.[6] Dispersant can be applied to spilled oil in order to soften the oil–water interface, allow-ing the formation of droplets of oil that are more likely to move down the water column rather than reach shore. However, the oil is not gone, only spread deeper in the water column, with unknown implications both for marine life and for the short- and long-term toxicity of combined disper-sants and crude. Although dispersants have been previously used in oil spills, the volume of use in the DWH spill was unprecedented.

Initial concerns were for responder and cleanup worker safety and for the toxicological effects in workers, visitors, and community members. Hydrocarbons, trace metals, and sulfur are of concern and vary depending on the source of the oil and its composition; respiratory, hepatic, renal, endocrine, neurologic, and hematologic effects can result from high doses, and benzene and polycyclic aromatic hydrocarbons (PAHs), present in crude and from the combustion process of burning it, are human carcinogens.[7] While some less-well characterized compounds and their possible effects are not understood, it appears that benzene evaporated before reaching shore—PAHs have since been found in soil.[7] There was also public concern about dispersants used. In 2011, various tests of the specific dispersant used were undertaken and their results published.[8]

Understanding of potential concerns was complicated by the fact that containment and cleanup groups consisted of both previously trained responders (e.g., members of the National Guard) and residents of the affected areas, many of whom were out of work because of the moratorium on offshore drilling and the closure of waters for fishing, shrimping, and oystering activity; this latter group was a major contributor to response efforts and was hired by British Petroleum,[4] who was responsible for the workplace conditions of those cleanup workers.[9] During response activities, the Occupational Safety and Health Administration, the National Institute for Occupational Safety and Health, the National Institute of Environmental Health Sciences, and other federal agencies played oversight and technical assistance roles for British Petroleum, as well as contributed staff for specific tasks ranging from worker training and education, observation of work, worker rostering, tracking injuries and illnesses, assessing hazards to health, advising on mitigation of hazards, and communicating with the public.[4]

From previous disasters of this magnitude (including the events of September 11, 2001, and the Exxon Valdez oil spill), we know that some of the most important and lasting health effects in communities are on behavioral health.[10] Research from other disasters provides some insight as to what ongoing concerns might be. After the Exxon Valdez spill, "highly exposed" cleanup workers as compared to those unexposed were 3.6 times more likely to suffer generalized anxiety disorder and 2.9 times as likely to have posttraumatic stress disorder 1 year later. Alaska Natives seemed especially vulnerable to effects of chemical exposure and were less likely to seek treatment.[11] In a geographic area still recovering from Hurricanes Katrina and Rita, repeated retraumatization is a concern. The entire Gulf region is heavily dependent on the natural resources of the area. Seafood and oil production, as well as tourist and restaurant industries, composed of many types of work settings (cruises, weddings, restaurants, hotels, bars) make up billions of dollars in economic activity annually in the five Gulf states.[1] Arata and colleagues noted that the chronic individual and community effects of technical disasters are worsened by compensation and litigation processes over time.[12] As of early 2015, litigation was ongoing.

Data gathered in National Commission and Institute of Medicine reports highlighted troubling trends in Gulf communities shortly after the spill.[1,7] A Gallup Survey conducted in August 2010 of 2,600 Gulf residents found that diagnoses of depressive illness had increased by 25% since the disaster and that their proprietary "well-being index" showed coastal residents to be more stressed, worried, and sad than people living inland.[13] A survey of adults living within 10 miles of the Louisiana and Mississippi coasts revealed that one-third believed their children were suffering mental or physical effects of the spill, with the greatest effect in families earning less than $25,000 annually. In that same survey, adults and children who were directly exposed to oil were twice as likely to report new mental health symptoms as those who were not.[14] The National Commission cited data from the Administration for Children and Families that showed an increase in calls to their National Domestic Violence Hotline from all Gulf states between April and June 2010.[1]

Furthermore, the Gulf region is extremely varied in population, complicating an understanding of symptomology and assessment of service needs. European Americans, African Americans, Native Americans, Cajuns, and communities of refugees from Vietnam, Laos, and Cambodia live and work in some of the areas hardest hit by the spill.[1] The approximately 25,000 Vietnamese fishers and tribal communities such as the United Houma Nation live on the coast and were still recovering from long-term damage to the Mississippi River Delta, four hurricanes in 3 years, and resulting loss of wetlands.[1] Cultural and linguistic challenges made accessing resources and making claims more challenging for these groups.[1]

As the National Commission report emphasized, "the lesson from the oil spill is that the nation was not well prepared for the possibility of widespread adverse effects on human health and mental well-being, especially among a particularly vulnerable citizenry."[1, p. 191] It further stated that "human health effects are the least-recognized fallout from the spill, and *those least-well addressed* in existing law and policies."[1, p. 174] The DWH spill, like all oil spill disasters, was viewed largely as an environmental disaster. The Oil Pollution Act of 1990 and other policies for hazardous substance releases offered few tools for addressing and paying for human health concerns within the broader population not directly involved in cleanup efforts. Likewise, plans for the roles of health agencies in the response efforts were not specified, nor was how funding for such efforts would be obtained. This posed a problem following the DWH spill—the Responsible Party was initially tasked to pay for *response*-related costs. Though the scope of expenditures that qualified for reimbursement by Responsible Parties was eventually expanded to include public health concerns and litigation continues for damages, that took time, and efforts at long-term health surveillance have been hampered by that lag.[6,15]

Economic damage and unemployment, along with social disruption, are associated with mental (e.g., anxiety, depression, posttraumatic stress) and behavioral (e.g., domestic violence, substance abuse, divorce, and family disruption) ill health. In addition to the influence on family economies, communities and the entire region have been affected. In fact, a recent study questioned our understanding of "exposure." The authors found that communities directly and indirectly exposed to oil itself in Alabama and Florida were not burdened in a statistically different way by psychological distress, adjustment challenges, neurocognitive function problems, or environmental worry—both groups showed clinically significant levels of depression and anxiety. However, those who suffered income loss as a result of the disaster had poorer mood disturbance results.[5] To further complicate matters, another study showed that community attachment, in many situations beneficial for positive behavioral and mental health, may in fact be associated with greater negative affective response in situations immediately following technological disaster, especially if the community in question is heavily dependent on the natural resources damaged by the disaster.[16]

The unprecedented scale of the disaster and the lack of relevant pre-disaster baseline data in Gulf communities hampered disease and injury surveillance efforts. The National Commission deemed long-term monitoring of cleanup and responder worker health as well as *community health* "warranted and scientifically important."[1, p. 195] It formally recommended the development of plans to address public health concerns during Spills of National Significance, and that charge specifically included medical screening, surveillance for chemical exposures, and mental health concerns in both cleanup workers and the larger community.[1] In 2010, the National Institute of Environmental Health Sciences undertook research to study the potential health effects of the oil spill over 10 years (Gulf Long-Term Follow-Up Study). Additional researchers continue to explore the ways in which this disaster may influence the health and well-being of Gulf populations.

SCENARIO

Jack has been hired by the Responsible Party and is leading one of the crews of people involved in the on-shore cleanup efforts at a beach in a hard-hit Gulf State. He does not know much about cleanup—before the spill he worked transporting materials that were used on the offshore rigs. He and the crew he is supervising have received training on how to do the work safely from a couple of national agencies whose work involves ensuring the safety and health of workers on the job. They have also been visiting the cleanup worksites to check in on how the crews are using that training. Jack has crew members who do not speak much English. Those workers received training in other languages, too, but it can still be difficult to communicate with them while they are working. Since the blowout several weeks earlier, others like him, hired to carry out response activities, have been working on stopping the leak and containing oil out on the water. Some local people who own boats are involved in cleanup, going out to do controlled oil burns, skim the waters, and lay boom. Jack has heard that, out there closer to the source of the oil, some people are concerned about inhaling chemicals from the crude and dispersant, and that some people got sick. That prompted the Responsible Party to request that a national research institute assess whether the people who got sick were sick from the chemicals.

The people from the research institute have been on shore, too, watching and asking questions about the way work is being done and how people feel. Oil cleanup requires difficult, physical work, whether on shore or off shore. Everyone is working long shifts, and physical discomfort is common among the people Jack is supervising. In the Gulf it is also very hot and humid, and the protective clothing the workers are supposed to wear makes it that much hotter—some of the workers would prefer not to wear it. Jack has also been told that giving the workers enough rest and plenty of water is essential, but there has been some tension when people in the community see the workers resting and wonder if cleanup work is really getting done.

At the same time, some workers report symptoms that they relate to exposure to the oil, tar balls, and dispersant used, such as dizziness or headaches. There is uncertainty about their health given all of the unknowns about the chemicals they are around. Many of the people working on cleanup are locals who are out of work because of the spill. There are also people who have come from other parts of the country and are temporarily in the area working on cleanup. Everyone in the area feels unsure and worried, and when the workers get tired, things can get tense. Jack is unsure how to handle all of these competing concerns about protective gear, heat, the workers' worries, the other people in the community, and all of the different agencies who seem to be in charge. Though Jack feels better that he has received training, and that the research people have been studying the work they are doing, he is not sure how he is supposed to interact with them because the Responsible Party hired him. Also, he is unsure whether he will be given the findings from the observations and the questions.

◆◆◆

Sonja works for one of the agencies collecting data about the response work being done and the symptoms the workers have. She has not been working for the agency very long, and this is her first major assignment. She is in charge of collecting symptom data from on-shore workers and putting them into a database for initial analyses. Because they are real field data, she is expecting them to be messy, and they are—she cannot believe how much missing exposure data there are, and how much work it takes her to get it all in order. Finally, she is able to make some comparisons about symptom reports between exposed and unexposed workers. These data will go into a broader report but will also need to be shared with community leaders and others. She does not have much experience communicating results to people in this way. This is an emotionally charged situation, and she is nervous about describing the practical implications of her calculations.

Fortunately, she knows some people who focus on risk communication at work. With her results in hand, she sits down with a group from that unit. They consider her findings and the base of public health evidence before fashioning a clear message, and they will work with her to decide how to talk to Jack and the other cleanup workers, in addition to others. The cleanup workers seem to be most concerned about chemical exposures from the oil and dispersants, but Sonja and her colleagues know that heat-related problems are likely to be a major concern for cleanup workers. By this point in the meeting, everyone is feeling a little overwhelmed, so they decide to put off talk about heat-related concerns until they can consult someone about health behavior and perception of risk in order to help them prioritize their messages.

◆◆◆

Janet sits silent in a staff meeting at the Gulf State Public Health Agency. As a senior employee of its environmental health department, she is among those state officials assigned to work on response and recovery after the oil spill under the direction of the unified command. Initially honored by this assignment, Janet has grown increasingly frustrated by the experience. Unfortunately, Gulf State has suffered several large and devastating hurricanes in the last few years. This time, as usual, the governor of her state declared a state of emergency and began response activities; such efforts were almost commonplace now. However, now there was a new wrinkle: under the NCP, in a Spill of National Significance, response efforts were to be managed at the federal level. Despite this, local authorities in Gulf State, used to more local control, proceeded with their own response to the point that local government leaders, with money from the Responsible Party, were initiating work parallel to the federal effort. Janet finds it difficult to keep track of who is in charge and what her role is. Sometimes in unified command meetings she does not feel she has the information she needs to report on progress. Equally often, she works to carry out tasks assigned to her by unified command only to be embarrassed to find those to whom she reaches out are already involved in state- or local-level efforts of similar type. She feels she cannot do her job as she would like, neither for Gulf State Public Health Agency nor as part of unified command. This makes her feel ineffective in front of the federal representatives and a bit marginalized by colleagues with whom she had worked for years.

◆◆◆

Bao, originally from Southeast Asia, now lives in a coastal area of Gulf State and works in outreach for a local nonprofit focused on community development. He has never been busier than since the oil spill. He became involved with the nonprofit in the aftermath of Hurricane Katrina. As a long-recognized but informal community leader, he was proud to be able to use his knowledge of the local Asian communities, cultures, and languages to serve as a bridge between them and the broader Gulf State community. He played many roles in his work, including that of translator and interpreter, while sometimes also providing outreach for health and social service organizations, or assisting community members in accessing those services. He and his colleagues had been troubled by the mental and behavioral ill health growing in the community after the disasters of recent years. He had made it a point to focus his efforts on how these needs could better be filled, and public health leaders in his area had already reached out to him following the oil spill. His organization and several others, the state health agency, and Gulf State universities are considering ways to support community behavioral and mental health.

Since the spill was deemed a Spill of National Significance, Bao had watched the pace of recovery work slow with confusion about leadership, and he observed that the response leaders were not always aware of the needs of his communities and that outreach and language services were sometimes lacking. Again, those with whom he worked frequently were not aware of available services, felt alienated by their cultural orientation, or were simply limited by language in their ability to access them. Bao is frequently called on as a source of information in such circumstances, so he is not surprised when Janet seeks his help in informing unified command of community needs. He has known Janet for years and likes her. Yet he is overwhelmed by the work already under way locally, and he is torn because he is stretched so thin and he perceives that the federally coordinated efforts are a slower, parallel version of efforts already in progress.

◆◆◆

In June, the national agency in charge of health and other human services informed Justin that he would be sent to the Gulf Coast to assess the public health situation there. Though surprised, because oil spills have usually been considered ecological problems, he knows that several federal health agencies are members of the National Response Team. He arrives in Gulf State and is surprised to learn that broader community health concerns, the roles of health agencies in the response efforts, and funding for their work appear not yet to have been fully considered in this particular national response plan. The Responsible Party has been tasked with response-related costs and is balking at the idea that health effects in the broader Gulf population would fall under its mandate.

Justin had attended recent workshops held by a large nonprofit institute to gather advice for decision makers about the disaster, which had established the mental and behavioral health needs of Gulf communities as high priorities, but a lack of previous planning and funds stymied immediate efforts. In fact, the parameters for determining eligible physical, mental, and behavioral conditions for compensation from the fund set up by the Responsible Party were being debated. As Justin talks to locals and learns more about the situation, he finds that state-level efforts to address mental and behavioral well-being are already under way. Yet Orwin from Gulf State Public Health Agency seems unaware of these activities or at least unconnected to them. Justin is surprised because he imagined she would push to connect the unified command with local programs aiming to address the broader health effects of this technological and ecological disaster.

Meanwhile, Joanna, a program coordinator in community health for the local health department responsible for serving an especially hard-hit locality, has been working on an application for funding from the State Public Health Agency for her area. She has been collaborating with her colleagues in behavioral health services on an intervention based on an existing model that would specifically serve coastal minority groups in her area. She wants to include both individual/clinical support services, such as counseling and surveillance of certain outcomes, and she wants to monitor and promote community cohesiveness and well-being. While the existing evidence suggests that the original intervention is efficacious and likely to be effective in her area, Joanna knows that her targeted project would be somewhat novel and that it could possibly be viewed as a new model for supporting mental health and community well-being after disasters. For that reason, she is especially concerned as to how the intervention will be planned, implemented, and evaluated.

Joanna schedules a meeting with her behavioral health colleague, Thierry, where they discuss their respective concerns. Thierry worries that the declining mental health of many individuals in the community may be affecting social connectedness and capital, and he wants to ensure that the intervention will address both, as well as monitor results over time prior to the final evaluation. He is also worried that if they do not tailor the original program sufficiently to the target groups' political, social, and cultural realities, it will not get off the ground, let alone help. Joanna perceives the need for at least 5 years of project funding and community engagement in order to determine whether the program might serve its purposes, but she is not sure how to design an evaluation to assess this. Together, they write a memo to the director of their local health unit discussing the major considerations that should go into how this intervention should be made locally relevant, implemented, and evaluated.

When Joanna and Thierry's boss receives their memo, she is initially annoyed. The health agency is on a very tight deadline for the funding proposal, and she feels that her employees have raised questions and concerns that, while important, cannot be easily or quickly addressed. She meets with them and expresses her concerns. She wants to gloss over those portions of the proposal, hope to get the funding, and worry about those issues later. Both Joanna and Thierry are intimidated. They know the proposal is important and that the community really needs the outreach and services that it could provide. With some trepidation, Joanna suggests to her boss that they try to talk to people from the nearby state university—she thinks that there are faculty members and a student response corps that might be able to help with this sort of work. To her surprise, her boss agrees and tells them to come up with important program and evaluation design questions they would like to pose to consultants.

◆◆◆

Jean works in administrative leadership for a local health department serving a different area, another of those extensively affected by the Gulf oil spill. At work, the team has talked at length since the spill occurred about the affect on the local population. The group does regular work to keep track of community health indicators and completed its first comprehensive community health needs assessment 3 years earlier. After the spill, though, Jean began to feel that the indicators he and his team had been using did not capture all of the effects that seemed important in terms of the population's health. It was not just the immediate effects of the disaster; the community's entire way of life had been disrupted, and though some things were returning to pre-spill conditions, Jean wondered how some groups might ever fully recover from the loss of jobs, way of life, and natural resources to which they were so intimately connected. Jean's county executive recently directed the agency to conduct a new comprehensive countywide health assessment and improvement initiative that would be grounded in state-of-the-art community health indicators. Jean thinks that this might be an opportunity to discuss with his boss the inclusion of other indicators that would reflect the special needs and circumstances associated with the Gulf oil spill. He feels a bit anxious about proposing changes, so in order to better prepare for the conversation, he begins to compile a list of proposed additions, a rationale for why these should be included, and potential data sources.

QUESTIONS FOR DISCUSSION

1. Discuss the ways in which the physical and social environments interact during an environmental disaster to influence human health.
2. What should be considered when thinking about the health and safety of cleanup workers and volunteers in the circumstances described by this case? How do the activities of the various groups make considerations different for each?
3. Discuss the types of exposures various populations in the aftermath and response to the spill might have to it. To which categories of hazards might different population groups be exposed?

4. Discuss the role of communication with the public in situations of disaster. How is the work of public health professionals helped or hindered by communication choices?

5. Can you think of factors that might compromise our understanding of the effects of the oil spill on human health and well-being?

6. How could the interactions among federal, state, local, and community organizations have been improved in this case study?

7. Identify five important program design and evaluation questions that Joanna and Thierry should pose to the university consultants.

8. Place yourself in Jean's position and propose and justify three community health indicators that should be included in the community health needs assessment. Assume that the leading health indicators for *Healthy People 2020* and the Institute of Medicine's community health assessment indicators in the chapter on health from an ecological perspective represent the initially proposed list of indicators for this effort. Your task is to identify three specific changes (modifications or additions) that you would make to the initially proposed list of indicators for this community health assessment process. For each of your three proposed indicators, explain what the indicator will measure (i.e., what concept is being measured—for example, infant mortality), provide a convincing rationale as to why this indicator would be an important addition to the process, and identify the specific measure of this concept that you plan to use (i.e., operational definition—for example, deaths in the first year of life per 1,000 live births). In addition to justifying your choices individually, explain how your three proposed indicators together will enhance the community assessment process.

9. Using the case study resources and any other Web- or print-based resources you deem necessary, analyze and compare the health systems (including the public health components) in Louisiana (a state hard hit by the Gulf oil spill) with one of the following states: New York, Massachusetts, California, Washington, Florida, Virginia, or Illinois. In your analysis, compare and contrast various measures of health status, resources, and risk characteristics in those two states. Then identify three important differences between the health systems in those two states, and explain the implications of these differences.

10. Assume that you are a program coordinator for a local health department serving a coastal area of a Gulf state and that you are implementing the targeted intervention proposed by Joanna in this case study. Identify three major obstacles or challenges (these can be social, ethical, political, cultural, legal, or distributional factors) to successful implementation of the project and explain how these anticipated risks can be mitigated.

REFERENCES

1. National Commission on the BP Deepwater Horizon Oil Spill and Offshore Drilling. *Deep Water: The Gulf Oil Disaster and the Future of Offshore Drilling—Report to the President.* http://www.gpo.gov/fdsys/pkg/GPO-OILCOMMISSION/content-detail.html. Accessed October 2011.

2. National Oil and Hazardous Substances Pollution Contingency Plan. 1994. 40 CFR § 300.323. (Spill of National Significance).

3. National Oil and Hazardous Substances Pollution Contingency Plan. 1994. 40 CFR § 300.

4. Michaels D, Howard J. Review of the OSHA-NIOSH response to the Deepwater Horizon oil spill: protecting the health and safety of cleanup workers. *PLOS Currents: Disasters.* 2012, July 18. Edition 1. doi:10.1371/4fa83b7576b6e

5. Grattan LM, Roberts S, Mahan WT Jr., et al. The early psychological impacts of the Deepwater Horizon oil spill on Florida and Alabama communities. *Environ Health Perspect.* 2011; *119*(6): 838–843.

6. McCoy MA, Salerno JA. *Assessing the Effects of the Gulf of Mexico Oil Spill on Human Health: A Summary of the June 2010 Workshop.* Washington, DC: National Academies Press; 2010.

7. Goldstein BD, Osofsky HJ, Lichtveld MY. The Gulf oil spill. *N Engl J Med.* 2011; *364*: 1334–1348.

8. Center's for Disease Control and Prevention. *Deepwater Horizon Response, Chemical Dispersant Research.* http://www.cdc.gov/niosh/topics/oilspillresponse/chemDispersant .html. Accessed January 25, 2012.

9. Occupational Safety and Health Act of 1970. 1970. (Public law no. 91-596).

10. Yun K, Lurie N, Hyde PS. Moving mental health into the disaster-preparedness spotlight. *N Engl J Med.* 2010; *363*: 1193–1195.

11. Palinkas LA, Petterson JS, Russell J, et al. Community patterns of psychiatric disorders after the Exxon Valdez oil spill. *Am J Psychiatry.* 1993; *150*(10): 1517–1523.

12. Arata CM, Picou JS, Johnson GD, et al. Coping with technological disaster: an application of the conservation of resources model to the Exxon Valdez oil spill. *J Trauma Stress.* 2000; *1*: 23–39.

13. Witters D. *Gulf Coast Residents Worse Off Emotionally After BP Oil Spill: Depression Diagnoses, Daily Stress and Worry All Increase for Gulf Residents.* http://www.gallup .com/poll/143240/gulf-coast-residents-worse-off-emotionally-oil-spill.aspx. Accessed September 28, 2010.

14. Abramson D, Redlener I, Stehling-Ariza T, et al. *Impact on Children and Families of the Deepwater Horizon Oil Spill: Preliminary Findings of the Coastal Population Impact Study.* New York: Columbia University Mailman School of Public Health; 2010. (Research brief 2010:8).

15. Institute of Medicine. *Research Priorities for Assessing Health Effects from the Gulf of Mexico Oil Spill: A Letter Report.* Washington, DC: National Academies Press; 2010.

16. Lee MR, Blanchard TC. Community attachment and negative affective states in the context of the BP Deepwater Horizon disaster. *Am Behav Sci.* 2012; *56*(1): 24–47.

ADDITIONAL REFERENCES CONSULTED

National Institute for Occupational Safety and Health. *Health Hazard Evaluation of Deepwater Horizon Response Workers.* Atlanta, GA: National Institute for Occupational Safety and Health; 2010.

Bioterrorist Attack on Food: A Tabletop Exercise

This exercise, developed by the Northwest Center for Public Health Practice,* is designed as an opportunity for public health personnel and their local emergency counterparts to gain skills and knowledge in preparing for and responding to a large-scale communicable disease event. Participants address a hypothetical bioterrorism incident in the form of an infectious disease outbreak to acquire this learning. The exercise enables participants to identify the communication, resources, data, coordination, and organizational elements associated with an emergency response. Discussion questions are embedded in the scenario as it unfolds.

LEARNING OBJECTIVES

Through review and discussion of this tabletop exercise, students will be able to:

- Understand measures that can be performed at the local level to prepare for a large-scale communicable disease or bioterrorism incident.

- Promote interagency collaboration/coordination regarding emergency preparation and responsiveness.

- Recognize the roles of a variety of public officials in a large-scale communicable disease or bioterrorism incident.

- Recognize the need for intense teamwork and communication to prepare for a large-scale communicable disease or bioterrorism incident.

- Identify gaps in local preparedness and ability to coordinate.

- Identify additional related training/learning needs (an assessment tool).

---

*Northwest Center for Public Health Practice, University of Washington, in conjunction with the Washington State Department of Health. Originally titled "Hands-on Training for Public Health Emergencies" and developed through funding from the Health Alert Network and the Bioterrorism Preparedness and Response Program at the Centers for Disease Control and Prevention.

INTRODUCTION

This exercise is aimed at identifying the policy questions that must be considered in responding to a bioterrorism event. The depicted exercise scenario will enable participants to understand and experience the shortcomings or gaps in their ability to identify and respond to policy issues (as opposed to operational procedures). Participants will be required to state policy questions such as these: Who should be responsible? Or what information is needed? Or when is public information given out? In essence, participants will be identifying *what* is required in responding to an incident and not necessarily *how* an agency will actually respond. It is important that the exercise identify policies required to respond effectively to the scenario rather than using only those policies that currently exist. Addressing those policies that need clarification or development will be helpful in eventually strengthening the overall response system and will identify areas in operational policies and procedures that need refinement.

PART 1

Storyboard 1

This incident affects four counties: Cedar, Dogwood, Pine, and Maple. The incident begins in Cedar County in the month of August.

Cedar County

- Total population: 150,000 residents.
- The major city, Watertown, has a population of 40,000 residents.
- There are two area hospitals; one is a children's hospital.
- There are numerous nursing homes and day care centers.
- International trade, tourism, agricultural products, and lumbering are the major industries.
- An economic trade group conference is scheduled to be held in Watertown in 3 weeks. About 100 members will be attending, including foreign economic officials.
- Residents are all served by a regional public water supply system.
- The Cedar County health department has a staff of 70 employees. The department has a full-time director of public health and a full-time health officer (MD). A full range of public health services, including environmental health, community health nursing, laboratory, and clinical public health services, are provided.

Dogwood County

- Located directly to the north of Cedar County.
- Total population: 35,000 residents.
- Noted for its numerous water recreational areas.

- About 10,000 residents are served by small or individual water supply systems.
- The Dogwood County health department has 25 total staff, including environmental health specialists and community health nurses. A health officer (MD) is part time.

Pine County

- Located directly to the south of Cedar County.
- Total population: 15,000 residents.
- Serves as a bedroom community to Cedar County. Many Pine County residents commute to work in Cedar County's major city.
- Residents receive public water supplied by Cedar County Regional Water Utility.
- The Pine County health department has a total of 14 staff members (5 are part time). Two are environmental health specialists and 10 are public health nurses. The remaining staff members provide administrative support. A health officer is a contract physician from the community.

The state health department is located in Maple County, 140 miles to the east of Cedar County. The state health department's public health laboratory and the state's university are also located in Maple County. The population of Maple County is 1 million.

Event 1

Day 1, Friday

Persons with gastrointestinal illness are beginning to contact their medical care providers through the nurse hotline and patient consultation lines. Individuals with gastrointestinal problems are calling or visiting area emergency rooms and urgent care centers on Friday afternoon and evening. The hospital's patient consultation line is experiencing an increased number of callers with symptoms including severe diarrhea, fever, chills, headache, nausea, vomiting, abdominal pain, and possibly bloody stools. All cases describe diarrhea as a symptom. Almost all report at least two or more of the additional symptoms. Illnesses have lasted 1 to 2 days without improvement. Most patients are middle-aged adults, but approximately 10% are over the age of 65. A total of 30 people are seen in hospital emergency rooms and urgent care centers by late Friday evening. (This means that a total of 400 individuals may be exhibiting similar symptoms but are not seeking medical care. The 30 cases, or 7.5% of the 400, visit a medical care provider for symptoms.) Stool samples are taken for six of the affected cases seen by a physician. Three individuals are hospitalized for dehydration or other gastrointestinal complications.

Day 2, Saturday Morning

Patients are still being seen in the emergency room and urgent care centers. By 10:00 a.m., the number of patients exhibiting similar symptoms is up to 45. The decision is made to notify the health department. There is some concern about the capacity of the clinics to handle the increasing number of patients seeking treatment.

Questions for you to consider and discuss as if you were part of the emergency preparedness response team follow. Please do not skip ahead in the story, but follow the events in the sequence they are presented here.

1. How do medical care providers decide when to contact health officials?
2. How do medical care personnel determine whom to contact?
3. How is the health department person contacted (after hours/non-business days)?
4. What does the health department do with this information? What additional information does the health department need? How does the medical care facility address its capacity needs?

Event 2

Day 2, Saturday Noon

By noon, the patient count is up to 60. The local health officer decides to convene a meeting to discuss next steps. A local pharmacist calls the local hospital to ask what is happening. The pharmacist reports that the store is almost out of antidiarrheal medicine because of heavy demand.

Questions for you to consider and discuss as if you were part of the emergency preparedness response team follow. Please do not skip ahead in the story, but follow the events in the sequence they are presented here.

1. Who should be involved in the meeting?
2. Would nontraditional partners, such as emergency management, be brought in at this time?
3. What should be discussed in the meeting?
4. What is the health department doing to collect additional information about cases?

Event 3

Day 2, Saturday Evening

The health department decides to begin interviewing cases.

Questions for you to consider and discuss as if you were part of the emergency preparedness response team follow. Please do not skip ahead in the story, but follow the events in the sequence they are presented here.

1. How do you proceed?
2. What additional information is needed for further investigation?

Event 4

Day 2, Saturday Evening

Medical care providers from Dogwood and Pine Counties are reporting a high number of patients complaining about severe gastrointestinal problems. By 5:00 p.m., the total patient count from all three counties is 75. Seventeen stool specimens have been taken. Six people have now been hospitalized.

Questions for you to consider and discuss as if you were part of the emergency preparedness response team follow. Please do not skip ahead in the story, but follow the events in the sequence they are presented here.

1. To whom do the medical care providers from Dogwood and Pine Counties report their information, particularly if key health department staff cannot be contacted?
2. How is information being shared between the health agencies?

Event 5

Day 2, Saturday Evening

Hospital personnel have confirmed to the news media a large number of people being seen with some type of "intestinal illness" but refer callers to the health department.

Questions for you to consider and discuss as if you were part of the emergency preparedness response team follow. Please do not skip ahead in the story, but follow the events in the sequence they are presented here.

1. How does the health department respond to the news media inquiries?
2. Does the health department have a designated public information officer?

Event 6

Day 2, Saturday Evening

At 5:00 p.m., a member of a tour group visiting the county reports to the health department that 35 out of 50 members have become ill with severe diarrhea, vomiting, and nausea. None have seen a doctor. All ate at local restaurants in the area for the past week. The group is primarily non-English speaking tourists from Southeast Asia.

Questions for you to consider and discuss as if you were part of the emergency preparedness response team follow. Please do not skip ahead in the story, but follow the events in the sequence they are presented here.

1. Which actions should be taken to respond to this information?
2. How are the issues of language translation handled?

PART 2

Storyboard 2

The focus of attention is being directed toward food service establishments in the three counties as a result of patient interview data. Numerous establishments are being identified as places where interviewed patients have eaten or have purchased foods in the past week. Many are restaurants; however, specialty grocery stores are also being frequently mentioned.

Twelve identified restaurants are in Cedar County. One is in Dogwood County. All restaurants serve a high volume and variety of customers. They range from well-known, moderately priced, national chain restaurants to popular, high-scale dining establishments. Company executives, business leaders, attorneys, and government officials often eat at the affected city establishments. All are popular with tourists visiting both counties. Four establishments serve ethnic foods. Two are Mexican. The other two are Asian. Three affected restaurants have a history of poor food handling practices, particularly hand washing and temperature violations. None of the establishments have had violations of foods from unapproved sources.

The three specialty grocery stores are highly popular and have a high turnover of food inventory. All are owned and operated by the same company. Two of the specialty stores are in Cedar County. The third is located in Dogwood County. All food service establishments are served by public water but from different water utilities.

Event 7

Day 3, Sunday Morning

Health department personnel interviewing cases are hearing about 12 restaurants being repeatedly named in Cedar County and one in Dogwood County. Three of the restaurants in Cedar County have had a history of food service violations. Several people becoming ill, however, have not eaten at any of the 13 named restaurants. Laboratory results on patients will not be available until the next day.

Questions for you to consider and discuss as if you were part of the emergency preparedness response team follow. Please do not skip ahead in the story, but follow the events in the sequence they are presented here.

1. What is the significance of this information?
2. Which actions are taken on the named restaurants, if any?
3. What information is shared with the news media, if any?

Event 8

Day 3, Sunday Morning

Many ill patients have not eaten at a restaurant in the past week; however, food items being commonly named include fresh salsa, pesto dishes, pizzas, Asian soups, and gourmet salads.

Questions for you to consider and discuss as if you were part of the emergency preparedness response team follow. Please do not skip ahead in the story, but follow the events in the sequence they are presented here.

1. What is the significance of this information?
2. How is this information shared with the public and first responders?

Event 9

Day 3, Sunday Morning

Remember that there is a large economic trade group conference scheduled in Watertown (Cedar County) in 3 weeks, as mentioned in Storyboard 1.

Hospital emergency rooms and medical clinics in the county are becoming overwhelmed with patients. Medical facilities are short staffed because many medical personnel are home ill with "gastrointestinal upset." There is concern among medical staff about spread of the illness within the hospital and the urgent care clinics.

Questions for you to consider and discuss as if you were part of the emergency preparedness response team follow. Please do not skip ahead in the story, but follow the events in the sequence they are presented here.

1. What is the procedure for added capacity to handle the high volume of patients?
2. What is the policy of infection control (and communication) within the medical care facilities?

Event 10

Day 3, Sunday Evening

The patient count is up to 250 after news reports on the disease outbreak. The source is not yet determined, but food is highly suspected, with attention focusing on fresh herbs. Most cases are middle-aged adults. The age range of cases is from 5 to 82 years.

Questions for you to consider and discuss as if you were part of the emergency preparedness response team follow. Please do not skip ahead in the story, but follow the events in the sequence they are presented here.

1. Which actions are being performed by the health department to determine the cause of the outbreak?

2. Which communication systems are in place?
3. Which resources are available to handle an influx of public calls? A phone bank?
4. Which state and national resources are called in?
5. What is the content of the food safety message to the public?
6. How and when does this message get out?
7. Who is dealing with the food industry in the three counties?

Event 11

Day 3, Sunday Evening

Early results of diagnostic tests indicate that *Shigella sonnei* is the causative agent.

Questions for you to consider and discuss as if you were part of the emergency preparedness response team follow. Please do not skip ahead in the story, but follow the events in the sequence they are presented here.

1. Which actions are needed in response to this result?

Shigellosis Fact Sheet

- Typical symptoms of Shigellosis include severe diarrhea often accompanied by fever, chills, headache, nausea, vomiting, abdominal pain, and possibly bloody stools. The incubation period is 1 to 7 days (usually 1 to 3 days). Fewer than 10% of cases seek medical care, and fewer have confirmatory stool cultures performed. Complications such as dehydration may result in hospitalization, but deaths are rare.

Event 12

Day 3, Sunday Evening

The city's mayor receives a message from an extremist group taking credit for "contaminating the food supply with an infectious bacterial agent." The group threatens to continue to do so unless the upcoming conference of economic trade group representatives is canceled. The mayor shares the message with the health department director and the chief of police.

Questions for you to consider and discuss as if you were part of the emergency preparedness response team follow. Please do not skip ahead in the story, but follow the events in the sequence they are presented here.

1. How should the health department handle this information?
2. Who should be involved in assessing this message?
3. Who is in charge?

Event 13

Day 3, Sunday Evening

An anonymous person calls the local newspaper and says she represents a group who wishes to take credit for "making people sick with food contaminated with botulism."

Questions for you to consider and discuss as if you were part of the emergency preparedness response team follow. Please do not skip ahead in the story, but follow the events in the sequence they are presented here.

1. What does the health department do with this information?

Events 14 and 15

Day 3, Sunday Evening

The health officer declares a public health emergency. The phone lines are jammed.

Questions for you to consider and discuss as if you were part of the emergency preparedness response team follow. Please do not skip ahead in the story, but follow the events in the sequence they are presented here.

1. Has an emergency operations center already been activated?
2. Where does the health department fit into the emergency operations center's command structure?

Event 16

Day 4, Monday Morning

The reported patient count is now more than 400. Eighty percent of cases are from the largest county. The remaining 20% come from the two adjacent counties. Thirty cases are restaurant workers. Affected cases range in age from 4 to 87 years. Thirty cases are hospitalized. Five are in serious condition.

Questions for you to consider and discuss as if you were part of the emergency preparedness response team follow. Please do not skip ahead in the story, but follow the events in the sequence they are presented here.

1. Which actions are taking place to prevent the outbreak from spreading?

Event 17

Day 4, Monday Morning

The state university microbiology laboratory located in another part of the state reports to the university campus security that numerous vials of *Shigella sonnei* are missing from the laboratory. The vials were last seen 7 days ago. A few vials from the original batch of the culture are still available. Campus security contacts the county sheriff. The county sheriff contacts its local health department (Maple County).

Questions for you to consider and discuss as if you were part of the emergency preparedness response team follow. Please do not skip ahead in the story, but follow the events in the sequence they are presented here.

1. What does the Maple County health department do after receipt of this information?
2. How is it shared with Cedar County?

PART 3

Storyboard 3

A terrorist group possesses 2 gallons of a liquid broth containing high concentrations of a disease-causing bacterial agent. The cultures of the bacterial agent have been secretly manufactured using stolen vials from a university laboratory. The infectious broth was surreptitiously sprayed onto produce at a food distribution warehouse in Cedar County over a 2-day period. The contaminated produce was then distributed to affected food establishments (13 restaurants and 3 specialty grocery stores): 12 local restaurants and 2 specialty grocery stores in Cedar County and 1 restaurant and a specialty grocery store in Dogwood County. Pine County food establishments were not affected. The produce was used for garnish and seasonings in a variety of dishes at the restaurants. The contaminated dishes were consumed in all 13 restaurants on Tuesday evening and Wednesday lunch and dinner. The produce was also purchased directly by consumers at the three local specialty grocery stores on Tuesday and Wednesday. Residents in all three counties became ill by consuming the contaminated products. Not all sick have visited their medical care provider.

Event 18

Day 4, Monday Evening

Business at area food establishments is dropping significantly.

Questions for you to consider and discuss as if you were part of the emergency preparedness response team follow. Please do not skip ahead in the story, but follow the events in the sequence they are presented here.

1. What is the message to food service operators? To food workers?
2. Who communicates food safety information to the public?

Event 19

Day 4, Monday Evening

News media from other states are calling for interviews or information.

Questions for you to consider and discuss as if you were part of the emergency preparedness response team follow. Please do not skip ahead in the story, but follow the events in the sequence they are presented here.

1. Who responds?
2. How is the response script developed?

Event 20

Day 4, Monday Evening

Re-interviewing of cases and working closely with restaurants to identify common ingredients indicates cilantro and basil as the most likely contaminated products.

Questions for you to consider and discuss as if you were part of the emergency preparedness response team follow. Please do not skip ahead in the story, but follow the events in the sequence they are presented here.

1. What is done with this information?

Event 21

Day 4, Monday Evening

An 86-year-old woman dies from complications resulting from Shigellosis. Her family threatens a lawsuit against the responsible agency.

Questions for you to consider and discuss as if you were part of the emergency preparedness response team follow. Please do not skip ahead in the story, but follow the events in the sequence they are presented here.

1. How are legal issues handled?

Event 22

Day 14, Friday—Recovery Period

Nothing more was ever heard from the extremists. No new infections are attributed to the identified food source; however, secondary cases continue to occur, including outbreaks in 3 day care centers. Public alarm has decreased, but people are still calling about food safety and concerned by the cases that continue to occur—the public does not understand the meaning of "secondary cases." The trade conference is still scheduled for 1 week from today.

Questions for you to consider and discuss as if you were part of the emergency preparedness response team follow.

1. How does the health department ensure the public that the outbreak is over and that the new cases are a result of secondary transmission?
2. Which recommendations should be given to the mayor about the risks of holding the annual conference of trade representatives?

Early 21st-Century Public Health Achievements

Previous editions of this text spotlighted a series of Centers for Disease Control and Prevention (CDC) reports on the Ten Great Public Health Achievements of the 20th Century. *This case study is adapted from a 2011 CDC article describing public health achievements in the first decade of the 21st century, many of which built on the CDC's initial series of reports. Although not presented in typical case-study format, this report bridges the history of public health practice in the United States over two centuries and offers insights into the challenges faced in the early decades of the new century.*

LEARNING OBJECTIVES

Through review and discussion of this case study, students will be able to:

- Describe the most important public health achievements of the first decade of the 21st century.

- Identify the forces and influences that have contributed to these achievements.

- Identify challenges and influences that may threaten continued progress for these achievements.

TEN GREAT PUBLIC HEALTH ACHIEVEMENTS IN THE UNITED STATES, 2001–2010*

During the 20th century, life expectancy at birth among U.S. residents increased by 62%, from 47.3 years in 1900 to 76.8 in 2000, and unprecedented improvements in population health status were observed at every stage of life.[1] In 1999, the *Morbidity and Mortality Weekly Report* (MMWR) published a series of reports highlighting 10 public health achievements that contributed to these improvements. This report assesses advances in public health during the first 10 years of the 21st century. Public health scientists at the Centers for Disease Control and Prevention (CDC) were asked to nominate noteworthy

---

*Reprinted from the Centers for Disease Control and Prevention. Ten great public health achievements: United States, 2001–2010. *MMWR*. 2011;*60*(19):619–623.

public health achievements that occurred in the United States during 2001 to 2010. From those nominations, 10 achievements, not ranked in any order, have been summarized in this report.

Vaccine-Preventable Diseases

The past decade has seen substantial declines in cases, hospitalizations, deaths, and healthcare costs associated with vaccine-preventable diseases. New vaccines (i.e., rotavirus, quadrivalent meningococcal conjugate, herpes zoster, pneumococcal conjugate, and human papillomavirus vaccines, as well as tetanus, diphtheria, and acellular pertussis vaccine for adults and adolescents) were introduced, bringing to 17 the number of diseases targeted by U.S. immunization policy. A recent economic analysis indicated that vaccination of each U.S. birth cohort with the current childhood immunization schedule prevents approximately 42,000 deaths and 20 million cases of disease, with net savings of nearly $14 billion in direct costs and $69 billion in total societal costs.[2]

The influence of two vaccines has been particularly striking. Following the introduction of pneumococcal conjugate vaccine, an estimated 211,000 serious pneumococcal infections and 13,000 deaths were prevented during 2000 to 2008.[3] Routine rotavirus vaccination, implemented in 2006, now prevents an estimated 40,000 to 60,000 rotavirus hospitalizations each year.[4] Advances also were made in the use of older vaccines, with reported cases of hepatitis A, hepatitis B, and varicella at record lows by the end of the decade. Age-specific mortality (i.e., deaths per million population) from varicella for persons aged < 20 years declined by 97%, from 0.65 in the prevaccine period (1990–1994) to 0.02 during 2005 to 2007.[5] Average age-adjusted mortality (deaths per million population) from hepatitis A also declined significantly, from 0.38 in the prevaccine period (1990–1995) to 0.26 during 2000 to 2004.[6]

Prevention and Control of Infectious Diseases

Improvements in state and local public health infrastructure, along with innovative and targeted prevention efforts, yielded significant progress in controlling infectious diseases. Examples include a 30% reduction from 2001 to 2010 in reported U.S. tuberculosis cases and a 58% decline from 2001 to 2009 in central line-associated blood stream infections.[7,8] Major advances in laboratory techniques and technology and investments in disease surveillance have improved the capacity to identify contaminated foods rapidly and accurately and prevent further spread.[9–12] Multiple efforts to extend HIV testing, including recommendations for expanded screening of persons aged 13 to 64 years, increased the number of persons diagnosed with HIV/AIDS and reduced the proportion with late diagnoses, enabling earlier access to life-saving treatment and care and giving infectious persons the information necessary to protect their partners.[13] In 2002, information from CDC predictive models and reports of suspected West Nile virus transmission through blood transfusion spurred a national investigation, leading to the rapid development and implementation of new blood donor screening.[14] To date, such screening has interdicted 3,000 potentially infected U.S. donations, removing them from the blood supply. Finally, in 2004, after more than 60 years of effort, canine rabies was eliminated in the United States, providing a model for controlling emerging zoonoses.[15,16]

Tobacco Control

Since publication of the first Surgeon General's Report on tobacco in 1964, implementation of evidence-based policies and interventions by federal, state, and local public health authorities has reduced tobacco use significantly.[17] By 2009, 20.6% of adults and 19.5% of youths were current smokers, compared with 23.5% of adults and 34.8% of youths 10 years earlier. However, progress in reducing smoking rates among youths and adults appears to have stalled in recent years. After a substantial decline from 1997 (36.4%) to 2003 (21.9%), smoking rates among high school students remained relatively unchanged from 2003 (21.9%) to 2009 (19.5%).[18] Similarly, adult smoking prevalence declined steadily from 1965 (42.4%) through the 1980s, but the rate of decline began to slow in the 1990s, and the prevalence remained relatively unchanged from 2004 (20.9%) to 2009 (20.6%).[19] Despite the progress that has been made, smoking still results in an economic burden, including medical costs and lost productivity, of approximately $193 billion per year.[20]

Although no state had a comprehensive smoke-free law (i.e., smoking prohibited in worksites, restaurants, and bars) in 2000, that number increased to 25 states and the District of Columbia by 2010, with 16 states enacting comprehensive smoke-free laws following the release of the 2006 Surgeon General's Report.[21] After 99 individual state cigarette excise tax increases, at an average increase of 55.5 cents per pack, the average state excise tax increased from 41.96 cents per pack in 2000 to $1.44 per pack in 2010.[22] In 2009, the largest federal cigarette excise tax increase went into effect, bringing the combined federal and average state excise tax for cigarettes to $2.21 per pack, an increase from $0.76 in 2000. In 2009, the Food and Drug Administration (FDA) gained the authority to regulate tobacco products.[23] By 2010, the FDA had banned flavored cigarettes, established restrictions on youth access, and proposed larger, more effective graphic warning labels that are expected to lead to a significant increase in quit attempts.[24]

Maternal and Infant Health

The past decade has seen significant reductions in the number of infants born with neural tube defects (NTDs) and expansion of screening of newborns for metabolic and other heritable disorders. Mandatory folic acid fortification of cereal grain products labeled as enriched in the United States beginning in 1998 contributed to a 36% reduction in NTDs from 1996 to 2006 and prevented an estimated 10,000 NTD-affected pregnancies in the past decade, resulting in a savings of $4.7 billion in direct costs.[25-27]

Improvements in technology and endorsement of a uniform newborn screening panel of diseases have led to earlier life-saving treatment and intervention for at least 3,400 additional newborns each year with selected genetic and endocrine disorders.[28,29] In 2003, all but four states were screening for only six of these disorders. By April 2011, all states reported screening for at least 26 disorders on an expanded and standardized uniform panel.[29] Newborn screening for hearing loss increased from 46.5% in 1999 to 96.9% in 2008.[30] The percentage of infants not passing their hearing screening who were then diagnosed by an audiologist before age 3 months as either normal or having permanent hearing loss increased from 51.8% in 1999 to 68.1% in 2008.[30]

Motor Vehicle Safety

Motor vehicle crashes are among the top 10 causes of death for U.S. residents of all ages and the leading cause of death for persons aged 5 to 34 years.[30] In terms of years of potential life lost before age 65, motor vehicle crashes ranked third in 2007, behind only cancer and heart disease, and account for an estimated $99 billion in medical and lost work costs annually.[31,32] Crash-related deaths and injuries are largely preventable. From 2000 to 2009, while the number of vehicle miles traveled on the nation's roads increased by 8.5%, the death rate related to motor vehicle travel declined from 14.9 per 100,000 population to 11.0, and the injury rate declined from 1,130 to 722; among children, the number of pedestrian deaths declined by 49%, from 475 to 244, and the number of bicyclist deaths declined by 58%, from 178 to 74.[33,34]

These successes largely resulted from safer vehicles, safer roadways, and safer road use. Behavior was improved by protective policies, including effective seat belt and child safety seat legislation; 49 states and the District of Columbia have enacted seat belt laws for adults, and all 50 states and the District of Columbia have enacted legislation that protects children riding in vehicles.[35] Graduated drivers' licensing policies for teen drivers have helped reduce the number of teen crash deaths.[36]

Cardiovascular Disease Prevention

Heart disease and stroke have been the first and third leading causes of death in the United States since 1921 and 1938, respectively.[37,38] Preliminary data from 2009 indicate that stroke is now the fourth leading cause of death in the United States.[39] During the past decade, the age-adjusted coronary heart disease and stroke death rates declined from 195 to 126 per 100,000 population and from 61.6 to 42.2 per 100,000 population, respectively, continuing a trend that started in the 1900s for stroke and in the 1960s for coronary heart disease.[40] Factors contributing to these reductions include declines in the prevalence of cardiovascular risk factors such as uncontrolled hypertension, elevated cholesterol, and smoking and improvements in treatments, medications, and quality of care.[41–44]

Occupational Safety

Significant progress was made in improving working conditions and reducing the risk for workplace-associated injuries. For example, patient lifting has been a substantial cause of low back injuries among the 1.8 million U.S. healthcare workers in nursing care and residential facilities. In the late 1990s, an evaluation of a best practices patient-handling program that included the use of mechanical patient-lifting equipment demonstrated reductions of 66% in the rate of workers' compensation injury claims and lost workdays and documented that the investment in lifting equipment can be recovered in fewer than 3 years.[45] Following widespread dissemination and adoption of these best practices by the nursing home industry, Bureau of Labor Statistics data showed a 35% decline in low back injuries in residential and nursing care employees between 2003 and 2009.

The annual cost of farm-associated injuries among youth has been estimated at $1 billion annually.[46] A comprehensive childhood agricultural injury prevention initiative was established to address this problem. Among its interventions was the development by the National Children's Center for Rural Agricultural Health and Safety of guidelines for parents to match chores with their child's development and physical capabilities. Follow-up data have demonstrated a 56% decline in youth farm injury rates from 1998 to 2009 (National Institute for Occupational Safety and Health, unpublished data, 2011).

In the mid-1990s, crab fishing in the Bering Sea was associated with a rate of 770 deaths per 100,000 full-time fishers.[47] Most fatalities occurred when vessels overturned because of heavy loads. In 1999, the U.S. Coast Guard implemented Dockside Stability and Safety Checks to correct stability hazards. Since then, one vessel has been lost and the fatality rate among crab fishermen has declined to 260 deaths per 100,000 full-time fishers.[47]

Cancer Prevention

Evidence-based screening recommendations have been established to reduce mortality from colorectal cancer and female breast and cervical cancer.[48] Several interventions inspired by these recommendations have improved cancer screening rates. Through the collaborative efforts of federal, state, and local health agencies, professional clinician societies, nonprofit organizations, and patient advocates, standards were developed that have significantly improved cancer screening test quality and use.[49,50] The National Breast and Cervical Cancer Early Detection Program has reduced disparities by providing breast and cervical cancer screening services for uninsured women.[49] The program's success has resulted from similar collaborative relationships. From 1998 to 2007, colorectal cancer death rates decreased from 25.6 per 100,000 population to 20.0 (2.8% per year) for men and from 18.0 per 100,000 to 14.2 (2.7% per year) for women.[51] During this same period, smaller declines were noted for breast and cervical cancer death rates (2.2% per year and 2.4%, respectively).[52]

Childhood Lead Poisoning Prevention

In 2000, childhood lead poisoning remained a major environmental public health problem in the United States, affecting children from all geographic areas and social and economic levels. Black children and those living in poverty and in old, poorly maintained housing were disproportionately affected. In 1990, five states had comprehensive lead poisoning prevention laws; by 2010, 23 states had such laws. Enforcement of these statutes, as well as federal laws that reduce hazards in the housing with the greatest risks, has significantly reduced the prevalence of lead poisoning. Findings of the National Health and Nutrition Examination Surveys from 1976 to 1980 and 2003 to 2008 reveal a steep decline, from 88.2% to 0.9%, in the percentage of children aged 1 to 5 years with blood lead levels ≥10 μg/dL. The risks for elevated blood lead levels based on socioeconomic status and race also were reduced significantly. The economic benefit of lowering lead levels among children by preventing lead exposure is estimated at $213 billion per year.[53]

Public Health Preparedness and Response

After the international and domestic terrorist actions of 2001 highlighted gaps in the nation's public health preparedness, tremendous improvements have been made. In the first half of the decade, efforts were focused primarily on expanding the capacity of the public health system to respond (e.g., purchasing supplies and equipment). In the second half of the decade, the focus shifted to improving the laboratory, epidemiology, surveillance, and response capabilities of the public health system. For example, from 2006 to 2010, the percentage of Laboratory Response Network labs that passed proficiency testing for bioterrorism threat agents increased from 87% to 95%. The percentage of state public health laboratories correctly subtyping *Escherichia coli* O157:H7 and submitting the results to a national reporting system increased from 46% to 69%, and the percentage of state public health agencies prepared to use Strategic National Stockpile material increased from 70% to 98%.[54] During the 2009 H1N1 influenza pandemic, these improvements in the ability to develop and implement a coordinated public health response in an emergency facilitated the rapid detection and characterization of the outbreak, deployment of laboratory tests, distribution of personal protective equipment from the Strategic National Stockpile, development of a candidate vaccine virus, and widespread administration of the resulting vaccine. These public health interventions prevented an estimated 5 to 10 million cases, 30,000 hospitalizations, and 1,500 deaths (CDC, unpublished data, 2011).

Existing systems also have been adapted to respond to public health threats. During the 2009 H1N1 influenza pandemic, the Vaccines for Children Program was adapted to enable provider ordering and distribution of the pandemic vaccine. Similarly, the President's Emergency Plan for AIDS Relief clinics was used to rapidly deliver treatment following the 2010 cholera outbreak in Haiti.

CONCLUSION

From 1999 to 2009, the age-adjusted death rate in the United States declined from 881.9 per 100,000 population to 741.0, a record low and a continuation of a steady downward trend that began during the last century. Advances in public health contributed significantly to this decline; seven of the 10 achievements described in this report targeted one or more of the 15 leading causes of death. Related *Healthy People 2010* data are available at http://www.cdc.gov/mmwr/preview/mmwrhtml/mm6019a5_addinfo.htm. The examples in this report also illustrate the effective application of core public health tools. Some, such as the establishment of surveillance systems, dissemination of guidelines, implementation of research findings, or development of effective public health programs, are classic tools by which public health has addressed the burden of disease for decades.

Although not new, the judicious use of the legal system, by encouraging healthy behavior through taxation or by shaping it altogether through regulatory action, has become an increasingly important tool in modern public health practice and played a major role in many of the achievements described in this report.[55] The creative use of the whole spectrum of available options, as demonstrated here, has enabled public health practitioners to respond effectively. Public health practice will continue to evolve to meet the new and complex challenges that lie ahead.

QUESTIONS FOR DISCUSSION

1. Which of the public health achievements of the first decade of the 21st century described in this case study are most important? Justify your selection(s).
2. Which forces and influences contributed the most to these achievements?
3. Which challenges and influences threaten continued progress for these achievements?

REFERENCES

1. National Center for Health Statistics. *Health, United States, 2010: With Special Feature on Death and Dying.* Hyattsville, MD: National Center for Health Statistics; 2011.
2. Zhou F. *Updated Economic Evaluation of the Routine Childhood Immunization Schedule in the United States.* Presented at the 45th National Immunization Conference. Washington, DC; March 28–31, 2011.
3. Pilishvili T, Lexau C, Farley MM, et al. Sustained reductions in invasive pneumococcal disease in the era of conjugate vaccine. *J Infect Dis.* 2010;*201*:32–41.
4. Tate JE, Cortese MM, Payne DC. Uptake, impact, and effectiveness of rotavirus vaccination in the United States: review of the first 3 years of postlicensure data. *Pediatr Infect Dis J.* 2011;*30*(1 Suppl):S56–S60.
5. Marin M, Zhang JX, Seward JF. Near elimination of varicella deaths in the US following implementation of the childhood vaccination program. *Pediatrics.* 2011;*128*(2):214–220.
6. Vogt TM, Wise ME, Bell BP, et al. Declining hepatitis A mortality in the United States during the era of hepatitis A vaccination. *J Infect Dis.* 2008;*197*:1282–1288.
7. Centers for Disease Control and Prevention. Vital signs: central line-associated blood stream infections: United States, 2001, 2008, and 2009. *MMWR.* 2011;*60*:243–248.
8. Centers for Disease Control and Prevention. Trends in tuberculosis: United States, 2010. *MMWR.* 2011;*60*:333–337.
9. Centers for Disease Control and Prevention. Ongoing multistate outbreak of *Escherichia coli* serotype O157:H7 infections associated with consumption of fresh spinach: United States, September 2006. *MMWR.* 2006;*55*:1045–1046.
10. Centers for Disease Control and Prevention. Multistate outbreak of Salmonella serotype Tennessee infections associated with peanut butter: United States, 2006–2007. *MMWR.* 2007;*56*:521–524.
11. Boxrud D, Monson T, Stiles T, et al. The role, challenges, and support of PulseNet laboratories in detecting foodborne disease outbreaks. *Public Health Rep.* 2010;*125*(Suppl 2):57–62.
12. Gottlieb SL, Newbern EC, Griffin PM, et al. Multistate outbreak of listeriosis linked to turkey deli meat and subsequent changes in US regulatory policy. *Clin Infect Dis.* 2006;*42*:29–36.
13. Centers for Disease Control and Prevention. Revised recommendations for HIV testing of adults, adolescents, and pregnant women in health-care settings. *MMWR.* 2006;*55*:RR–14.
14. Pealer LN, Marfin AA, Petersen LR, et al. Transmission of West Nile virus through blood transfusion in the United States in 2002. *N Engl J Med.* 2003;*349*:1236–1245.

15. Blanton JD, Hanlon CA, Rupprecht CE. Rabies surveillance in the United States during 2006. *J Am Vet Med Assoc.* 2007;*231*:540–556.

16. Rupprecht CE, Barrett J, Briggs D, et al. Can rabies be eradicated? *Dev Biol.* 2008;*131*:95–121.

17. U.S. Department of Health, Education, and Welfare, Public Health Service. *Smoking and Health: Report of the Advisory Committee to the Surgeon General of the Public Health Service.* Washington, DC: U.S. Department of Health Education and Welfare, Public Health Service; 1964.

18. Centers for Disease Control and Prevention. Trends in the prevalence of tobacco use: national YRBS, 1991–2009. Atlanta, GA: Centers for Disease Control and Prevention; 2010.

19. Centers for Disease Control and Prevention. Vital signs: current cigarette smoking among adults aged ≥18 years: United States, 2009. *MMWR.* 2010;*59*:1135–1140.

20. Centers for Disease Control and Prevention. Smoking-attributable mortality, years of potential life lost, and productivity losses: United States, 2000–2004. *MMWR.* 2008;*57*:1226–1228.

21. Centers for Disease Control and Prevention. State smoke-free laws for worksites, restaurants, and bars: United States, 2000–2010. *MMWR.* 2011;*60*:472–475.

22. Centers for Disease Control and Prevention. *State Tobacco Activities Tracking and Evaluation (STATE) System.* http://www.cdc.gov/tobacco/statesystem. Accessed May 17, 2011.

23. U.S. Government Printing Office. *Family Smoking Prevention and Tobacco Control Act.* Washington DC: U.S. Government Printing Office; 2009. (Public law no. 111-31).

24. Centers for Disease Control and Prevention. CDC grand rounds: current opportunities in tobacco control. *MMWR.* 2010;*59*:487–492.

25. Centers for Disease Control and Prevention. Spina bifida and anencephaly before and after folic acid mandate: United States, 1995–1996 and 1999–2000. *MMWR.* 2004;*53*:362–365.

26. Centers for Disease Control and Prevention. CDC grand rounds: additional opportunities to prevent neural tube defects with folic acid fortification. *MMWR.* 2010;*59*:980–984.

27. Grosse SD, Ouyang L, Collins JS, et al. Economic evaluation of a neural tube defect recurrence-prevention program. *Am J Prevent Med.* 2008;*35*:572–577.

28. Centers for Disease Control and Prevention. Using tandem mass spectrometry for metabolic disease screening among newborns: a report of a work group. *MMWR.* 2001;*50*:RR–3.

29. Centers for Disease Control and Prevention. Impact of expanded newborn screening: United States, 2006. *MMWR.* 2008;*57*:1012–1015.

30. Centers for Disease Control and Prevention. *Summary of Infants Screened for Hearing Loss, Diagnosed, and Enrolled in Early Intervention, United States, 1999–2008.* Atlanta, GA: Centers for Disease Control and Prevention.

31. Centers for Disease Control and Prevention. *Injury Prevention and Control: Data and Statistics (WISQARS).* http://www.cdc.gov/injury/wisqars/index.html. Accessed May 17, 2011.

32. Naumann RB, Dellinger AM, Zaloshnja E, et al. Incidence and total lifetime costs of motor vehicle-related fatal and nonfatal injury by road user type, United States, 2005. *Traffic Inj Prev.* 2010;*11*:353–360.

33. National Highway Traffic Safety Administration. *Traffic Safety facts, 2009 Data: Children.* Washington, DC: U.S. Department of Transportation; 2010. (Report no. DOT HS 811-387).

34. National Highway Traffic Safety Administration. *Traffic Safety Facts 2009.* Washington, DC: U.S. Department of Transportation; 2010. (Report no. DOT HS 811-402).

35. Insurance Institute for Highway Safety. *Child Passenger Safety.* Arlington, VA: Insurance Institute for Highway Safety, Highway Loss Data Institute; 2011.

36. Baker SP, Chen L-H, Li G. *Nationwide Review of Graduated Driver Licensing*. Washington, DC: AAA Foundation for Traffic Safety; 2007.

37. Centers for Disease Control and Prevention. *Leading Causes of Death, 1900–1998*. http://www.cdc.gov/nchs/data/dvs/lead1900_98.pdf. Accessed May 17, 2011.

38. Xu JQ, Kochanek KD, Murphy SL, et al. Deaths: final data for 2007. *Natl Vital Stat Rep*. 2010;*58*(19):1–136.

39. Kochanek KD, Xu JQ, Murphy SL, et al. Deaths: preliminary data for 2009. *Natl Vital Stat Rep*. 2010;*59*(4):1–51.

40. Centers for Disease Control and Prevention. Decline in deaths from heart disease and stroke: United States, 1900–1999. *MMWR*. 1999;*48*:649–656.

41. Institute of Medicine. *A Population-Based Policy and Systems Change Approach to Prevent and Control Hypertension*. Washington, DC: National Academies Press; 2010.

42. Centers for Disease Control and Prevention. *Health, United Sates, 2009: With Special Feature on Medical Technology*. Atlanta, GA: Centers for Disease Control and Prevention; 2010.

43. Centers for Disease Control and Prevention. Use of a registry to improve acute stroke care: seven states, 2005–2009. *MMWR*. 2011;*60*:206–210.

44. Roger VL, Go AS, Lloyd-Jones DM, et al. Heart disease and stroke statistics–2011 update: a report from the American Heart Association. *Circulation*. 2011;*123*: e18–e209.

45. Bureau of Labor Statistics. *Table R6. Incidence Rates for Nonfatal Occupational Injuries and Illnesses Involving Days Away from Work per 10,000 Full-Time Workers by Industry and Selected Parts of Body Affected by Injury or Illness, 2003*. http://www.bls.gov/iif/oshwc/osh/case/ostb1384.pdf. Accessed May 17, 2011.

46. Zaloshnja E, Miller TR, Lee BC. Incidence and cost of nonfatal farm youth injury, United States, 2001–2006. *J Agromedicine*. 2011;*16*:6–18.

47. Centers for Disease Control and Prevention. Commercial fishing deaths: United States, 2000–2009. *MMWR*. 2010;*59*:842–845.

48. Centers for Disease Control and Prevention. *The Guide to Community Preventive Services*. Atlanta, GA: Centers for Disease Control and Prevention; 2011.

49. Centers for Disease Control and Prevention. *Breast Cancer*. http://www.cdc.gov/cancer/breast/index.htm. Accessed May 17, 2011.

50. Centers for Disease Control and Prevention. Colorectal cancer test use among persons aged ≥50 years-United States, 2001. *MMWR*. 2003;*52*:193–196.

51. Kohler BA, Ward E, McCarthy BJ, et al. Annual report to the nation on the status of cancer, 1975–2007, featuring tumors of the brain and other nervous system. *J Natl Cancer Inst*. 2011;*103*:714–736.

52. Edwards BK, Ward E, Kohler BA, et al. Annual report to the nation on the status of cancer, 1975–2006, featuring colorectal cancer trends and impact of interventions (risk factors, screening, and treatment) to reduce future rates. *Cancer*. 2010;*116*: 544–573.

53. Grosse SD, Matte TD, Schwartz J, et al. Economic gains resulting from the reduction in children's exposure to lead in the United States. *Environ Health Perspect*. 2002;*110*: 563–569.

54. Centers for Disease Control and Prevention. *Justification of Estimates for Appropriation Committees: Fiscal Year 2011*. Atlanta, GA: Centers for Disease Control and Prevention; 2011.

55. Centers for Disease Control and Prevention. Law and public health at CDC. *MMWR*. 2006;*55*(Suppl 2):29–33.

Developing a Program Intervention

This case study offers an opportunity to consider the role of coalitions in public health policy development and advocacy and the basics steps necessary to develop an effective public health intervention.[1]

LEARNING OBJECTIVES

Through review and discussion of this case study, students will be able to:

- Describe the role of coalitions in modern public health practice.
- Discuss the characteristics of successful coalitions.
- Delineate the key steps in designing a program intervention.

PART 1: COALITION BUILDING

Patricia Hogan serves as the director of the Center for Health Promotion, one of the units of the Office of Community Health within the Lincoln State Department of Public Health. Her office is within a few blocks of the state capitol building, which lies in the heart of the city of Jackson Springs, the capital of Lincoln.

Data indicate that the number of deaths in the state attributable to injury continues to be a problem. The fourth leading cause of death in terms of numbers of deaths, injury accounts for more years of potential life lost before age 65 than any other cause among Lincoln residents each year. Resources in state government are increasingly scarce. To maximize available resources, Patricia convinces the agency director that an injury coalition should be formed.

The Lincoln Injury Coalition would be composed of organizational and individual representatives from throughout Lincoln with an interest in injury control and an influence on potentially affected groups of people. Ideally, this broad participation would not only bring diversity of perspective but would also ensure buy-in from or commitment by involved organizations to project goals as these are developed. The role of the Lincoln Injury Coalition would be to determine, on the basis of presentations of data concerning the burden of injury in Lincoln, which populations in the state are at greatest risk of death from injuries and how these groups might best be reached with preventive services.

The coalition would help develop a statewide injury control plan, set priorities in areas of greatest concern, and determine future interventions. The annual budget allocated to cover planning and other activities of the Lincoln Injury Coalition is $100,000.

Patricia Hogan and her coworkers at the state health department have had some experience setting up and working with coalitions on tobacco control and maternal and child issues in the past. Contact with legislators is not always easy in Lincoln because of both political and geographic considerations.

QUESTIONS FOR DISCUSSION

1. Why should the Lincoln Injury Coalition be formed? What do you see as the potential advantages and drawbacks of working with a coalition for this purpose?
2. How can Patricia Hogan and the state health department build on prior successful involvement with coalitions?
3. What is the ideal size for such a coalition? Which factors might help determine size?
4. Who should be invited to coalition meetings? How should members be recruited? Which other facts should be considered when planning coalition membership? Should members represent organizations or participate on the basis of individual leadership in their fields? Should they be agency heads?
5. Are there organizations that should not be represented on the Lincoln Injury Coalition?
6. Assuming that the decision is made to develop such a coalition, who should be in charge?
7. Should Lincoln State Department of Public Health staff serve as coalition members? Why or why not? Should they be in charge of the coalition? Should they staff the coalition?
8. Which powers and authorities should be given to the coalition? How might decision making within the coalition take place? What are the advantages and disadvantages of different styles of decision making?
9. Which geographic factors particular to Lincoln might need to be considered when planning coalition meetings?
10. What can you expect to be the coalition's major expenses? How might these be reduced?
11. How would you evaluate the coalition's effectiveness?

PART 2: PROGRAM DEVELOPMENT

The statewide injury-control initiative has resulted in a newly funded program in the state of Lincoln. In the meantime, Patricia

Hogan has taken a new position with the planning unit of the largest local health department in the state. A community-wide planning group has proposed priorities for the health department's Health Improvement Plan at the request of the mayor. Domestic violence emerged as one of the priorities and the health department proposes using funds from the new statewide program in conjunction with local resources to address the city's domestic violence problem. To that end, the mayor and city council have committed to an appropriation of $1 million from state and local sources for the next fiscal year to begin an intervention program to address domestic violence. The overall goal is to reduce mortality and morbidity related to domestic violence in the city. All of the available resources are to be directed toward this goal.

QUESTIONS FOR DISCUSSION

1. **Task A: Develop a health problem statement and a desired outcome objective for domestic violence in a specific community.**
   (a) Characterize the current state of the art for control of this health problem.
   (b) Develop a carefully designed problem statement that includes the magnitude and extent of the problem, population at risk, and pertinent trends.
   (c) Determine the resources available to address the problem and any additional resources that might be needed.
   (d) Develop a desired outcome objective for the health problem.
2. **Tasks B and C: Develop an intervention strategy and impact objectives.** After completing the following activities, record your work in a suitable format.
   (a) Analyze the health problem in terms of the factors most amenable to intervention.
   (b) Identify the two most important determinants, and for each, two major contributing factors.
   (c) After completion, this logic model should describe potential pathways through which domestic violence-related mortality and morbidity can be reduced. Record your two determinants and their contributing factors in a suitable format. (Refer back to the chapter on health from an ecological perspective for a description and illustration of this approach.)
   (d) Develop an intervention strategy that would address one or both determinants for the health problem. To do so, select one determinant and its associated contributing factors for which to develop an impact objective and at least two process objectives. Consider the state of the art and available resources in

developing your objectives. Record your impact objective and the two process objectives.

(e) Examine the projected impact objective and the associated process objectives. On the basis of these objectives, evaluate the desired outcome objective and modify it as needed to develop the expected outcome objective. Record the expected outcome objective.

3. **Task D: Develop a work plan.** After completing the following activity, develop a summary of the work plan to achieve each process objective in a suitable format. For each of the process objectives identified previously, specify the major tasks (activities) that must be performed by program personnel to achieve the objective such that:

(a) The tasks are in logical sequence and will lead to the achievement of the process objective.

(b) The person(s) or position(s) generally responsible for each task is identified.

(c) Necessary deadlines are specified.

(d) The budget of $1 million is not exceeded.

4. **Task E: Develop an evaluation strategy.** Prepare a summary report of the evaluation plan, addressing questions such as these: What is the evidence that this intervention approach will really work? and How will we know that this valid approach is really working in this situation?

(a) Describe how you will evaluate each of the following: activities, process objectives, impact objective, and outcome objective. For each evaluation process include information on items to be measured or counted, sources of information, and periodicity of monitoring.

(b) Assume that you achieve all of your process objectives and that your outcome objective is 80% achieved and 40% achieved. Discuss the appropriate actions based on these evaluation scenarios.

5. **Task F: Develop an executive summary.** You may develop your executive summary in any way that you choose, but it should summarize the problem (why is this important?), the approach (what will be accomplished?), and how progress and success will be tracked. The executive summary should be developed in a format suitable for submission to the health committee of the city council and should be brief (suggested length for the executive summary is about 500 words).

REFERENCES

1. Adapted from Centers for Disease Control and Prevention. *Translating Science Into Practice*. Atlanta, GA: Centers for Disease Control and Prevention; 1991. (Case study).

GLOSSARY

ACCESS

The potential for entry or actual entry of a population into the health system. Entry is dependent on the wants, resources, and needs that individuals bring to the care-seeking process. The ability to obtain wanted or needed services may be influenced by many factors, including travel distance, waiting time, available financial resources, and availability of a regular source of care.

ACCREDITATION

For public health agencies, accreditation is a process that measures the performance of the organization against a set of nationally recognized, practice-focused, and evidence-based standards. The Public Health Accreditation Board recognizes (i.e., accredits) public health agencies that meet these standards.

ACTIVITIES

Specific tasks that must be completed for a program's processes to achieve their targets.

ACTIVITY MEASURES

Indicators of whether a program's activities are successfully completed.

ACTUAL CAUSE OF DEATH

A primary determinant or risk factor associated with a pathologic or diagnosed cause of death. For example, tobacco use would be the actual cause for deaths from many lung cancers.

ADJUSTED RATE

The adjustment or standardization of rates is a statistical procedure that removes the effect of differences in the composition of populations. Because of its marked effect on mortality and morbidity, age is the variable for adjustment used most commonly. For example, an age-adjusted death rate for any cause permits a better comparison between different populations and at different times because it accounts for differences in the distribution of age.

ADMINISTRATIVE LAW

Rules and regulations promulgated by administrative agencies within the executive branch of government that carry the force of law. Administrative law represents a unique situation in which legislative, executive, and judicial powers are carried out by one agency in the development, implementation, and enforcement of rules and regulations.

AFFORDABLE CARE ACT

The common name for the Patient Protection and Affordable Care Act of 2010 (Public Law 111-148), which is the federal statute incorporating many health reform provisions affecting health insurance policies, coverage, cost, and quality of care. This legislation is also known as Obamacare as it was proposed by the Obama administration and signed into law by President Obama.

AGE-ADJUSTED MORTALITY RATE

The expected number of deaths that would occur if a population had the same age distribution as a standard population, expressed in terms of deaths per 1,000 or 100,000 persons.

APPROPRIATENESS

Health interventions for which the expected health benefit exceeds the expected negative consequences by a wide enough margin to justify the intervention.

ASSESSMENT

One of the three core functions of public health. Assessment calls for regularly and systematically collecting, analyzing, and making available information on the health of a community, including statistics on health status, community health needs, and epidemiologic and other studies of health problems.

ASSESSMENT PROTOCOL FOR EXCELLENCE IN
PUBLIC HEALTH (APEXPH)

A tool and process for local health department involvement in community health improvement initiatives. APEXPH includes organizational self-assessment and community health assessment components. APEXPH was the predecessor to the Mobilizing for Action through Planning and Partnerships (MAPP) process.

ASSETS

Resources available to achieve a specific end, such as community resources that can contribute to community health-improvement efforts or emergency-response resources, including human, to respond to a public health emergency.

ASSOCIATION

The relationship between two or more events or variables. Events are said to be associated when they occur more frequently together than one would expect by chance. Association does not necessarily imply a causal relationship.

ASSURANCE

One of the three core functions of public health. It involves assuring constituents that services necessary to achieve agreed-upon goals are provided by encouraging action on the part of others, requiring action through regulation, or providing services directly.

ATTRIBUTABLE RISK

The theoretical reduction in the rate or number of cases of an adverse outcome that can be achieved by elimination of a risk factor. For example, if tobacco use is responsible for 75% of all lung cancers, the elimination of tobacco use will reduce lung cancer mortality rates by 75% in a population over time. The risk of lung cancer attributable to tobacco use is 75%.

BEHAVIORAL RISK FACTORS SURVEILLANCE SYSTEM (BRFSS)

A national data collection system supported in part by the Centers for Disease Control and Prevention to assess the prevalence of behaviors that affect health status. Through individual state efforts, BRFSS coordinates the collection, analysis, and distribution of survey data on seat belt use, hypertension, physical activity, smoking, weight control, alcohol use, mammography screening, cervical cancer screening, and AIDS, as well as other health-related information.

BIOSURVEILLANCE

The process of gathering, integrating, interpreting, and communicating essential information that might relate to disease activity and threats to human, animal, or plant health. For public health workers, biosurveillance activities range from standard epidemiological practices to advanced technological systems, utilizing complex algorithms.

BIOTERRORISM

The threatened or intentional release of biologic agents (viruses, bacteria, or their toxins) for the purpose of influencing the conduct of government or intimidating or coercing a civilian population to further political or social objectives. These agents can be released by way of air (as aerosols), food, water, or insects.

BUDGET

A financial tool for systematically converting the objectives of an organization into a plan for acquiring revenues and/or controlling expenditures.

CAPACITY

The capability to carry out the core functions of public health (also see Infrastructure).

CAPITATION

A method of payment for health services in which a provider is paid a fixed amount for each person served, without regard to the actual number or nature of services provided to each person in a set period of time. Capitation is the characteristic payment method in health maintenance organizations.

CASE DEFINITION

Standardized criteria for determining whether a person has a particular disease or health-related condition. Criteria often include clinical and laboratory findings, as well as personal characteristics (age, gender, location, time period, etc.). Case definitions are often used in investigations and for comparing potential cases.

CASE MANAGEMENT

The monitoring and coordinating of services rendered to individuals with specific problems or who require high-cost or extensive services.

CASUALTY

Any person suffering physical and/or psychological damage that leads to death, injury, or material loss.

CAUSALITY

The relationship of causes to the effects they produce; several types of causes can be distinguished. A cause is termed necessary when a particular variable must always precede an effect. This effect need not be the sole result of the one variable. A cause is termed sufficient when a particular variable inevitably initiates or produces an effect. Any given cause may be necessary, sufficient, both, or neither.

CAUSE OF DEATH

For the purpose of national mortality statistics, every death is attributed to one underlying condition, based on the information reported on the death certificate and using the international rules for selecting the underlying cause of death from the reported conditions.

CENTERS FOR DISEASE CONTROL AND PREVENTION (CDC)

The CDC, based in Atlanta, Georgia, is the federal agency charged with protecting the nation's public health by providing direction in the prevention and control of communicable and other diseases and responding to public health emergencies. The CDC's responsibilities as the nation's prevention agency have expanded over the years in response to contemporary threats to health, such as injury, environmental and occupational hazards, behavioral risks, chronic diseases, and emerging communicable diseases, such as the Ebola virus.

CENTERS FOR MEDICARE AND MEDICAID SERVICES

The government agency within the U.S. Department of Health and Human Services that directs the Medicare and Medicaid programs (Titles XVIII and XIX of the Social Security Act) and conducts the research to support these programs.

CERTIFICATION

A process by which an agency or association grants recognition to another party who has met certain predetermined qualifications specified by the agency or association.

CERTIFIED IN PUBLIC HEALTH (CPH)

The credential awarded by the National Board of Public Health Examiners after an individual successfully passes the national credentialing test.

CHRONIC DISEASE

A disease that has one or more of the following characteristics: it is permanent, leaves residual disability, is caused by a nonreversible pathologic alteration, requires special training of the patient for rehabilitation, or may be expected to require a long period of supervision, observation, or care.

CLINICAL PRACTICE GUIDELINES

Systematically developed statements that assist practitioner and patient decisions about appropriate health services for specific clinical conditions.

CLINICAL PREVENTIVE SERVICES

Clinical services provided to patients to reduce or prevent disease, injury, or disability. These are preventive measures (including screening tests, immunizations, counseling, and periodic physical examinations) provided by a health professional to an individual patient.

COALITION

Formal partnerships involving two or more groups working together to achieve specific goals according to a common plan; sometimes referred to as consortia.

COMMUNITY

A group of people with common characteristics. Communities can be defined by location, race, ethnicity, age, occupation, interest in particular problems or outcomes, or other common bonds. Ideally, there should be available assets and resources, as well as collective discussion, decision making, and action.

COMMUNITY HEALTH-IMPROVEMENT PROCESS

A systematic effort that assesses community needs and assets, prioritizes health-related problems and issues, analyzes problems for their causative factors, develops evidence-based intervention strategies based on those analyses, links stakeholders to implementation efforts through performance monitoring, and evaluates the effect of interventions in the community.

COMMUNITY HEALTH NEEDS ASSESSMENT

A formal approach to identifying health needs and health problems in the community. A variety of tools or instruments may be used; the essential ingredient is community engagement and collaborative participation.

COMMUNITY PREVENTIVE SERVICES

Population-based interventions to reduce or prevent disease, injury, or disability. Community preventive services target populations, such as the entire population or some subset of that population, rather than individuals.

COMPREHENSIVE EMERGENCY MANAGEMENT

A broad style of emergency management, encompassing prevention, preparedness, response, and recovery.

CONDITION

A health condition is a departure from a state of physical or mental well-being. An impairment is a health condition that includes chronic or permanent health defects resulting from disease, injury, or congenital malformations. All health conditions except impairments are coded according to an international classification system based on their duration. There are two types of conditions: acute and chronic.

CONSEQUENCE MANAGEMENT

An emergency management function includes measures to protect public health and safety, restore essential government services, and provide emergency relief to governments in the event of terrorism.

CONTAMINATION

An accidental release of hazardous chemicals or nuclear materials that pollutes the environment and places humans at risk.

CONTRIBUTING FACTOR

A risk factor (causative factor) that is associated with the presence and/or level of a determinant. Direct contributing factors are linked with the level of determinants; indirect contributing factors are linked with the level of direct contributing factors.

CORE FUNCTIONS

Three basic roles for public health for ensuring conditions in which people can be healthy, as identified in the Institute of Medicine's landmark report, *The Future of Public Health*. These are assessment, policy development, and assurance.

COST-BENEFIT ANALYSIS

An economic analysis in which all costs and benefits are converted into monetary (dollar) values, and results are expressed as dollars of benefit per dollars expended.

COST-EFFECTIVENESS ANALYSIS

An economic analysis assessed as a health outcome per cost expended.

COST-UTILITY ANALYSIS

An economic analysis assessed as a quality-adjusted outcome per net cost expended.

COUNTERMEASURES

A measure or action that is taken to counter or offset another measure. Countermeasures are designed or selected for their precision and specificity in preventing undesired outcomes from occurring.

COVERT RELEASES

An unannounced release of a biologic agent that causes illness or other effects. If undetected, a covert release has the potential to spread widely before it is discovered.

CREDENTIALING

A review and approval process that distinguishes someone who is recognized for a particular status from others who are not. For public health workers, the Certified in Public Health (CPH) credential is awarded by the National Board of Public Health Examiners.

CRISIS MANAGEMENT

Administrative measures that identify, acquire, and plan the use of resources needed to anticipate, prevent, and/or resolve a threat to public safety (such as terrorism).

CRUDE MORTALITY RATE

The total number of deaths per unit of population reported during a given time interval, often expressed as the number of deaths per 1,000 or 100,000 persons.

CULTURAL COMPETENCE

The ability to communicate with and provide services to an individual or a group with full respect for the culturally associated values, preferences, language, and experiences of the group.

DECISION ANALYSIS

An analytic technique in which probability theory is used to obtain a quantitative approach to decision making.

DECONTAMINATION

The removal of hazardous chemicals or nuclear substances from the skin and/or mucous membranes by showering or washing the affected area with water or by rinsing with a sterile solution.

DEMOGRAPHICS

Characteristic data, such as size, growth, density, distribution, and vital statistics, that are used to study human populations.

DEMONSTRATION SETTINGS

A population- or clinic-based environment in which prevention strategies are field tested.

DETERMINANT

A primary risk factor (causative factor) associated with the presence and/or level of health problem (i.e., the level of the determinant influences the level of the health problem).

DISABILITY LIMITATION

An intervention strategy that seeks to arrest or eradicate disease and/or limit disability and prevent death.

DISASTER

Any event, typically occurring suddenly, that causes damage, ecological disruption, loss of human life, or deterioration of health and health services and that exceeds the capacity of the affected community on a scale sufficient to require outside assistance.

DISASTER SEVERITY SCALE

A scale that classifies disasters by the following parameters: the radius of the disaster site, the number of dead, the number of wounded, the average severity of the injuries sustained, the impact time, and the rescue time. By attributing a numeric score to each of the variables from 0 to 2, with 0 being the least severe and 2 the most severe, a scale with a range of 0 to 18 can be created.

DISCOUNTING

A method of adjusting for the value of future costs and benefits. Expressed as a present dollar value, discounting is based on the time value of money (i.e., a dollar today is worth more than it will be a year from now, even if inflation is not considered).

DISEASE MANAGEMENT

A set of strategies that focuses on a specific disease or condition (such as diabetes) and attempts to reduce the burden of disease by identifying and proactively monitoring high-risk populations, assisting patients and providers to adhere to treatment plans that are based on proven interventions, promoting provider coordination, increasing patient education, and preventing avoidable medical complications.

DISTRIBUTIONAL EFFECTS

The manner in which the costs and benefits of a strategy affect different groups of people based on various demographics, geographic location, and other descriptive factors.

EARLY CASE FINDING AND TREATMENT

An intervention strategy that seeks to identify disease or illness at an early stage so that prompt treatment will reduce the effects of the process.

EFFECTIVENESS

The improvement in health outcome that a strategy can produce in typical community-based settings; also, the degree to which objectives are achieved, such as for a program or service.

EFFICACY

The improvement in health outcome effect that a strategy can produce in expert hands under ideal circumstances.

EMERGENCY

Any natural or man-made situation that results in severe injury, harm, or loss to humans or property.

EMERGENCY MANAGEMENT AGENCY

The federal, state, or local agency, under the authority of the highest elected official, that coordinates the efforts of the health department, housing and social service agencies, and public safety agencies (such as police) during an emergency or disaster.

EMERGENCY MEDICAL SERVICES (EMS) SYSTEM

The coordination of the pre-hospital system (including public access, 911 dispatch, paramedics, and ambulance services) and the in-hospital system (including emergency departments, hospitals, and other definitive care facilities and personnel) to provide emergency medical care.

EMERGENCY OPERATIONS CENTER (EOC)

The site from which civil governmental officials (such as municipal, county, state, or federal) direct emergency operations in a disaster.

EPIDEMIC

The occurrence of a disease or condition at higher than normal levels in a population.

EPIDEMIOLOGY

The study of the distribution of determinants and antecedents of health and disease in human populations. The ultimate goal is to identify the underlying causes of a disease and then apply findings to disease prevention and health promotion.

ESCHERICHIA COLI (E. COLI) O157:H7

A bacterial pathogen that can infect humans and cause severe bloody diarrhea (hemorrhagic colitis) and serious renal disease (hemolytic uremic syndrome).

ESSENTIAL PUBLIC HEALTH SERVICES

A formulation of the processes used in public health to prevent epidemics and injuries, protect against environmental hazards, promote healthy behaviors, respond to disasters, and ensure quality and accessibility of health services. Ten essential services have been identified:

1. Monitoring health status to identify community health problems
2. Diagnosing and investigating health problems and health hazards in the community
3. Informing, educating, and empowering people about health issues
4. Mobilizing community partnerships to identify and solve health problems
5. Developing policies and plans that support individual and community health efforts

6. Enforcing laws and regulations that protect health and ensure safety
7. Linking people to needed personal health services and ensuring the provision of health care when otherwise unavailable
8. Ensuring a competent public health and personal healthcare workforce
9. Evaluating effectiveness, accessibility, and quality of personal and population-based health services
10. Conducting research for new insights and innovative solutions to health problems

EVACUATION

The organized removal of civilians from a dangerous or potentially dangerous area.

EVIDENCE-BASED PUBLIC HEALTH

Key components of evidence-based public health include making decisions on the basis of the best available scientific evidence, using data and information systems systematically, applying program-planning frameworks, engaging the community in decision making, conducting sound evaluation, and disseminating what is learned. Three types of evidence have been presented on the causes of diseases and the magnitude of risk factors, the relative effect of specific interventions, and how and under which contextual conditions interventions were implemented.

EXERCISES

A generic term for a range of activities undertaken by an agency or a group of agencies within or between communities to test readiness to respond to emergencies or to evaluate response plans or success of training and development programs. Exercises fall into five basic categories: orientation, drill, tabletop exercise, functional exercise, and full-scale exercise.

FEDERALLY FUNDED COMMUNITY HEALTH CENTER

An ambulatory healthcare program (defined under Section 330 of the Public Health Service Act), usually serving a catchment area that has scarce or nonexistent health services or a population with special health needs, and sometimes known as a neighborhood health center. Community health centers attempt to coordinate federal, state, and local resources in a single organization capable of delivering both health and related social services to a defined population. Although such a center may not directly provide all types of health care, it usually takes responsibility to arrange all medical services for its patient population.

FEDERAL RESPONSE PLAN

The plan that coordinates federal resources in disaster and emergency situations in order to address the consequences when there is need for federal assistance under the authority of the Stafford Disaster Relief and Emergency Assistance Act.

FIELD MODEL

A framework for identifying factors that influence health status in populations. Initially, four fields were identified: biology, lifestyle, environment, and health services. Extensions of this approach have also identified genetic, social, and cultural factors and have related these factors to a variety of outcomes, including disease, normal functioning, well-being, and prosperity in an ecological model of health.

FOODBORNE ILLNESS

Illness caused by the transfer of disease organisms or toxins from food to humans.

GENERAL WELFARE PROVISIONS

Specific language in the Constitution of the United States that empowers the federal government to provide for the general welfare of the population. Over time, these provisions have been used as a basis for federal health policies and programs.

GEOCODING

A technique that specifies the geographic location where a specific event occurs. Public health agencies may use geocoding to detect geographic clusters of disease or concentrations of health disparity, for example.

GOALS

For public health programs, goals are general statements expressing a program's aspirations or intended effect on one or more health problems, often stated without time limits.

GOVERNMENTAL PRESENCE AT THE LOCAL LEVEL

A concept that calls for the assurance that necessary services and minimum standards are provided to address priority community health problems. This responsibility ultimately falls to local government, which may use local health departments or other means for its execution.

HARM REDUCTION

A set of practical strategies reflecting individual and community needs that meet individuals with risk behaviors where they are to help them reduce any harms associated with their risk behaviors.

HAZARD

A possible source of harm or injury.

HAZARD VULNERABILITY ANALYSIS

A systematic approach to recognizing hazards that may affect a population, community, or organization. The risks associated with each hazard are analyzed to prioritize planning, mitigation, response, and recovery activities. A hazard vulnerability analysis serves as a needs assessment for emergency preparedness and response activities.

HEALTH

The state of complete physical, mental, and social well-being and not merely the absence of disease or infirmity. It is recognized, however, that health has many dimensions (anatomic, physiologic, and mental) and is largely culturally defined. The relative importance of various disabilities will differ, depending on the cultural milieu and on the role of the affected individual in that culture.

HEALTH DISPARITY

The difference in health status between two groups, such as the health disparity in mortality between men and women, or the health disparity in infant mortality between African American and white infants.

HEALTH EDUCATION

Any combination of learning opportunities designed to facilitate voluntary adaptations of behavior (in individuals, groups, or communities) conducive to good health. Health education encourages positive health behavior.

HEALTH IMPACT ASSESSMENT

A systematic process that uses an array of data sources and analytic methods, and considers input from stakeholders, to determine the potential effects of a proposed policy, plan, program, or project on the health of a population and the distribution of those effects within the population. Health impact assessments provide recommendations on monitoring and managing those effects.

HEALTH MAINTENANCE ORGANIZATIONS

Entities that manage both the financing and provision of health services to enrolled members. Fees are generally based on capitation, and health providers are managed to reduce costs through controls on utilization of covered services.

HEALTH PLANNING

Planning concerned with improving health, whether undertaken comprehensively for an entire community or for a particular population, type of health services, institution, or health program. The components of health planning include data assembly and analysis, goal determination, action recommendation, and implementation strategy.

HEALTH POLICY

Social policy concerned with the process whereby public health agencies evaluate and determine health needs and the best ways to address them, including the identification of appropriate resources and funding mechanisms.

HEALTH PROBLEM

A situation or condition of people (expressed in health outcome measures such as mortality, morbidity, or disability) that is considered undesirable and is likely to exist in the future unless something is done to address it.

HEALTH PROBLEM ANALYSIS

A framework for analyzing health problems to identify their determinants and contributing factors so that interventions can be targeted rationally toward those factors most likely to reduce the level of the health problem.

HEALTH PROMOTION

An intervention strategy that seeks to eliminate or reduce exposures to harmful factors by modifying human behaviors. Any combination of health education and related organizational, political, and economic interventions designed to facilitate behavioral and environmental adaptations that will improve or protect health. This process enables individuals and communities to control and improve their own health. Health promotion approaches provide opportunities for people to identify problems, develop solutions, and work in partnerships that build on existing skills and strengths.

HEALTH PROTECTION

An intervention strategy that seeks to provide individuals with resistance to harmful factors, often by modifying the environment to decrease potentially harmful interactions. These population-based services and programs control and reduce the exposure of the population to environmental or personal hazards, conditions, or factors that may cause disease, disability, injury, or death. Health protection also includes programs that ensure that public health services are available on a 24-hour basis to respond to public health emergencies and coordinate responses of local, state, and federal organizations.

HEALTH REGULATION

Monitoring and maintaining the quality of public health services through licensing and discipline of health professionals, licensing of health facilities, and enforcement of standards and regulations.

HEALTH STATUS INDICATORS

Measurements of the state of health of a specified individual, group, or population. Health status may be measured by proxies such as people's subjective assessments of their health; by one or more indicators of mortality and morbidity in the population, such as longevity or maternal and infant mortality; or by the incidence or prevalence of major diseases (communicable, chronic, or nutritional). Conceptually, health status is the proper outcome measure for the effectiveness of a specific population's health system, although attempts to relate effects of available medical care to variations in health status have proved difficult.

HEALTH SYSTEM

As used in this text, the health system is the sum total of the strategies designed to prevent or treat disease, injury, and other health problems. The health system includes population-based preventive services, clinical preventive and other primary medical care services, and all levels of more sophisticated treatment and chronic care services.

HEALTHY COMMUNITIES 2020

A framework for developing and tailoring community health objectives so that these could be tracked as part of the initiative to achieve the year 2020 national health objectives included in *Healthy People 2020*.

HEALTHY PEOPLE 2020

The national disease prevention and health promotion agenda that includes more than 1,200 national health objectives to be achieved by the year 2020, addressing improved health status, risk reduction, social determinants of health, and utilization of preventive health services.

IMPACT OBJECTIVE

The level of a determinant to be achieved through the processes and activities of an intervention strategy. Impact objectives are generally intermediate in term (2 to 5 years) and must be measurable and realistic.

INCIDENCE

A measure of the disease or injury in the population, generally the number of new cases occurring during a specified time period.

INCIDENT COMMAND SYSTEM (ICS)

The model for command, control, and coordination of a response to an emergency providing the means to coordinate the efforts of multiple agencies and organizations.

INDICATOR

A measure of health status or a health outcome.

INFANT MORTALITY RATE

The number of live-born infants who die before their first birthday per 1,000 live births, often broken into two components, neonatal mortality (deaths before 28 days per 1,000 live births) and post-neonatal mortality (deaths from 28 days through the rest of the first year of life per 1,000 live births).

INFECTIOUS DISEASE

A disease caused by the entrance into the body of organisms (such as bacteria, protozoans, fungi, or viruses) that then grow and multiply there, often used synonymously with communicable disease.

INFRASTRUCTURE

The systems, competencies, relationships, and resources that enable performance of public health's core functions and essential services in every community. Categories include human, organizational, informational, and fiscal resources.

INPUTS

Sometimes referred to as capacities, the human resources, fiscal and physical resources, information resources, and system organizational resources necessary to carry out the core functions of public health.

INTERVENTION

A generic term used in public health to describe a program or policy designed to have an effect on a health problem. For example, a mandatory seat belt law is an intervention designed to reduce the incidence of automobile-related fatalities. The five categories of health interventions are health promotion, specific protection, early case finding and prompt treatment, disability limitation, and rehabilitation.

LEADING CAUSES OF DEATH

Those diagnostic classifications of disease that are most frequently responsible for deaths, such as the top 10 causes of death.

LEADING HEALTH INDICATORS

A panel of health-related measures that reflect the major public health concerns in the United States. They were selected to track progress toward achievement of the *Healthy People 2010* goals and objectives. They address 10 public health concerns: physical activity, overweight and obesity, tobacco use, substance abuse, responsible sexual behavior, mental health, injury and violence, environmental quality, immunizations, and access to health care.

LIFE EXPECTANCY

The number of additional years of life expected at a specified point in time, such as at birth or at age 45 or 65 years.

LOCAL HEALTH DEPARTMENT (LHD)

Synonymous with the term *local public health agency* (LPHA); functionally, a local (county, multicounty, municipal, town, other) health agency, operated by local government, often with oversight and direction from a local board of health, that carries out public health's core functions throughout a defined geographic area. It is sometimes defined as an agency serving less than an entire state that carries some responsibility for health and has at least one full-time employee and a specific budget.

LOCAL HEALTH JURISDICTION (LHJ)

A unit of local government (county, multicounty, municipal, town, other), often with oversight and direction from a local board of health, with an identifiable local health department that carries out public health's core functions through-out a defined geographic area.

LOCAL PUBLIC HEALTH AUTHORITY

The agency charged with responsibility for meeting the health needs of the community. Usually this is the policy/governing body and its administrative arm, the local health department. The authority may rest with the policy/governing body, may be a city/county/regional authority, or may consist of a legislative mandate from the state. Some local public health authorities have independence from all other governmental entities, whereas others do not.

LOCAL PUBLIC HEALTH SYSTEM

The collection of public and private organizations having a stake in and con-tributing to public health at the local level. It involves far more than the local health department.

MANAGED CARE

A system of administrative controls intended to reduce costs through man-aging the utilization of services. Managed care can also mean an integrated system of health insurance, financing, and service delivery that focuses on the appropriate and cost-effective use of health services delivered through defined networks of providers and with allocation of financial risk.

MEASURE

An indicator of health status or a health outcome, used synonymously with indicator in this text.

MEDICAID

A federally aided and state-operated and administered program that provides basic medical services to eligible low-income populations; established through amendments as Title XIX of the Social Security Act in 1965. It does not cover all of the poor, however, but only persons who meet specified eligibility criteria. Subject to broad federal guidelines, states determine the benefits covered, program eligi-bility, rates of payment for providers, and methods of administering the program.

MEDICAL RESERVE CORPS

A locally based team of health professionals and other personnel who provide surge capacity for emergencies.

MEDICARE

A national health insurance program for older persons established through amendments to the Social Security Act in 1965 that were included in Title XVIII of that act.

MENTAL HEALTH

Mental health is sometimes thought of as simply the absence of a mental ill-ness but is actually much broader. Mental health is a state of successful mental functioning, resulting in productive activities, fulfilling relationships, and the ability to adapt to change and cope with adversity. Mental health is indispensable to personal well-being, family and interpersonal relationships, and one's contribution to society.

META-ANALYSIS

A systematic, quantitative method for combining information from multiple studies to derive the most meaningful answer to a specific question. Assessment of different methods or outcome measures can increase power and account for bias and other effects.

MIDLEVEL PRACTITIONERS

Nonphysician healthcare providers, such as nurse practitioners and physician assistants.

MISSION

For public health, ensuring conditions in which people can be healthy.

MITIGATION

Measures taken to reduce the harmful effects of a disaster or emergency by attempting to limit the effect on human health and economic infrastructure.

MOBILIZING FOR ACTION THROUGH PLANNING AND PARTNERSHIPS (MAPP)

A voluntary process for organizational and community self-assessment, planned improvements, and continuing evaluation and reassessment. MAPP is the second generation of such tools, following the Assessment Protocol for Excellence in Public Health (APEXPH), which appeared in the early 1990s. The MAPP process focuses on community-wide public health practice, including a health department's role in its community and the community's actual and perceived problems. It provides for a community health-improvement process to assess health needs, sets priorities, develops policy, and ensures that health needs are met.

MORBIDITY

A measure of disease incidence or prevalence in a given population, location, or other grouping of interest.

MORTALITY

Expresses the number of deaths in a population within a prescribed time. Mortality rates may be expressed as crude death rates (total deaths in relation to total population during a year) or as death rates specific for diseases and sometimes for age, gender, or other attributes (e.g., the number of deaths from cancer in white males in relation to the white male population during a given year).

NATIONAL HEALTH EXPENDITURES

The amount spent for all health services and supplies and health-related research and construction activities in the United States during the calendar year.

NATIONAL HEALTH SECURITY STRATEGY

An ongoing assessment and enhancement of public health and medical capabilities for emergency preparedness and response to all forms of threats and events with health effects.

OBAMACARE

See Affordable Care Act.

OBJECTIVES

Targets for achievement through interventions. Objectives are time limited and measurable in all cases. Various levels of objectives for an intervention include outcome, impact, and process objectives.

OPERATIONAL DEFINITION OF A FUNCTIONAL LOCAL HEALTH DEPARTMENT

A set of standards based on the essential public health services framework that describes the responsibilities that everyone can expect their local health department to fulfill regardless of where they live.

OUTCOME OBJECTIVE

The level to which a health problem is to be reduced as a result of an intervention. Outcome objectives are often long term (2 to 5 years) and are measurable and realistic.

OUTCOMES

Sometimes referred to as results of the health system. These are indicators of health status, risk reduction, and quality-of-life enhancement. Outcomes are long-term objectives that define optimal, measurable future levels of health status; maximum acceptable levels of disease, injury, or dysfunction; or prevalence of risk factors.

OUTPUTS

Health programs and services intended to prevent death, disease, and disability and to promote quality of life.

PERFORMANCE IMPROVEMENT

The active use of performance data or measures in making management decisions, integrating four fundamental components: applying appropriate standards, measuring performance against those standards, reporting and interpreting those measurements, and making change based on the results of the performance measurements.

PERFORMANCE MEASUREMENT

The process of tracking work produced and results achieved, often as part of a performance improvement or performance management system.

PERSONAL HEALTH SERVICES

Diagnosis and treatment of disease or provision of clinical preventive services to individuals or families in order to improve individual health status.

POLICE POWER

A basic power of government that allows for restriction of individual rights to protect the safety and interests of the entire population.

POLICY DEVELOPMENT

One of the three core functions of public health. Policy development involves serving the public interest by leading in developing comprehensive public health policy and promoting the use of the scientific knowledge base in decision making.

POPULATION-BASED PUBLIC HEALTH SERVICES

Interventions aimed at disease prevention and health promotion that affect an entire population and extend beyond medical treatment by targeting underlying risks, such as tobacco, drug, and alcohol use; diet and sedentary lifestyles; and environmental factors.

POPULATION HEALTH

The physical, mental, and social well-being of defined groups of individuals and the differences or disparities in health between and among population groups.

POSTPONEMENT

A form of prevention in which the time of onset of a disease or injury is delayed to reduce the prevalence of a condition in the population.

PREPAREDNESS

All measures and policies taken before an event occurs that allow for prevention, mitigation, and readiness.

PREVALENCE

A measure of the burden of disease or injury in a population, generally the number of cases of a disease or injury at a particular point in time or during a specified time period. Prevalence is affected by both the incidence and the duration of disease in a population.

PREVENTED FRACTION

The proportion of an adverse health outcome that has been eliminated as a result of a prevention strategy.

PREVENTION

Anticipatory action taken to prevent the occurrence of an event or to minimize its effects after it has occurred. Prevention aims to minimize the occurrence of disease or its consequences. It includes actions that reduce susceptibility or exposure to health threats (primary prevention), detect and treat disease in early stages (secondary prevention), and alleviate the effects of disease and injury (tertiary prevention). Examples of prevention include immunizations, emergency response to epidemics, health education, modification of risk-prone behavior and physical hazards, safety training, workplace hazard elimination, and industrial process change.

PREVENTIVE STRATEGIES

Frameworks for categorizing prevention programs, based on how the prevention technology is delivered—provider to patient (clinical preventive services), individual responsibility (behavioral prevention), or alteration in an individual's surroundings (environmental prevention)—or on the stage of the natural history of a disease or injury (primary, secondary, and tertiary).

PRIMARY MEDICAL CARE

Clinical preventive services, first-contact treatment services, and ongoing care for commonly encountered medical conditions. Basic or general health care focuses on the point at which a patient ideally seeks assistance from the medical care system. Primary care is considered comprehensive when the primary provider takes responsibility for the overall coordination of the care of the patient's health problems, whether these are medical, behavioral, or social. The appropriate use of consultants and community resources is an important part of effective primary health care. Such care is generally provided by physicians but can also be provided by other personnel, such as nurse practitioners or physician assistants.

PRIMARY PREVENTION

Prevention strategies that seek to prevent the occurrence of disease or injury, generally through reducing exposure or risk factor levels. These strategies can reduce or eliminate causative risk factors (risk reduction).

PROCESS MEASURES

Steps in a program logically required for the program to be successful.

PROCESS OBJECTIVE

The level to which a contributing factor is to be reduced as a result of successfully carrying out a program's activities.

PUBLIC HEALTH

Activities that society undertakes to ensure the conditions in which people can be healthy. These include organized community efforts to prevent, identify, and counter threats to the health of the public.

PUBLIC HEALTH ACCREDITATION BOARD

The organization that establishes performance standards for public health agencies and coordinates the process of measuring those standards and recognizing (i.e., accrediting) those agencies that meet these standards. Also see Accreditation.

PUBLIC HEALTH AGENCY

A unit of government (federal, state, local, or regional) charged with preserving, protecting, and promoting the health of the population through ensuring delivery of essential public health services.

PUBLIC HEALTH IN AMERICA

A document developed by the Core Functions Project that characterizes the vision, mission, outcome aspirations, and essential services of public health. See also Essential Public Health Services.

PUBLIC HEALTH ORGANIZATION

A nongovernmental entity (nonprofit agency, association, corporation, etc.) participating in activities designed to improve the health status of a community or population.

PUBLIC HEALTH PRACTICE

The development and application of preventive strategies and interventions to promote and protect the health of populations.

PUBLIC HEALTH PRACTICE GUIDELINES

Systematically developed statements that assist public health practitioner decisions about interventions at the community level.

PUBLIC HEALTH PRACTICES

Those organizational practices or processes that are necessary and sufficient to ensure that the core functions of public health are being carried out effectively. Ten public health practices have been identified:

1. Assess the health needs of the community.
2. Investigate the occurrence of health risks and hazards in the community.
3. Analyze identified health needs for their determinants and contributing factors.
4. Advocate and build support for public health.
5. Establish priorities from among identified health needs.
6. Develop comprehensive policies and plans for priority health needs.
7. Manage resources efficiently.
8. Ensure that priority health needs are addressed in the community.
9. Evaluate the effects of programs and services.
10. Inform and educate the public.

PUBLIC HEALTH PROCESSES

Those collective practices or processes that are necessary and sufficient to ensure that the core functions and essential services of public health are being carried out effectively, including the key processes that identify and address health problems and their causative factors and the interventions intended to prevent death, disease, and disability and to promote quality of life.

PUBLIC HEALTH SERVICE

U.S. Public Health Service, as reorganized in 1996. It now includes the Office of Public Health and Science (which is headed by the Assistant Secretary for Health and includes the Office of the Surgeon General), eight operating agencies (Health Resources and Services Administration, Indian Health Service, Centers for Disease Control and Prevention, National Institutes of Health, Food and Drug Administration, Substance Abuse and Mental Health Services Administration, Agency for Toxic Substances and Disease Registry, and Agency for Healthcare Research and Quality), and the Regional Health Administrators for the 10 federal regions of the country.

PUBLIC HEALTH SYSTEM

That part of the larger health system that seeks to ensure conditions in which people can be healthy by carrying out public health's three core functions. The system can be further described by its inputs, practices, outputs, and outcomes.

PUBLIC HEALTH WORKER

An individual who is contributing to at least one essential public health service with greater than 50% of his or her time and effort, whether employed by, staff to, or contracting with employers or agencies, full or part time.

PUBLIC HEALTH WORKFORCE

The public health workforce includes individuals with the following characteristics:

- Employed by an organization engaged in an organized effort to promote, protect, and preserve the health of a defined population group. The group may be public or private, and the effort may be secondary or subsidiary to the principal objectives of the organization.
- Performing work made up of one or more specific public health services or activities.
- Occupying positions that conventionally require at least 1 year of postsecondary specialized public health training and that are (or can be) assigned a professional occupational title.

QUALITY-ADJUSTED LIFE YEARS (QALYS)

A measure of health status that assigns to each period of time a weight, ranging from 0 to 1, corresponding to the health-related quality of life during that period. These are then summed across time periods to calculate QALYs. For each period, a weight of 1 corresponds to optimal health, and a weight of 0 corresponds to a health state equivalent to death.

QUALITY OF CARE

The degree to which health services for individuals increase the likelihood of desired health outcomes and are consistent with established professional standards and judgments of value to the consumer. Quality also may be seen as the degree to which actions taken or not taken maximize the probability of beneficial health outcomes and minimize risk and other undesired outcomes, given the existing state of medical science and art.

RAPID NEEDS ASSESSMENT

A variety of epidemiologic, statistical, and anthropological techniques designed to provide information about an affected community's needs after a disaster or other public health emergency.

RATE

A mathematical expression for the relationship between the numerator (number of deaths, diseases, disabilities, services, etc.) and denominator (population at risk), together with specification of time. Rates make possible a comparison of the number of events between populations and at different times. Rates may be crude, specific, or adjusted.

RECOVERY

Actions of responders, government, and victims that help return an affected community to normal by stimulating community cohesiveness and governmental involvement. The recovery period falls between the onset of an emergency and the reconstruction period.

REHABILITATION

An intervention strategy that seeks to return individuals to the maximum level of functioning possible.

RESPONSE

The phase in a disaster or public health emergency when relief, recovery, and rehabilitation occur.

RISK

The probability that exposure to a hazard will lead to a negative consequence.

RISK ASSESSMENT

A determination of the likelihood of adverse health effects to a population after exposure to a hazard.

RISK FACTOR

A behavior or condition that, on the basis of scientific evidence or theory, is thought to influence susceptibility to a specific health problem.

RISK RATIO/RELATIVE RISK

The ratio of the risk or likelihood of the occurrence of specific health outcomes or events in one group to that of another. Risk ratios provide a measure of the relative difference in risk between the two groups. Relative risk is an example of a risk ratio in which the incidence of disease in the exposed group is divided by the incidence of disease in an unexposed group.

SCREENING

The use of technology and procedures to differentiate those individuals with signs or symptoms of disease from those less likely to have the disease. If necessary, further diagnosis and, if indicated, early intervention and treatment can then be provided.

SECONDARY MEDICAL CARE

Specialized attention and ongoing management for common and less frequently encountered medical conditions, including support services for people with special challenges caused by chronic or long-term conditions. Services provided by medical specialists who generally do not have their first contact with patients (e.g., cardiologists, urologists, and dermatologists). In the United States, however, there has been a trend toward self-referral by patients for these services, rather than referral by primary care providers.

SECONDARY PREVENTION

Prevention strategies that seek to identify and control disease processes in their early stages before signs and symptoms develop (screening and treatment).

SOCIAL-ECOLOGICAL MODEL

A framework for considering the multiple determinants of health and the linkages and relationships among those determinants.

SOCIAL-ECOLOGICAL PERSPECTIVE

A perspective on health that involves knowledge of the ecological model of determinants of health and an attempt to understand a specific problem or situation in terms of that model.

SOCIAL MARKETING

A program planning process that applies commercial marketing concepts and techniques in order to promote voluntary behavioral change. Social marketing facilitates the acceptance, rejection modification, abandonment, or maintenance of specific behaviors by specific groups often called target audiences.

SPAN OF HEALTHY LIFE

A measure of health status that combines life expectancy with self-reported health status and functional disabilities to calculate the number of years in which an individual is likely to function normally.

SPECIFIC RATE

Rates vary greatly by race, gender, and age. A rate can be made specific for gender, age, race, cause of death, or a combination of these.

STATE CHILD HEALTH INSURANCE PROGRAM (SCHIP)

Title XXI of the Social Security Act, jointly financed by the federal and state governments and administered by the states. Within broad federal guidelines, each state determines the design of its program, eligibility groups, benefit packages, payment levels for coverage, and administrative and operating procedures. SCHIP provides a capped amount of funds to states on a matching basis based on state expenditures under approved plans.

STATE HEALTH AGENCY

The unit of state government that has leading responsibility for identifying and meeting the health needs of the state's citizens. State health agencies can be freestanding or units of multipurpose health and human service agencies.

STRATEGIC NATIONAL STOCKPILE

Formerly known as the National Pharmaceutical Stockpile, a collection of pharmaceuticals, medical supplies, and equipment that can be immediately deployed to meet state and local needs during a public health emergency.

STRATEGIC PLANNING

A disciplined process aimed at producing fundamental decisions and actions that will shape and guide what an organization is, what it does, and why it does what it does. The process of assessing a changing environment to create a vision of the future; determining how the organization fits into the anticipated environment, based on its mission, strengths, and weaknesses and then setting in motion a plan of action to position the organization.

SURVEILLANCE

Systematic monitoring of the health status of a population through collection, analysis, and interpretation of health data in order to plan, implement, and evaluate public health programs, including determining the need for public health action.

SYNDROMIC SURVEILLANCE

The collection and analysis of statistical data on health trends, such as symptoms reported by people seeking care in emergency rooms or other health-care settings, or even sales of flu medications, to detect disease outbreaks earlier than would otherwise be possible through conventional surveillance efforts.

TERTIARY MEDICAL CARE

Subspecialty referral care requiring highly specialized personnel and facilities. Services provided by highly specialized providers (e.g., neurologists, neurosurgeons, thoracic surgeons, and intensive care units). Such services frequently require highly sophisticated equipment and support facilities. The development of these services has largely been a function of diagnostic and therapeutic advances attained through basic and clinical biomedical research.

TERTIARY PREVENTION

Prevention strategies that prevent disability by restoring individuals to their optimal level of functioning after a disease or injury is established and damage is done.

TRIAGE

The selection and categorization of victims of a disaster or other public health emergency as to their need for medical treatment according to the degree of severity of illness or injury, as well as the availability of medical and transport facilities.

VULNERABILITY

The susceptibility of a population to a specific type of event, generally associated with the degree of possible or potential loss from a risk that results from a hazard at a given intensity. Vulnerability can be influenced by demographics, the age and resilience of the environment, technology, and social differentiation and diversity, as well as regional and global economics and politics.

WAIVER

States must obtain waivers of current federal Medicaid law provisions from the Centers for Medicare and Medicaid Services to enroll their Medicaid population in managed care plans or to deviate otherwise from law.

WEAPONS OF MASS DESTRUCTION

Any device, material, or substance used in a manner, in a quantity or type, or under circumstances evidencing intent to cause death or serious injury to persons or significant damage of property.

YEARS OF POTENTIAL LIFE LOST (YPLL)

A measure of the effect of disease or injury in a population that calculates years of life lost before a specific age (often age 65 or 75 years). This approach places additional value on deaths that occur at earlier ages.

Index

Note: Italicized page locators indicate figures; tables are noted with a *t*.